Aesthetic Treatments for the Oncology Patient

Aesthetic Treatments for the Oncology Patient

Edited by

Paloma Tejero, MD, PhD
Universidad de Alcalá
Alcalá de Henares
Madrid, Spain

Hernán Pinto, MD, PhD, MSc, CETC
i2e3 Biomedical Research Institute
Barcelona, Spain

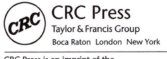

CRC Press
Taylor & Francis Group
Boca Raton London New York

CRC Press is an imprint of the
Taylor & Francis Group, an **informa** business

First edition published 2021
by CRC Press
6000 Broken Sound Parkway NW, Suite 300, Boca Raton, FL 33487-2742

and by CRC Press
2 Park Square, Milton Park, Abingdon, Oxon, OX14 4RN

© 2021 Taylor & Francis Group, LLC

CRC Press is an imprint of Taylor & Francis Group, LLC

ISBN: 978-1-138-30557-1 (hbk)
ISBN: 978-0-203-72888-8 (ebk)

Typeset in Times LT Std
by Nova Techset Private Limited, Bengaluru & Chennai, India

Contents

v

Contributors

Dario Acuña-Castroviejo
Biomedical Research Center
Health Sciences Technology Park
University of Granada
and
Faculty of Medicine
Department of Physiology
University of Granada
and
CIBERFES
Biosanitary Research Institute
Granada Hospital Complex
Granada, Spain

Rosa María Rodríguez Arias
CB
Madrid, Spain

Agustín Arroyo Bielsa
Angiology and Vascular Surgery Unit
Hospital Vithas Nuestra Señora de América
Madrid, Spain

Karina Díaz Bustamante
Universidad Católica de Cuenca
Cuenca, Ecuador

Emma Iglesias Candal
Oral and Maxilofacial Surgery
Svenson Group
Madrid, Spain

José Luis Ciucci
Department of Anatomy
School of Medicine
University of Buenos Aires
Buenos Aires, Argentina

Marta Yuste Colom
Hospital Clinic Barcelona
Barcelona, Spain

Ana Isabel Cobo Cuenca
Faculty of Phisiotherpy and Nursing of Toledo
Multidisciplinary Care Research Group (IMCU)
Toledo, Spain

Eglee Montilla de Somaza
HM Hospitales
Madrid, Spain

Juana Deltell
San & Del Medicina Estética
Madrid, Spain
Spanish School of Aesthetic Medicine
Barcelona, Spain

and
University of Alcalá de Henares
Madrid, Spain

B. N. Díaz
IES Pérez de Ayala
Oviedo, Spain

Paloma Domingo
Vodder Center Physiotherapy
Madrid, Spain

Germaine Escames
Biomedical Research Center
Health Sciences Technology Park
University of Granada
and
Faculty of Medicine
Department of Physiology
University of Granada
and
CIBERFES
Biosanitary Research Institute
Granada Hospital Complex
Granada, Spain

Margarita Esteban
Aesthetic Medical Dra
Esteban Bilbao
Vitoria, Pamplona, Spain

Beatriz I Fernandez-Gil
Biomedical Research Center
Health Sciences Technology Park
University of Granada
Granada, Spain

Javier Florido
Biomedical Research Center
Health Sciences Technology Park
University of Granada
Granada, Spain

Mario Gisbert
Asociación Española de Micropigmentación
Madrid, Spain

Ana Guerra-Librero
Biomedical Research Center
Health Sciences Technology Park
University of Granada
and
CIBERFES
Biosanitary Research Institute
Granada Hospital Complex
Granada, Spain

Iris Luna-Boquera
Department of Endocrinology and Clinical Nutrition
Hospital Universitario Quironsalud
Universidad Europea de Madrid
Madrid, Spain

María Elena Fernández Martín
Clinic Ortega & Gasset
Madrid, Spain

Laura Martinez-Ruiz
Biomedical Research Center
Health Sciences Technology Park
University of Granada
Granada, Spain

Ángela García Matas
Relais Termal
Chaine de Thermal Centers
Madrid, Spain

Andrea Lourdes Mendoza
Kinesióloga
Buenos Aires, Argentina

Sheila K. Mota Antigua
Mediestetic Clinics
Madrid and Toledo, Spain

M. Lourdes Mourelle
Research Group FA2
Department of Applied Physics
University of Vigo
Vigo, Galicia, Spain

Emilce Insua Nipoti
Universidad Autónoma de Madrid
Regenerative and Antiaging Medicine of Universidad
    Complutense de Madrid
Pineal Medical Center
Lipedema Area of Medivas Clinic
Madrid, Spain

Hernán Pinto
i2e3 Biomedical Research Institute
Barcelona, Spain

Rosa Revert
Aesthetic Medicine
and
Pediatry and AP, Osasunbidea
Pamplona, Navarra, Spain

Ángela Río
Phisyotherapy
Universidad Europea
Sanamanzan Physiotherapy Center
Madrid, Spain

Raquel Benlloch Rodríguez
Department of Radiation Oncology
Hospital Universitario Puerta de Hierro
Madrid, Spain

Cesar Rodríguez-Santana
Biomedical Research Center
Health Sciences Technology Park
University of Granada
Granada, Spain

Eva Ruiz
Medical Oncology
Fundación Jiménez Díaz
Madrid, Spain

Iryna Russanova
Biomedical Research Center
Health Sciences Technology Park
University of Granada
and
Faculty of Medicine
Department of Physiology
University of Granada
and
CIBERFES
Biosanitary Research Institute
Granada Hospital Complex
Granada, Spain

Manuela Sánchez-Cañete
Médica San & Del
Aesthetic Medicine
Madrid, Spain

Adriana Schwartz
International Medical OZONE Federation
Madrid, Spain

Paloma Tejero
Universidad de Alcalá
Alcalá de Henares
Madrid, Spain

Victoria Zamorano Triviño
Mediestetic Valdemoro
Mediestetic
Madrid, Spain

Carmen Yélamos
Clinical Psycology
Psycooncologist Asociación Española Contra el Cáncer (AECC)
    and Genesis Care
Madrid, Spain

Silvia Gabriela Ortiz Zamorano
Family and Community Medicine
Escorial Hospital
Mediestetic
Madrid, Spain

1

The Oncological Patient and Aesthetic Medicine: The Bonded Approach

Paloma Tejero and Hernán Pinto

Aesthetic Medicine is a new field of medicine, in which different specialists share the objective of building and reconstructing the physical balance of the individual. Treatment of physical aesthetic alterations and unsightly sequelae of diseases or injuries, coupled with the prevention of aging, are perhaps two of the most emblematic areas of aesthetic medicine intervention [1].

J.J. Legrand
General Secretary of the International
Union of Aesthetic Medicine (UIME)

Introduction

The incidence of cancer is increasing gradually in the populations of developed countries. According to the Europe against Cancer Program, in the next few years, two out of every three Europeans will have cancer [2]. Globocan [3] published that the number of new cases in 2018, worldwide, was 18,078,957. Population estimates indicate that the number of new cases will probably increase by 70% in the coming decades, reaching approximately 24 million cases in the year 2035 [4].

Despite having increased in incidence, survival has also increased. Approximately 67% of cancer survivors are currently living with a diagnosis of cancer made 5 or more years previously. All this is due to an increasingly early diagnosis, to the coordination of several medical specialties in the diagnosis, and to the use of increasingly effective treatment protocols.

The current guidelines of the American Society of Clinical Oncology (ASCO), the European Society for Medical Oncology (ESMO), and the World Health Organization (WHO) define the need to approach the oncological patient from the point of view of "continuous care," defined as the integral attention to patients in their complete reality—biological, psychological, familial, work, and social [5]. Continuous care is applicable throughout the evolutionary process of cancer and its different stages.

Often, "the line between beauty and health is extremely fine" [7]. The classic phrase, "the face is the mirror of the soul," explains that our state of mind, how we feel, and also our state of health can be reflected in our image. The face is also our business card that distinguishes us as a person different from others, which is why cancer is a stigmatizing disease for many patients, not only because of its direct effects, as in skin or head and neck tumors, but also because of the aftermath of many of their treatments.

The Oncological Patient

The number of cancer patients, or of those with a history of having an oncological disease, who require medical consultation for aesthetic reasons, is increasing rapidly.

As the overall death rate from cancer has declined, the number of cancer survivors has increased. Currently, 5% of the population are cancer survivors [8]. These trends show that progress is being made against the disease, but there is still a lot of work to be done. It is currently estimated that more than 30% of cancer cases could be avoided with healthy habits, but while smoking rates (smoking is a leading cause of cancer) have declined, the population is aging, and cancer rates increase with age. Additionally, obesity, a risk factor for many types of cancer, is on the rise [10].

In 2011, Tarsilo Ferro and Josep M. Borras [11] warned that "A snowball is growing in health services: surviving patients with cancer." Many of today's oncology patients will evolve into chronic patients who need to achieve quality of life standards that are part of what we call "the challenges of survival": they want to live not only longer but also in the best possible way. The greater life expectancy and improved results from oncology treatment lead the oncological patient increasingly to demand medical-aesthetic cosmetic and reparative treatments that minimize adverse effects and stigmas linked to their disease. In a paper published in 2010, in the *Latin American Journal of Nursing*, that aimed to identify the stress factors present in the lives of women in the period of 1–5 years postdiagnosis, "the results indicated conflicts with self-image, alteration in the sensation of self-sufficiency, fear in relation to the evolution of the illness, the feeling of guilt for the disorder generated in the family, the experience of disturbing social situations, and the desire to return to professional occupation" [9].

Patients experience a strong emotional impact when receiving the news of their diagnosis; their personal, work, and social life change radically in a short time. In addition, they have to face aggressive treatments and the side effects of these treatments that tend to cause significant physical deterioration leading to loss of self-esteem. A low mood increases the levels of cortisol in the blood, damaging the immune system, affecting the state of well-being and health. Oncologists, and the medical community in general, increasingly recognize that treating the patient in a holistic way improves the results of treatment. This is where the role of aesthetic medicine is fundamental in oncology, since it intervenes at several levels: in prevention, during treatment (chemotherapy, radiotherapy, hormonotherapy, immunotherapy, and postsurgery), and in minimizing side effects (alterations in the skin and nails, mucositis, burns, alopecia, loss of eyebrows, vaginal dryness, lymphedema, weight loss, nausea and vomiting, sleep problems, problems in sexual relations, digestive disorders, etc.).

We know that the maintenance and improvement of quality of life is one of the key objectives of the care received by the patient. Since the 1990s, the evaluation of and the search for improvement of the quality of life of these patients have increased significantly. Quality of life is currently one of the key variables in oncology, as important as other medical variables (survival or response to treatment) [12], and it should guide therapeutic behavior, which must always be multidisciplinary. The preservation of a good self-image for the patient has a fundamental role in enabling the patient to avoid stigmatization (as the consequences of cancer on the skin, the self-image, and the body functions all betray its presence) and to enhance self-esteem and thus also to favor the immune response and adaptation to changes linked to the disease. Today no one doubts the therapeutic power of self-image [13] and the role that aesthetic medicine has to have in the continuum of the disease.

One aspect that we cannot forget is the number of patients diagnosed at young ages in whom the maintenance of an ability to work is essential for their lives. According to Stone [14], in 2017, 63% of cancer survivors continued to work or returned to work after treatment. Among this population, the ability to work and the challenges encountered in the workplace by these cancer survivors have not been well established, but we do know that the possibility of reducing labor productivity due to decreased capacity—functional, cognitive, and physical (changes in appearance, scars, etc.) changes caused by cancer and its treatments—significantly affects the reintegration of the patient into work and causes insecurity, anguish, and fear in a patient.

Aesthetic Medicine

Physical beauty has become so relevant in Western culture that many people consider physical appearance a major factor in their lives. The number of patients requiring medical consultation is increasing rapidly for aesthetic reasons. Aspects such as acceptance and its impact on self-esteem are considered increasingly important in the process of social adaptation. A dysmorphophobic, negative perception of one's appearance can lead to pathologies (dysmorphisms and dysmorphobias). Psychosomatic disorders resulting from low self-esteem due to aesthetic reasons are frequent and cannot be ignored by doctors, who will have to respond to the aesthetic needs of their patients, seeking *health* according to WHO, which defines it as "a state of complete physical, mental and social well-being and not only the absence of affections or illnesses"; so, without a doubt, we have to prepare ourselves to work as a team. Beauty, based on a concept of health, is a social good, and therefore beneficial for everyone. Beauty thus understood reaches both healthy individuals and those with pathologies.

Aesthetic medicine began in France in the early 1970s, establishing the French Society of Aesthetic Medicine, founded by Dr. J.J. Legrand, and soon spread to Italy, Belgium, and Spain. Its main objective was to meet social needs and demands that the official medical specialties did not treat, in that they were limited to diseases. In 1976, these four national societies created the UIME (Union Internationale de Medecine Esthetique) based in Paris, which currently has members in 32 European and non-European countries, with the aim of gathering all over the world, in a single scientific program, doctors of different specialties but with a common interest in the problems related to aesthetic medicine [15].

The General Assembly of the Medical Collegial Organization of Spain approved in 2004 the need to create a National Register of Aesthetic Medicine Doctors and approved the proposal of the organizations consulted to define *aesthetic medicine* as the "combination of prescriptions, actions, techniques and medical and/or surgical procedures—the latter limited to the skin, the cutaneous compartments, the subcutaneous cellular tissue and the superficial venous system—devoted to the promotion of health, prevention, diagnosis, and treatment of aspects that are inaesthetic (or judged as such by the patient), constitutional or acquired; and to the treatment of the states of general discomfort that are a consequence of physiological aging" [6].

Aesthetic medicine progresses hand in hand with antiaging medicine and regenerative medicine, constituting itself as a basic pillar in the well-being of our society. "Aesthetic Medicine is a new field of medicine, in which different specialists share the objective of building and reconstructing the physical balance of the individual. Treatment of physical aesthetic alterations and unsightly sequelae of diseases or injuries, together with the prevention of aging, are perhaps two of the most emblematic areas of aesthetic medicine intervention" [7].

The Oncological Patient and Aesthetic Medicine

At present, a focus on the multidisciplinary approach for comprehensive care of oncological patients is the way forward [19], allowing us as physicians to provide information, preventive measures, and treatment of symptoms and adverse effects associated with oncological therapies. We pursue the desire for the patient to be treated comprehensively, since oncological diseases affect all aspects of the patient's life. We seek to promote multidisciplinary follow-up and treatment, which include a greater diversity of specialists, counting on oncology units that have an aesthetic doctor and other health professionals who can help to alleviate those adverse effects now expected to be among the effects of antitumor therapies and not simply of narrow clinical interest. The perception by the patients of their image and their psychosocial state are aspects that can act positively or negatively in the prognosis and in their survival. Thanks to the emergence of new therapies, which are increasingly personalized, better knowledge of tumor biology, and the early diagnosis of many tumors, cancer has become, in an increasing number of cases, a disease with a high survival rate, where the patient is a survivor who demands a return to normalcy, seeking to recover his or her physical appearance, needing to correct or improve the consequences that the adverse effects of his or her treatment may have caused [18].

We also seek to emphasize the importance of nutrition and micronutrition as well as physical exercise in the different stages of the disease, knowing the positive impact they have on the survival of this group. We want to make known the importance of the "healing power of self-image." We must not forget that it influences not only self-esteem but also the response of a patient through different mechanisms, such as an improved state of mind, better personal relationships, and acceptance of treatments; all these aspects imply a better prognosis, as has been demonstrated particularly in patients with breast cancer [17].

In the oncological patient, the performance of the aesthetic physician is extremely important in prevention, early diagnosis, and recovery after the oncological treatment.

Aesthetic doctors should play an important role in the prevention of new neoplasms by proposing hygiene-dietary recommendations such as those included in the European Code Against Cancer: do not smoke; avoid obesity; perform physical activity; increase the consumption of fruits and vegetables; limit the consumption of fats of animal origin; moderate alcohol consumption; use sunscreen; apply the rules of radiological protection; undergo tests for early detection of cancer of the uterus, breast, colon, and prostate from a certain age; and participate in vaccination programs against human papillomavirus (HPV) and hepatitis B virus (HBV).

Aesthetic medicine can also play an important role in the early detection of cancer, since some of the symptoms associated with this disease can often be detected when taking the clinical history of a patient, such as a persistent pain over time; a nodule; a wound or ulcer that does not heal; a spot or mole that changes shape, size, or color; a lesion that has appeared on the skin and increases in size; bleeding or abnormal hemorrhages; persistent cough or hoarseness; changes in urinary or intestinal habits or unjustified weight loss; among others. In these cases, the cause of these signs and symptoms should be studied and the patient referred to the oncologist to confirm the diagnosis and prescribe the appropriate treatment.

After diagnosis and oncological treatment, these patients will also need periodic oncological checkups, psychological care, and the support of aesthetic medicine specialists. Aesthetic medicine specialists have the necessary tools (soft tissue fillers, peel, lasers, botulinum toxin) to tackle all the most important disorders within the aesthetic field, but they should only be managed with knowledge, experience, and evidence. This knowledge must be adapted specifically to the oncological patient. It is necessary to work on the practical adaptation of protocols and guidelines on how and when to act to make them accord with the demands of our patients and their situations in the continuum of the disease. To do this, we must know patients' needs and prepare and train physicians to give them adequate responses.

This constitutes an exciting challenge that has generated the need to create the master's degree in Quality of Life and Medical-Aesthetic Care of the Oncology Patient at the University of Alcalá de Henares [16]. Its main objective is to unify criteria allowing a multidisciplinary and personalized approach to the patient that has brought together the different professionals involved in patient care, such as oncologists, radiotherapists, psychologists, plastic surgeons, dermatologists, aesthetic doctors, pharmacists, urologists, gynecologists, immunologists, endocrinologists, physiotherapists, beauticians, and so on, to quantify the care and treatments that the oncological patient needs, integrating all the knowledge in order to achieve a broad and detailed vision of the different treatment plans with efficacy and safety.

Professional and patient associations (e.g., Spanish Society of Medical Oncology [SEOM], Spanish Society of Radiation Oncology, National Institutes of Health [NIH], Spanish Association Against Cancer [AECC], Spanish Group of Cancer Patients [GEPAC], Group of Oncoaesthetic Medicine Experts [GEMEON], etc.) have developed and made available to patients and their families action guides and manuals in which information is offered on the possible effects of oncological treatments on the skin, hair, mucous membranes, or nails, and tips, medical-aesthetic products, and treatments that will help in the care of the self-image. However useful these may be, it requires personalized attention and a professional with specific training in the topics to undertake the correct advice, care, and monitoring for these patients.

We could speak then of a new discipline—"oncoaesthetics"—directed to improving the quality of life of oncological patients, avoiding stigmatization, favoring self-esteem, improving self-image, and enhancing at the same time the immune system. This discipline helps patients to love themselves, to take care of themselves, and to accept themselves, emerging stronger from that process. When talking about quality of life, we refer to the global health of the patient, not only to the absence of illness but also to positive physical, psychological, and social well-being, and strength to face life again.

Conclusions

Aesthetic oncology medicine is a young discipline, but not lacking in scientific rigor; there are already research publications that guarantee the safety of the different medical-aesthetic treatments that can be offered to this type of patient, as well as what can be considered a necessary part of the multidisciplinary units of comprehensive care for oncological patients.

As Dr. Jean-Jacques Legrand, General Secretary of UIME, said: "Today and in the near future, aesthetic medicine and Anti-Aging Medicine offer our patients, who now live longer, better well-being with aesthetic treatments of aging of the skin and treatments for general aging. Aesthetic medicine is on the rise, but all doctors must be trained correctly, so the future will be bright" [1].

REFERENCES

1. Legrand J-J. Aesthetic Medicine, the booming medical activity. *Aesthetic Med.* April/June 2016;2(2).
2. Las cifras del cáncer en España. Sociedad Española de Oncología Médica (SEOM), 2016. at: http://www.seom.org/en/prensa/ el-cancer-en-espanyacom/105460-el-cancer-en-espana-2016 *Fuente*: http://www.seom.org (accessed 04 29, 2019).
3. All cancers excl. non-melanoma skin cancer: source, Globocan 2018; Accessed at: http://globocan.iarc.fr/Default.aspx
4. Ferlay J, Steliarova-Foucher E, Lortet-Tieulent J et al. Cancer incidence and mortality patterns in Europe: Estimates for 40 countries in 2012. *Eur J Cancer.* 2013 Apr;49(6):1374–403.
5. Manual SEOM de cuidados contínuos: accessed at https:// www.seom.org/seomcms/images/stories/recursos/sociosy-profs/documentacion/manuales/cuidCont/cuidadosContin-uos01-20.pdf

4

Aesthetic Treatments for the Oncology Patient

6. Libro Blanco de la SEME. Sociedad Española de Medicina Estética. Accessed at: http://www.seme.org/area_seme/libro-blanco.php (accessed 07 29, 2018).

7. Romanelli F. EDITORIAL. *Aesthetic Med.* April/June 2016;2(2).

8. https://www.cancer.gov/espanol/cancer/naturaleza/estadisticas; (accessed 08 04, 2018).

9. Da Silva G, Dos Santos MA. Factores estresantes del post-tratamiento del cáncer de mama: Un enfoque cualitativo. *Rev Latino-Am.* Enfermagem Artículo Originale 18(4):[09 pantallas] jul.-ago. 2010. Accessed at: http://www.scielo.br/scielo.php?pid=S0104-11692010000400005&script=sci_arttext&tlng=es

10. https://www.seom.org/seomcms/images/stories/recursos/NP_Dia_Mundial_del_Superviviente_de_Cancer.pdf

11. Ferro T, Borras J. Una bola de nieve está creciendo en los servicios sanitarios:los pacientes supervivientes con cáncer. *Gac Sanit.* 2011;25(3):240–5.

12. Arraras Urdaniz JA. La calidad de vida en el paciente oncologico. Accessed at: http://www.unedpamplona.es/documentos/admin/archivos/LECCION_INAUGURAL_EVALUACION_DE_CALIDAD_DE_VIDA_EN_EL_PACIENTE_ONCO

13. Sanchez C. apuntes master en Calidad de vida y cuidados medico-esteticos del paciente Oncológico. Accessed at:

https://www.formacionmbl.com/actualidad/articulos-relacionados/fundacion-angela-navarro.html

14. Stone D, Ganz P, Pavlish C, Robbins W. Young adult cancer survivors and work: A systematic review. *J Cancer Surviv Res Practice.* 2017;11(6):765–81.

15. https://www.aestheticmedicinejournal.org/?page_id=409; (accessed 12 24, 2018).

16. http://www.uah.es/es/estudios/Master-en-Calidad-de-Vida-y-Cuidados-Medico-Esteticos-del-Paciente-Oncologico/ EDCM – Marzo 2016 (1/7), also available at: http://www.ine.es/prensa/np963.pdf

17. Kroenke C, Michael Y, Poole E et al. Postdiagnosis social networks and breast cancer mortality in the After Breast Cancer. Pooling Project. *Cancer.* April 1, 2017;123(7):1228–37.

18. Burg MA, Adorno G, Lopez ED et al. Current unmet needs of cancer survivors: Analysis of open-ended responses to the American Cancer Society Study of cancer survivors II. *Cancer.* 2015;121(4):623–30. 10.1002/cncr.28951.

19. *Unidades asistenciales del área del cáncer. Estándares y recomendaciones de calidad y seguridad.* Informes, estudios e investigación. Ministerio de Sanidad, Servicios Sociales e Igualdad, 2013. (accessed 04 29, 2017) at: http://www.msssi.gob.es/organizacion/sns/planCalidadSNS/docs/Cancer_EyR.pdf

2

Challenges for Oncology: Prevention, Palliation, and Survival

Eva Ruiz

Prevention

Cancer is one of the most important public health problems worldwide. Given the important role that various external factors have in the development of cancer, strategies aimed at promoting prevention can help reduce the incidence and mortality figures.

There are two fundamental aspects of cancer prevention to consider. The first is primary prevention, which attempts to reduce the incidence of the disease by avoiding exposure to certain causal factors that are necessary for or favor the beginning of oncological disease. Secondary prevention attempts to detect tumors in healthy people as soon as possible so that, through appropriate intervention at an early stage, the natural history of the disease can be modified.

The World Health Organization (WHO) estimates that between 30% and 50% of cancer cases are preventable. Therefore, it is necessary to reduce the risk factors and apply preventive scientific-based strategies [1]. Currently, about one-third of cancer deaths are due to the five main behavioral and dietary risk factors: tobacco use, alcohol consumption, high body mass index, reduced intake of fruit and vegetables, and lack of physical activity. The European Code Against Cancer 2019 [2] focuses on measures that every citizen should take to help prevent cancer. There are 12 points:

1. Do not smoke; do not consume any form of tobacco.
2. Guarantee smokeless homes; support antismoking policies in the workplace.
3. Maintain a healthy weight.
4. Exercise every day; limit the time you spend sitting.
5. Eat healthily.
   - Eat lots of whole grains, legumes, fruits, and vegetables
   - Limit hypercaloric foods (high in sugar or fat) and avoid sugary drinks
   - Avoid processed meat; limit the consumption of red meat and foods with a lot of salt
6. Limit alcohol consumption, although it is best for cancer prevention to avoid alcoholic beverages.
7. Avoid excessive sun exposure, especially in children; use sunscreen; do not use UVA booths.
8. At work, protect yourself from carcinogenic substances by following the instructions in the regulations on occupational health and safety.
9. Find out if you are exposed to radiation from high natural radon levels in your home and take steps to reduce them.
10. For women:
    - Breastfeeding reduces the risk of cancer in the mother; if possible, the baby should be breastfed.
    - Hormone replacement therapy (HRT) during menopause increases the risk of certain types of cancer; limit treatment with HRT.
11. Make sure your children participate in vaccination programs against hepatitis B virus (HBV; newborns) and human papillomavirus (HPV).
12. Participate in organized cancer screenings [4]:
    - Colorectal (male and female)
    - Breast (female)
    - Cervical (female)

Primary prevention consists of reducing or avoiding exposure to factors clearly related to the beginning of cancer. It includes health promotion activities also, not only avoiding exposure to carcinogenic factors. These are the most important factors in the primary prevention of cancer [6]:

- Tobacco in any of its forms is responsible for 30% of mortality from cancer, and it is considered the most important risk factor to developing cancer and is the leading isolated and preventable cause of mortality worldwide. Lung, oral cavity, larynx, pharynx, esophagus, stomach, liver, pancreas, kidney, ureter, colon, rectum, bladder, cervix, leukemia, hepatoblastoma, and childhood leukemia have been linked to tobacco. Tobacco smoke released into the environment by smokers is also harmful to people who inhale it ("passive smokers"). It causes a small increase in the risk of lung cancer (estimated at 1%) in this subset. Important measures of primary prevention are antismoking policies, which should be considered in the long term, avoiding access to the habit, enhancing abandonment, and making relapse difficult. Determined and persistent medical advice to quit smoking has proven to be one of the most useful and efficient measures to gain years and quality of life. This continuous information to the population constitutes a valuable resource to facilitate citizens adopting healthy decisions.

- Alcohol also plays a causal role in the development of squamous carcinomas of the oral cavity, pharynx, larynx, esophagus (these tumors have the most evidence available, especially when also related to tobacco), liver, colon, rectum, and breast. There is evidence of a probable link with stomach and pancreatic cancers, and it is considered to be involved in 3% of cancer deaths in developed countries. In addition, the simultaneous consumption of alcohol and tobacco, due to its synergistic effect, significantly increases the risk of cancer of the respiratory and upper digestive tracts (up to 35 times). People who smoke and drink increase the risk of cancer by 10–100 times in comparison with nonsmokers or nondrinkers.

- Overweight and obesity are responsible for 20% of total cancer cases worldwide. The WHO in its World Cancer Report 2018 concludes that the increase in body fat intake boosts the risk of cancer of the esophagus, colon, pancreas, endometrium, and kidney, as well as breast cancer in postmenopausal women. Similarly, a study carried out by the International Agency for Research on Cancer (IARC) working group in 2016 concludes, with the available evidence from observational studies, that the absence of excess body fat has a preventive effect on the occurrence of the following neoplastic diseases: esophageal adenocarcinoma, gastric cancer located in the cardias, colorectal cancer, hepatocellular cancer, endometrial, ovarian, bladder, pancreas, renal cells, thyroid, breast cancer in postmenopausal women, multiple myeloma, and meningioma.

- The concept of a healthy lifestyle, in summary, would include the following aspects: maintain a regular body weight (body mass index [BMI]: 18.5–24.9 kg/m^2), avoid foods that promote weight gain (sugary drinks and fast food), carry out some physical activity for at least 30 minutes a day, breastfeed (for women; if possible), eat mainly foods of plant origin, limit the consumption of red meat, avoid processed meats, and limit consumption of alcoholic beverages. The contribution diet makes to the development of cancer is well known; there are some foods or nutrients clearly related to some types of cancer. However, with epidemiological studies of this type, it is very difficult to attribute the risk to a particular food or dietary component. In general, an abundant consumption of cereals, legumes, fruits, and vegetables is beneficial to reduce the risk of cancer, particularly of digestive tumors. Likewise, the preservation of salted or smoked foods increases the risk of gastric cancer, accompanied by *Helicobacter pylori* infection, and the contamination of some foods with aflatoxins (dried fruit and nuts) increases the risk of liver cancer. For some cancers (colorectal, breast, and endometrial cancers), there is a preventive effect from regular physical activity regardless of weight control.

- Ultraviolet radiation (UVR) is the most important carcinogen in different types of skin cancer. We can receive it through natural sources (sun exposure) or through exposure to artificial sources (UVA booths).

The incidence of melanoma doubled in Europe between the 1960s and 1990s, and this is attributed to the significant increase of intense sun exposure. The incidence of nonmelanoma skin cancers (basal cell and spinocellular carcinomas) has also increased in all European countries; although much less life-threatening than melanoma, these tumors represent 95% of all skin cancers. The individuals at highest risk are those with very light skin, particularly (but not exclusively) redheads and individuals with freckles and a tendency to burn with sun exposure. Currently, the primary prevention of skin cancer through photoprotection or the reduction of sun exposure is the best weapon to control the problem. It is advisable to avoid sun exposure around noon; wear clothing, hat, and glasses to reduce body exposure to sunlight; and remain in shadowed areas with the same objective. Sun exposure should be moderated, to reduce throughout the course of life and avoid extreme exposures and intense tanning. Excessive exposure to the sun is more harmful during childhood and adolescence than during adulthood. Some studies have revealed that sunburn that occurs before age 15 is a risk factor for melanoma. Solariums and ultraviolet lamps have the same harmful effect on the skin as natural sunlight and should be avoided at all times.

- Environmental factors (including both occupational and environmental risks) generate an average of 19% of cancer globally. Of those that are known, there are some natural ones, such as arsenic, radon, or solar radiation, but more artificial ones (the product of human activities), such as dioxins, electromagnetic radiation, or urban air pollution. In general terms, preventive measures will depend more on legislative and regulatory actions than on changes in people's individual behavior; generally, coordination between different administrations is required. There are criteria related to the classification, packaging, and labeling of dangerous chemical substances and preparations (Royal Decrees 363/95 and 255/03), and for the protection of workers against risks related to exposure to carcinogens in labor (RD 665/97).

- Radon is a natural radioactive gas that is produced in the Earth's crust. It cannot be detected by humans because it has no color or smell, but it can be measured due to its radioactivity. It is present especially in areas with more natural uranium in the soil and rocks. Radon exposure increases the risk of lung cancer. This risk is proportional to the concentration of radon in the air and the duration of exposure. In addition, this risk is more likely to increase in smokers and former smokers. There are maps that can be used to know if a house is in an area at higher or lower risk of having high levels of radon. Nevertheless, only a small number of cancers might be caused by radiation.

- Women who breastfeed their babies for a prolonged period of time have a lower risk of breast cancer, compared to women who do not breastfeed. The longer a woman breastfeeds, the higher the protection against breast cancer. The risk reduction is approximately 4% for every 12 months of breastfeeding. This adds to the risk reduction known for having a baby. Similarly, prolonged breastfeeding helps women reduce long-term weight gain and also promotes the return to prepregnancy weight.

- The use of HRT increases the risk of some types of cancer, such as breast cancer, endometrial cancer, and ovarian cancer. The cancer risk pattern depends on the type of therapy and on its hormonal composition (estrogens alone or in combination with progestogens).

- Vaccination is one of the tools available for primary prevention of some cancers. HBV and HPV vaccines are recommended. The infection caused by HBV is a problem of global public health, approximately 5% of the population is chronically infected, causing the deaths of 600,000 people every year. This virus causes liver damage, and the longer the infection lasts (chronic HBV), the higher are the chances of developing liver cancer. Newborns must be vaccinated within the first 24 hours of birth, as recommended by the WHO. With the three-dose schedule, protection against infection is induced in more than 95% of breastfed babies, children, and adolescents, and in more than 90% of healthy adults under 40 years of age.

- HPV infection is the most prevalent sexually transmitted infection. Although in most cases it is cured by the immune system, in a small percentage it can remain as a chronic infection and contribute to tumors, mainly cervical, vulvar and vaginal cancers in women, and anal and throat cancers in men and women, as well as penile cancer in men. Vaccination against HPV can prevent infection by virus subtypes that cause approximately 70% of cervical cancers. However, this vaccination is only effective for people who have not yet been infected by it. For this reason, it is recommended to vaccinate girls before they are sexually active. WHO recommends vaccination for girls between the ages of 9 and 13 years. Despite vaccination, it is still important for women to participate in cervical cancer screening programs [7].

From the public health perspective, primary prevention measures should be considered as a priority since they are very effective, especially in the long term. There are still some types of cancer in which the causes are not well established. For this reason, primary preventive measures must be completed with early diagnostic activities that must be implemented on a population basis and against certain pathological processes. This is known as *secondary prevention* [8].

The objectives of secondary prevention are as follows:

1. Decrease prevalence
2. Reduce mortality rates
3. Improve cancer prognosis
4. Avoid sequelae and disabilities

Secondary prevention techniques are as follows:

1. Provide health education to the population
2. Conduct studies of selective detection
3. Search for clinical cases (case finding)
4. Conduct population screening (screening)

The main objective of health education in relation to secondary prevention is to raise public awareness and strengthen the active participation of primary care physicians in public information. These physicians need to explain to the public that they need to recognize particular signs that should prompt an individual to consult a doctor (lumps; a wound that does not heal; a mole that changes shape, size, or color; abnormal blood loss; persistent problems such as hoarseness or cough; changes in bowel habits; urinary disorders; or abnormal weight loss). This would allow the population to collaborate in the early detection of some tumors.

Another way to make an early diagnosis is through selective clinical detection or opportunistic screening, performed in asymptomatic people who go to the health system for another reason. This is particularly beneficial since it expedites the diagnosis, improving the likelihood of survival.

Population screening, selective population detection, screening, or early diagnosis can be defined as the set of activities applied to large unselected populations that aim to detect the disease before it manifests clinically and thus be able to start treatment early with the purpose of improving the prognosis [4]. A disease susceptible to entering a screening program must meet the following conditions [5]:

- It must be frequent and serious, so that it is perceived as a social problem by the population.
- It must be clearly differentiable from normality; its clinical course must be known, and its symptoms must be clearly defined.
- Treatment in the presymptomatic stage should reduce mortality or serious complications (if this is the effect) more markedly than treatment after the onset of symptoms. If such treatment does not reduce mortality or the incidence of serious illness, it should at least improve the patient's quality of life.
- It must be a treatable and controllable disease as a mass phenomenon.

The population susceptible of being included in a screening program must meet the following requirements:

- It must be at high risk for the disease, that is, have a high prevalence of the disease.
- It must be a population with good community relations and cooperative attitudes.
- Demographic data on this population must be available so that the resources needed to execute the screening program can be correctly planned.

The diagnostic test to be used in the screening differs in a series of characteristics from those routinely used in the care diagnosis and must have the following characteristics:

- It must be acceptable by the population, even if it may be difficult to participate.

- It must be reproducible and valid. (Logically, it must first be reproducible, that is, it must provide the same results under similar conditions, before its validity can be estimated.)

It is important to consider all these aspects since a screening program involves economic, psychological, and social costs from carrying out unnecessary diagnostic tests and for false positives and their psychological cost. The relationship between cost and effectiveness should be part of the evaluation of any screening program before recommending its application.

The effectiveness of cancer screening has been clearly demonstrated in three cancers: breast, cervical, and colorectal cancers. There are some cancers in which the existing evidence does not allow us to give a clear answer about the effectiveness of population screening, although the research is in progress, such as prostate cancer or lung cancer, among others.

However, there are high-risk groups for developing cancer that may benefit from screening activities other than those proposed, as is the case in hereditary syndromes predisposing certain individuals to cancer [3].

1. *Breast cancer screening*:
   - Women 45–50–69 years.
   - Screening test: Mammography.
   - Screening interval: 2 years (individualize according to findings on mammography, BI-RADS score, and risk factors).
2. *Cervical cancer screening*:
   - Asymptomatic women who are or have been sexually active, between ages 25 and 65 years.
   - Screening test: Cervical cytology every 3 years versus HPV test every 5 years.
   - Screening interval: 3–5 years.
3. *Colorectal cancer screening*:
   - Men and women 50–69 years.
   - Screening test: Fecal occult blood (SOH) versus colonoscopy.
   - Screening interval: 2 (SOH) and 10 years (colonoscopy). Individualize according to results.

Palliation

Continuous care or supportive care treatments are aimed at improving symptoms through full, active care and continued coverage of a patient's psychological/emotional, social, spiritual, and physical needs. Several studies have shown that this type of care is beneficial for patients and their families because it reduces pain, breathlessness or shortness of breath, nausea and other digestive disorders, anxiety, fear, and depression, and thereby contributes to improved quality of life of patients [9].

Initially, palliative or supportive care was synonymous with end-of-life care. Currently, these actions are considered as complementary to therapies specifically aimed at treating cancer and should be applied jointly from the moment of diagnosis of the disease. Several studies have shown that the early integration of supportive treatment and antitumor therapy not only increased the quality of life and mood of patients with lung cancer, which was probably extrapolated to other diseases, it was also able to significantly improve the prognosis of patients [10,11].

Therefore, this type of care is included not only in the final stage of life but also in the diagnosis and treatment process. It is important that patients know that they can access these services at any time, not only when deciding to end an active cancer treatment or when it is not possible to continue it.

In recent years, effective treatments have been developed that have improved the evolution of many cancers. Along with these, good supportive care, including the biopsychosocial field and the support of families are crucial for these treatments to be feasible and applicable in clinical practice. Thus, one of the objectives of comprehensive care is to reduce complications and support the administration of treatments such as chemotherapy. In fact, individualized support therapy has allowed an increasing number of patients to benefit from these advances against cancer by comprehensively handling a very variable problem that includes the following:

- Prevention and treatment of infections
- Prevention and treatment of thromboembolic disease
- Prevention and management of chemotherapy toxicities, such as anemia, neutropenia, mucositis, diarrhea, vomiting, etc.
- Skeletal health care, including the prevention of fractures and other bone events
- Recommendations on lifestyle, physical exercise, cardiovascular health, nutrition, and types of diet
- Confrontation of diagnosis and psychological symptoms such as depression, anxiety, fear, and insomnia
- Optimization of the treatment of previous diseases such as diabetes, chronic bronchitis, or heart failure
- Preservation of fertility in young patients who have not fulfilled their desire to be parents
- Development of outpatient treatment strategies, aimed at streamlining the use of hospital resources and improving the quality of life and well-being of patients and families
- Treatment of the elderly, fragile patients, and other special populations
- Recommendations based on the evidence of "alternative" therapies (better called "integrative medicines" that should complement cancer treatment and never replace it)
- Palliation of symptoms associated with cancer
- Approach the patient and family as a unit that shares decision-making with the doctor

This continuous care often requires specialized multiprofessional teams that provide a higher level of patient support with an active and rehabilitative aim. These support or palliative care units will usually be able to deal with more complex medical problems, difficult-to-control symptoms, or social or family problems. The doctors in these units, as well as those in primary care, work in collaboration with the oncologist to try to improve the situation, and the units may have other specialists such as a psycho-oncologist, social worker, palliative care nurse, and so on. As much as possible, this care takes place at home, in the company of loved ones, in an environment as familiar as possible for the patient seeking to safeguard his or her dignity and autonomy. However, if at any time the symptoms cannot be treated at home or care cannot be performed at home, especially in the final stages of life, it is possible to have care in a hospice. The goal is to help patients live as comfortably as possible during the last days.

Survival

All cancer patients wait for the day when the doctor says the treatment has finally been completed. At that point, the end of cancer treatment marks the beginning of a new journey: survival.

According to WHO, in 2016 it was estimated that there were 15.5 million cancer survivors in the United States, and this number is expected to increase to about 20.3 million by 2026. Currently, more than 50% of adult patients diagnosed with cancer live at least 5 years [10]. To a great extent, those who presented with tumors in early stages have a life expectancy similar to the general population. In childhood tumors, the number of patients with a 5-year survival rate rises to 73%. The most frequent tumors among survivors are as follows:

- *Men*: Prostate cancer, colorectal cancer, and melanoma
- *Women*: Breast cancer, colorectal cancer, and uterine cancer

Cancer survivors have specific social and health needs that in many cases are not covered, since health professionals are often not familiar with survival problems. In 1985, Fitzhugh Mullan, a cancer survivor doctor, described the situation of abandonment and disorientation that patients feel when they finish cancer treatment. Now teams of professionals are recognizing that they need to better prepare patients for this next phase of life. As an example, pediatric oncologists lead survival initiatives, thanks to the long-term survival of children with cancer [2].

Once the treatment is finished, there is a transition experience from the concerns related to the prognosis and the treatment to new concerns about the future. In this phase, there are new milestones to overcome. One of them is the risk of cancer recurrence. It should be explained how follow-up plans will be organized and what symptoms should act as alarms so that cancer survivors and health professionals will be able to detect symptoms early. In addition, psychological support is necessary since fear of the disease is a frequent symptom and should be addressed from the beginning. However, this is also the time for survivors to recover completely, both physically and spiritually, from the treatments received and their consequences in order to achieve a true state of health and well-being. It is also important to talk about the "late effects" of treatment (side effects that may not be apparent until years later) and the general plan for follow-up and prevention visits. The most frequent late effects are as follows:

- Anxiety and depression
- Changes in cognitive function
- Fatigue
- Lymphedema
- Symptoms related to menopause
- Alterations of the hair, skin, and mucosae
- Neuropathy
- Pain
- Sexual dysfunction (woman/man)
- Loss of fertility
- Sleep disorders

It is necessary to develop formal survival plans that can provide attention to patients and their families and thus increase their quality of life. This will improve the training of professionals, and multidisciplinary groups can be created. A cancer survivor care plan should include the following:

- Training on side effects, follow-up, and possible treatments. Immediate side effects such as skin and hair disorders, digestive disorders, and so on, should be monitored. Certain drugs, such as anthracyclines, can cause late heart damage, and bleomycin can cause a reduction in lung capacity.
- Schedule of appointments for follow-up tests.
- Medical and nursing reports to be able to communicate to the same doctors the diagnosis, date of diagnosis, and treatment received.
- Rehabilitation programs.
- Emotional support programs for patients and families.
- Support for social reintegration and work.
- Recommendations for a healthy lifestyle.
- Genetic counseling and screening plans for children and family members.
- Research plans in long-term cancer survivors.

It is necessary to create easy-to-understand tools for patients and their families and caregivers that facilitate the life and survival of cancer patients.

"One day you will realize that you are not one more survivor, but a brave warrior who never gave up." World Breast Cancer Day 2019.

REFERENCES

1. European Cancer Leagues. Accessed Oct 2019. www.europeancancerleagues.org
2. Sociedad Española de Oncología Médica (SEOM), Plan Integral de Atención a los Largos Supervivientes de Cáncer, 2013. Accessed Oct 2019 http://www.seom.org/
3. Castells X, Sala M, Ascunce N et al. Description of cancer screening in Spain. DESCRIC project. 2007.
4. GBD 2015 Risk Factors Collaborators. Global, regional, and national comparative risk assessment of 79 behavioural, environmental and occupational, and metabolic risks or clusters of risks, 1990–2015: A systematic analysis for the Global Burden of Disease Study 2015. *Lancet*. 2016 Oct;388(10053):1659–724.
5. Plummer M, de Martel C, Vignat J, Ferlay J, Bray F, Franceschi S. Global burden of cancers attributable to infections in 2012: A synthetic analysis. *Lancet Glob Health*. 2016 Sep;4(9):e609–16. doi: 10.1016/S2214-109X(16)30143.

6. Cerdá T, Elizaga NA, Garcia A. *Implantación y evaluación de programas poblacionales de cribado.* Sociedad Española de Epidemiología; 2006.

7. Wild C, Espina C. Cancer Prevention Europe. 2019. *Molecular Oncology* https://doi.org/10.1002/1878-0261.12455

8. Guia Cuidados Paliativos. *SECPAL*, 2019. Accessed Oct 2019. www.secpal.com

9. Protocolos de la Sociedad Catalano-Balear de Cuidados Paliativos (SEPCAL). 1993. SEPCAL. Accessed Oct 2019. www.sepcal.com

10. Gómez-Batiste Alentorn X, Roca Casas J, Pladevall Casellas C, Gorchs Font N, Guinovart Garriga C. Atención Domiciliaria. In: López y RM, Maymo N, Eds. *Monografías Clínicas en Atención Primaria.* Barcelona: Ed. DOYMA, 1991: 131–49.

11. Salud OM. *Plan Integral de Atención a los Largos Supervivientes del Cáncer.* 2019. Accessed Oct 2019. www.who.int

3

Cancer as a Chronic Disease

Eva Ruiz

Introduction

The term *cancer* comprises a large group of diseases that are characterized by the development of abnormal cells, which divide, grow, and spread without control in any part of the body.

Cancer continues to be one of the leading causes of morbidity and mortality worldwide. According to GLOBOCAN data estimates [1], the incidence keeps growing, having increased from 14 million cases worldwide in 2012 to 18.1 million in 2018. Prospective population statistical studies indicate that cancer incidence will continue to increase in the next two decades, likely reaching 29.5 million in 2040 and potentially becoming the leading cause of death worldwide, particularly in developed countries. This effect is probably the consequence of increasing population; aging (age is an underlying risk factor in the development of cancer); exposure to risk factors such as tobacco, alcohol, pollution, obesity, sedentary lifestyle, among many others; and in some types of cancer, such as colorectal, breast, cervical, or prostate cancer, the increase in early detection. Of note, the most frequently diagnosed tumors in 2018 were lung, breast, colon and rectum, prostate, and stomach.

In contrast to its incidence, cancer mortality in developed countries has experienced a sharp decline in recent decades. These trends reflect improvements in survival as a consequence of more aggressive preventive activities, early diagnostic campaigns, and, especially, therapeutic advances (although the last ones, particularly relevant in recent years, will be more reliably reflected in the epidemiological data of the upcoming years) and, in men, the decrease in smoking prevalence. This decrease is not uniform in all tumors, since, for example, mortality in women due to lung cancer has experienced an increase in recent years due to the later incorporation of women into the smoking habit.

The survival of all cancer patients in Spain shows similar trends compared to its neighboring countries, standing at 53% at 5 years after diagnosis. Some countries in Europe, such as the United Kingdom, have doubled their survival rates in the last 40 years, showing a slightly higher expectancy with 50% of cancer survivors at 10 years after diagnosis, overall. This is a reflection of the increased survival for which screening policies may have an impact, like breast and colon cancer, while for the rest of cancer types, it remains similar within the European Union [2].

Therefore, cancer remains one of the leading causes of morbidity and mortality globally, with approximately 9.6 million cancer-related deaths in 2018, according to data provided by the World Health Organization (WHO). The tumors responsible for the highest number of deaths worldwide were lung cancer (18.4% of total cancer deaths), colorectal cancer (9.2%), stomach cancer (8.2%), and liver cancer (8.2%).

In any case, one of the most important aspects to consider is that according to the data published by WHO in its 2014 World Cancer Report [3], about a third of cancer deaths are due to the five most important avoidable factors. Among them, tobacco use (responsible for up to 33% of tumors worldwide, and up to 22% of cancer deaths), infections (especially relevant in developing countries, in which they are responsible for up to 25% of tumors), alcohol intake (responsible for up to 12% of tumors), sedentary lifestyle, and inadequate diets (insufficient amount of fruit and vegetable) are the more frequent ones [2–7].

We could infer that, likely thanks to advances in preventive medicine, diagnostic methods, and new therapeutic approaches, and as a direct consequence of increased incidence and survival rates, cancer is becoming a chronic disease.

Defining and Battling Cancer

The type of cancer is defined by many aspects, such as the tissue or organ of origin, the degree of differentiation of the conforming cells, and molecular and genetic characteristics, among others. From a strict perspective, there can be as many types of cancers as there are patients, each one with its specific molecular and cellular alterations. Thanks to technological, scientific advances, the molecular profile of each tumor can be subclassified in much more detail, using next-generation sequencing techniques, which can grant a comprehensive description of the genetic mutations of the tumor in a quick and reliable way. This amount of information allows not only the diagnosis and classification of the tumor, but, more importantly, the application of newly developed targeted treatments, opening the path for personalized medicine [8].

Regarding cancer spread, we can find oncological disease in a localized or locally advanced stage with invasion of contiguous organs, referred to as "local invasion"; in these cases, the treatments are aimed at the eradication of the disease thanks to combined systemic therapies (including chemotherapy, immunotherapy, targeted therapies, etc.) and/or radiotherapy. Once the treatment with curative intent is completed, the patient must subsequently carry out medical and multidisciplinary follow-up with the aim of detecting possible recurrences of the disease, controlling side effects that have occurred, and advising preventive healthy lifestyles.

Likewise, tumor cells can invade blood and lymph vessels and travel through the system to distant organs or tissues in which they can be implanted and continue to increase. These new sources of disease are named *metastases*, or *disseminated disease* or *distant recurrence*.

The term *advanced cancer* involves a tumor that has extended beyond the organ where it originated, usually leading to a situation where curation of the disease is difficult to achieve. Localized tumors that invade an extensive area and are only with difficulty removable by regional approaches also fit this characteristic. Thanks to the new combined therapies and treatments, the number of tumors with advanced disease that can be cured is higher; however, most advanced-stage cancers are still not curable but can become chronic, with continuous treatment that can control the disease for months or years. As with other chronic diseases, such as heart disease or diabetes, the goal of cancer treatment is to help patients live as well as possible for as long as possible, preventing the disease from growing, spreading, or progressing. In the past, many people did not live long with metastatic cancer. Today, especially with the new era of targeted therapies and immunotherapy, patients can be treated for a prolonged period of time and with good living standards.

The treatment used for cancer as a chronic condition depends on the type and origin of the primary tumor, specific mutations predicting response to therapy, aggressiveness or distribution of metastases, previously received treatments, age, performance status, and patient preferences. Monotherapy regimens or drug combinations may be used, based on classical chemotherapy, hormonal therapy, targeted therapies, or immunotherapy [9].

Chemotherapy remains the main tool. Its goal is to eliminate all cells that are in division, since the tumor cells have uncontrolled cell division mechanisms activated. This is where the side effects appear, since they are not specific to tumor cells, and they can potentially affect any cell in the body. It is given on a regular basis, usually intravenously (central catheter or "port-a-cath") and depends on the type of drug or treatment scheme. It acts at the systemic level; this means that chemotherapy can kill cancer cells that have spread (metastasized) to parts of the body distant from the original (primary) tumor.

Hormone therapy, also called hormonal treatment, is a form of medical cancer treatment that uses drugs that act by modifying hormones (preventing their synthesis or altering their effects on certain cells) to slow the growth of certain tumors—tumors that have hormonal receptors in their cells and, therefore, are hormone dependent and can be treated with hormone therapy. These are usually breast and prostate cancers [10].

Targeted therapy stops the action of the molecules that are key to the growth of cancer cells and the differences of normal cells; therefore, it affects cancer cells more than normal cells. The specific action of targeted therapy differs from traditional chemotherapy, which affects all rapidly growing cells; it has a better safety profile than chemotherapy but is not exempt from side effects, especially at the skin and digestive levels (diarrhea) [11].

Immunotherapy, unlike the other available treatments, is not aimed at destroying tumor cells but stimulates the patient's immune system so that it attacks and destroys the tumor. Immunotherapy is relatively specific since the immune system recognizes abnormal tumor cells and not healthy ones, limiting the toxicity. Another advantage is the immune system's memory that allows it to continue recognizing the tumor as "abnormal," favoring a prolonged action that can result in prolonged survival, a fundamental characteristic of this treatment. However, the activation of the immune system can trigger immune-related side effects that can affect any organ and become serious or precipitate the exacerbation of underlying autoimmune diseases. Despite these potential limitations, immunotherapy and precision medicine are currently the main therapeutic revolutions in oncology, since they have drastically changed the prognosis of some tumor types and increased survival [12].

These treatments can be administered intravenously (by reservoir when potentially vesicant chemotherapies are used or peripherally) or orally, with increasingly simple and shorter-duration regimens that give patients more autonomy.

During the treatment, different scenarios can be proposed: that the disease progresses despite the treatment, or remains stable, or decreases in size, or disappears. This is what oncologists define as progression, stabilization, partial response, or complete response. Some types of cancer are more likely to become chronic, such as leukemias, lymphomas, and prostate and breast cancers. In these cases, when the disease is under control and in response, maintenance treatments are performed. For example, men with prostate cancer can sometimes be treated with hormonal therapies for several years. Treatment may be suspended if the cancer is in remission and restarted if it relapses or recurs (reappears). It is also common for cancers to stop responding to treatments, as new mutations and escape routes occur in tumor cells, allowing them to evade and become resistant to therapies. In these cases, when the disease progresses, a different treatment can be recommended, with a different mechanism of action leading to cancer patients receiving several subsequent lines of treatment throughout their disease. Sometimes it is necessary to stop an effective treatment or switch to another treatment for side effects that are not tolerated or that may be irreversible and permanent, such as neuropathy or cardiac damage.

In this sense, a frequent question that patients ask oncologists is: How long will the treatment last? The answer is usually not clear. There is no specific schedule, and it depends on each patient, but in advanced cases, treatment often lasts for life since the disease cannot be cured, just as a patient with insulin-dependent diabetes receives insulin in a chronic lifetime manner. There are other factors to consider, such as the type of cancer, the type of treatment and treatment plan, how well the treatment is controlling the cancer, how the drug is being tolerated and what side effects it produces (not just physical ones, but also emotional), how advanced or aggressive the cancer is, and, most importantly, the patient's preferences.

In the chronic cancer scenario, those patients who have presented a localized disease in which a radical curative treatment was performed but who may subsequently need prolonged treatment to prevent their return, could also be included. The term for this scenario where a treatment is administered after radical approaches with the intent of preventing its reappearance is *adjuvant treatment*; for example, patients with early stage breast cancer whose disease has been cured by surgery or radiotherapy may receive continuous hormonal therapy, even for life, to decrease the risk of recurrence.

Living with chronic cancer (controlled, but not cured) can be difficult, on psychological, physical, and financial levels, especially when you have to "normalize" a life with nontoxic treatments, routine checkups, and the uncertainty of what will happen. That is why it is important to carry out early, complete, and multidisciplinary medical care in order to help control the disease, manage the challenges of survival, and maintain a good quality of life. In order to meet this challenge, it is recommended to develop treatment plans in dedicated multidisciplinary centers. The essential points to consider for medical professionals who treat patients with chronic cancer are as follows [13–15]:

- To provide information about the disease—Where to go and how to treat the symptoms, the phases, and the possible evolutions of the disease, what to expect regarding survival and quality of life. In this way, patients can understand their situation better and make truly "informed choices."

- Develop an assistance plan—Report on the treatment to be performed; its management, frequency, and duration; what kind of symptomatic improvements should be expected; and when the routine controls will be carried out with complementary tests (analytical, imaging tests, etc.), as there will be time to reevaluate the disease, and physicians will be able to know the effectiveness of the treatments. This information should improve adherence to treatment, which has been shown to be more effective and beneficial for the patient.

- Inform about the possible side effects of the treatment and ideas to control them and improve their health. In addition, sometimes doses and schedules can be altered; new treatments could even be considered. The patient must always know how and when to reach the professionals before leaving the treatment.

- Try to choose and adjust treatments to conform to the patient's schedules and availability of transfers, allowing a better quality of life and autonomy.

- Consider rehabilitation options—A wide range of treatments and services can be included, such as physiotherapy, pain management, nutritional planning, exercise, and emotional counseling, which can keep the patient as independent and productive as possible.

- Make healthy lifestyle changes—Recommend not smoking and provide the patient with the required tools to achieve this, limit alcohol consumption, eat well, control stress, and stay physically active, exercise.

- Support in the social and family atmosphere—Advise on financial resources, the costs of medical treatment; consider social assistance.

- Emotional support—Patients with chronic cancer experience borderline emotional situations, from diagnosis, during treatment, and in the last moments of their illness. They can go through moments of anger, fear, anxiety, sadness, and uncertainty. It is important to talk about their concerns, even when the treatment is working well. Doctors should help to manage the uncertainty of not knowing what to expect or what will happen next. There are different ways to help patients: experts in oncological psychology, support groups, support partnerships through a cancer organization, and relaxation techniques and stress management, such as meditation, yoga, or deep breathing.

- Support for caregivers—When the treatment lasts for months or even years, patient caregivers who provide physical, emotional, and practical care, such as accompanying them during treatments or medical checkups, may experience symptoms such as fatigue, sleep problems, depression, and anxiety. Therefore, health-care teams can also suggest ways to help caregivers cope with it.

Advances in oncology have managed to turn cancer into a chronic condition, increasing survival and quality of life, but it also often remains an incurable disease. We must bear in mind that many, even most, patients will present a progressive disease despite the treatments, especially in the final stages, where most therapies will be ineffective and only worsen the patient's situation. They may also have uncontrolled symptoms or intolerable side effects that may need attention. Patients could also reject continuation of therapy, as an informed choice, and doctors need to be able to accept and allow these decisions. For these reasons, palliative care and symptom control must be an integral part of the disease from the early stages.

> Living with cancer is different from living after cancer. And it's becoming more common every day. (American Cancer Society)

REFERENCES

1. Cancer IA. *Global Cancer Observatory*. 2019. https://gco.iarc.fr/

2. Bray F, Ferlay J, Soerjomataram I, Siegel RL, Torre LA, Jemal A. 2018. Global cancer statistics 2018: GLOBOCAN estimates of incidence and mortality worldwide for 36 Cancers in 185 Countries. *CA Cancer J Clin* 2018;68(6):394–424. https://onlinelibrary.wiley.com/doi/full/10.3322/caac.21492

3. Ferlay J, Colombet M, Soerjomataram I, Mathers C, Parkin DM, Piñeros M, Znaor A, Bray F. Estimating the global cancer incidence and mortality in 2018: GLOBOCAN sources and methods. *Int J Cancer.* 2019;144(8):1941–1953. doi: 10.1002/ijc.31937. PubMed PMID: 30350310

4. Steliarova-Foucher E, O'Callaghan M, Ferlay J et al. *European Cancer Observatory: Cancer Incidence, Mortality, Prevalence and Survival in Europe.* Version 1.0 (September 2012) European Network of Cancer Registries, International Agency for Research on Cancer. Disponible en: http://eco.iarc.fr, último acceso el 16/01/2016.

5. WHO Cancer Mortality Database. [accessed Jan 2019]. http://www-dep.iarc.fr/WHOdb/WHOdb.htm

6. Instituto Nacional de Estadística (INE). Defunciones según la causa de muerte, año 2017. https://www.ine.es/prensa/edcm_2017.pdf

7. REDECAN. Red Española de Registros de Cáncer. http://redecan.org/es/index.cfm

8. Javier Puente DG. *Sociedad Española Oncología Médica*. (06 de Marzo de 2017). https://seom.org/

9. Treatment To. *American Cancer Society*. (accessed Jan 2019). Obtenido de cancer.org

10. Zamora DP. *Sociedad Española Oncologia Médica*. (22 de enero de 2013). seom.org

11. Jorge DA. *Sociedad Española Oncología Médica*. (05 de Abril de 2013). seom.org

12. Remon J. *Sociedad Española Oncología Médica*. seom.org. (14 de noviembre de 2019).

13. Cancer LW. *Information from ASCO*. 2018; cancer.net

14. Condition MC. *National Comprehensive Cncer Network*. 2019; nccn.org

15. Illness MC. *American Cancer Society*. 2019; cancer.org

4

Clinical Record: Oncological Screening

Raquel Benlloch Rodríguez

General Concepts

At present, cancer constitutes one of the most significant diseases worldwide—a big public health problem and one of the main causes of morbidity/mortality. Early diagnosis, or diagnosis at the early stages, is essential in order to achieve a higher cure rate and, therefore, a reduction in mortality.

Population screening is a secondary prevention measure, defined as a set of actions performed on the general population in order to detect the disease in its latent phase, before it manifests clinically, improving treatment efficacy in relation to the scenario in which the disease has been diagnosed at a more advanced stage. Supplementary tests that allow a presumed diagnosis are usually used, which identify the population group that is more at risk of suffering the disease and, therefore, will benefit from undergoing more specific tests that can confirm the diagnostic suspicion.

Screening can be classified as mass or *nonselective screening*, which focuses on the entire population; *selective screening*, intended for certain high-risk groups; and individual or *opportunistic screening*, which the doctor performs on the patient.

To be part of a screening program, a disease or condition must meet a series of criteria that justify its application. These criteria, established in 1968 by Wilson and Jugner [1], include aspects related to the disease and screening tests. In general terms, the criteria to be met are as follows:

- The disease must be considered a public health problem.
- Its natural history, from the latent phase to the clinical phase, must be properly known.
- The latent phase must be recognizable and defined.
- There must be a test for its diagnosis.
- It must have an efficient treatment. Furthermore, in the preclinical phase, the treatment must show a higher benefit with respect to that conducted once the symptoms have appeared.
- Facilities for diagnosis and treatment must be available.
- There must be a defined population.
- The investigation of a case must be a continuous process, not a unique event.
- Screening tests must be valid and reproducible, reliable, accepted by the population, assessable, and cost-effective, in such a way that the expenses (including diagnosis and treatment of diagnosed patients) are well-balanced with the potential cost entailed by population health care.

Screening tests may yield four potential results (Table 4.1): true positives (TP), false positives (FP), true negatives (TN), and false negatives (FN). One of the most significant parameters to evaluate the validity of the test is the positive predictive value (PPV), which reflects the proportion of subjects with a positive screening test and the disease. This parameter must be elevated, for which two key aspects are required: *high sensitivity*, that is, the test must be able to properly identify a sick subject; and *high prevalence* of the disease, that is, the object of the diagnosis [2].

It must be taken into account that population screenings are conducted on asymptomatic people, and there still could be adverse effects; a person with an FP result, that is, a positive screening test but no diagnosis of cancer, is subject to more aggressive tests, which in turn can trigger a state of anxiety or distress secondary to the uncertainty of the process. A person with an FN result, that is, a negative screening test who actually has the disease, may have the wrong assurance of being healthy and not be vigilant about initial symptoms.

Within the assessment of population screening programs, another aspect to take into account is the potential existence of bias. The three most common biases are as follows.

1. *Lead-Time Bias*: The latency period is the time interval between the moment an occult disease can be detected and the occurrence of symptoms or signs. In this type of bias, the screening test anticipates the time of diagnosis, that is, it shortens the latency period during which the disease would have been detected through the occurrence of signs or symptoms but does not improve survival.

TABLE 4.1

Assessment of Screening Test Validity

Result of the Screening Test	State of the Disease	
	Sick	**Healthy**
Positive	TP	FP
Negative	FN	TN

Sensitivity (S): TP/TP+FN
Positive predictive value (PPV): TP/TP+FP

Specificity (Sp): TN/TN+FP
Negative predictive value (NPV): TN/TN+FN

Abbreviations: FN, false negative; FP, false positive; TN, true negative; TP, true positive.

The disease is detected at a stage in which the treatment has an efficacy rate similar to what it would have if administered after symptoms appear, or it does not improve the prognosis of the disease, resulting in the subject's death whether the screening test has been conducted or not. This bias can misrepresent an improvement of survival rates in the group undergoing screening.

2. *Length-Time Bias*: Screening tests more easily detect those cancers with slow evolution and longer duration, which usually have a more indolent course and are less aggressive. For this reason, this bias makes it difficult to compare results from screening-detected cancers with those diagnosed using tests other than screening.

3. *Overdiagnosis*: The purpose of screening programs is to diagnose cancers in the initial stages of the disease. However, there may be cases in which its evolution is so slow that there are no clinical manifestations, and the subject dies due to other causes, in a way that the detection of the disease does not benefit the patient at all.

Recommendations for screening tests must take into account both their benefits and potential adverse effects, with the application of strict criteria that ensure their quality. To justify conducting a screening program, it is advisable to develop randomized clinical trials that evaluate the reduction of cancer-specific mortality as the main end point. However, conduction of these studies is restricted by the need for large samples of patients, long duration, and high costs.

Population Screening Based on Type of Cancer

Scientific societies and health-care organizations recommend carrying out massive population screenings of mainly three types of cancer: breast, colorectal, and cervical. There are other tumors, such as lung cancer, for which massive population screening is not justified due to the lack of scientific evidence, but the potential efficacy of conducting computed tomography (CT) scans in risk groups is under research. Regarding prostate cancer, some published articles have shown an increase in early detection rates, but there are currently no published randomized clinical trials that have objectified a reduction in mortality; despite this fact, some scientific societies recommend that males undergo prostate-specific antigen (PSA) testing once a year beginning at 50 years of age. The *Official Journal of the European Union* (EU), published in 2003, includes all the recommendations about cancer screening for the EU member countries [3], with the purpose of developing and implementing effective strategies that can help in the early detection of cancer.

The characteristics of massive screening programs based on the type of tumor are described later.

Screening in Breast Cancer

Introduction

Breast cancer is the most common nondermatological tumor in women, both worldwide and in Europe. It constitutes a public health problem, since 8% of European women are at risk of suffering breast cancer before the age of 75 [4]. In 2012, breast cancer was estimated to represent 25% (1,676,500 of diagnosed cases) of all cancers in women worldwide. Although men can also present with breast cancer, its incidence is estimated to be lower than 1%.

Based on the information provided by the Spanish Network of Cancer Registries (REDECAN) [5], the last publication of which dates back to 2014, the total number of new cases in Spain was estimated at 26,354, with a gross rate of 135.8, compared with rates adjusted to the world and European population of 72.9 and 98.9 per 100,000 people, respectively.

The implementation of population screening programs, which has enabled an increase in the number of patients diagnosed at the early stages, as well as great diagnostic and therapeutic advances in recent years, has resulted in an increase in survival rates, estimated at 82.8% for patients diagnosed between 2000 and 2007, according to data provided by EUROCARE-4 [6].

Given its high incidence and survival rates, it constitutes the most prevalent tumor among women [5]. Despite being the main cause of mortality due to cancer in women, a reduction in mortality of around 2% a year has been demonstrated.

Screening and Diagnostic Methods

Breast cancer screening programs started several decades ago, being implemented in Spain from 1990. Early diagnosis is considered the best strategy to improve the prognosis of this disease, since the main known risk factors (age, sex, family, and personal history, etc.) cannot be modified.

The surveillance program includes breast self-examination and clinical examinations as procedures complementing mammography, although it is true that recent studies show that breast self-examination in itself has no efficacy at all as an early detection method [7].

Mammography represents the gold standard, since it is the most effective test to detect lesions in their initial phases. The presence of abnormal findings in mammography often makes it necessary to conduct additional projections, or to use other diagnostic tests such as ultrasound, which are also used to guide punctures or biopsies of the lesion in order to obtain a definitive diagnosis.

In recent years, full-field digital mammography has been proposed as an alternative to conventional mammography due to potential improvements that have been demonstrated for the early detection of breast cancer, mainly in cases of breast thickness or young women. Although more comparative and cost-effective studies are required to confirm its benefits, it appears that this imaging modality will gain importance in the future.

Computer-aided detection (CAD) systems have been used in both conventional and digital mammography, which help radiologists to interpret images by improving the efficacy of lesion detection.

There are currently no other imaging tests recommended for breast cancer screening. Young patients with high risk of cancer due to family history may benefit from an ultrasound scan as a screening method to supplement mammography [8]. In the group of high-risk patients, in turn, magnetic resonance imaging (MRI) shows promising results in published articles [9], being the imaging technique of choice in those women with breast implants.

There is strong scientific evidence proving the efficacy of mammography as a screening test for breast cancer. Multiple randomized clinical trials have been published, which show a reduction in mortality of 20%–32% [10–14] that varies based on age, follow-up years, and test periodicity within the screening protocol.

The Health Insurance Plan (HIP) of New York was the first randomized study to assess the efficacy of mammography and breast examination in breast cancer screening. This study included 62,000 women aged between 40 and 64 years old, demonstrating a reduction in mortality due to breast cancer of 30% at 10 years [10] and of 23% at 18 years [11]. These positive results favored the development of a multicenter project known as the Breast Cancer Detection Demonstration Project (BCDDP) [12], conducted between 1973 and 1980, which included 280,000 women. The results from this study confirmed the information obtained previously; additionally, a clear increase in tumor detection due to the quality improvement of mammograms was demonstrated.

Several studies have been conducted since then, which have helped to establish the utility of breast cancer screening with the use of mammograms.

A significant reduction in mortality has been clearly observed in the group of patients over 50 years old [10,13]. Screening in women aged 40–49 years has been debated due to the lack of clear evidence; however, meta-analyses and clinical trials show a comparable benefit in this group of patients [14,15].

Screening Recommendations

In 2003, the Council of the European Union (EU) established a series of recommendations about breast cancer screening, including the carrying out of screening mammograms in patients from 50 years of age every 2 years, according to the European Guidelines for Quality Assurance in Mammography Screening. In Spain, most autonomous communities perform screenings in women aged between 50 and 69 years, although some communities have reduced the age of onset to 45 years [16] and perform screenings once a year. Furthermore, a monthly physical self-examination has been recommended for women over 50 years, and a physical examination every 3 years for women aged 20–50 years, and once a year for women over 50 years.

There is controversy among several scientific societies concerning the age of onset to recommend breast cancer screening. There is a general consensus that sets this age at 50 years old; however, many scientific societies, such as the American Cancer Society (ACS), the National Cancer Institute (NCI), or the American College of Radiology (ACR) recommend starting at 40 years old.

In women at high risk of suffering breast cancer (with family history or presence of mutations in susceptibility genes, like *BRCA1* and *BRCA2*), currently there is no consolidated scientific evidence, but there are studies that recommend starting screening before the age of 40 [17].

Concerning when to stop conducting screenings, there are currently studies in which the age to perform screening tests has been extended to 75 years old with positive results [18]. For this reason, several scientific societies, such as the ACS, do not recommend restricting the age to perform mammography but believe that patients' life expectancy should be considered.

Screening in Colorectal Cancer

Introduction

Colorectal cancer (CRC) is a very important health problem. It represents almost 10% of all cancers, ranking third worldwide (1,360,500 new cases in 2012). If we consider both sexes together, it is the second most common cancer in Europe and ranks first in Spain, being the second cause of death [5]. The accumulated risk of developing CRC throughout life is higher than 5% [19]. The incidence in European countries shows a tendency to rise, which has been mainly attributed to the influence of risk factors and the implementation of screening programs. The risk of death due to CRC is estimated to be 2.7% [19].

Survival depends on the stage at which the disease is diagnosed. In localized stages, there is a 90% chance of a 5-year survival, 65% if there is regional involvement, and 9% if the disease has spread [20], so early diagnosis significantly improves the prognosis of the disease. With the start of the screening programs and the diagnostic and therapeutic advances, a reduction in mortality rates has been demonstrated [21].

Screening and Diagnostic Methods

Several scientific societies recommend screening programs for CRC. The purpose of screening is to identify asymptomatic subjects with initial stages of CRC and/or precursor lesions and prevent its further development.

There are several screening tests for the early diagnosis of CRC.

1. *Fecal occult blood test (FOBT)*: This is based on the detection of occult blood in feces, which can indicate the presence of large polyps or CRC. A positive result requires conducting additional tests, such as colonoscopy, in order to determine the origin of the bleeding.

   The method usually used for its detection is through a chemical process (cFOBT), a procedure that has been widely studied as a screening method. Currently, new FOBTs have been developed based on the determination of human globin through specific antibodies (iFOBT). This test has the advantage of not requiring diet restrictions or medications prior to performing the test, but it is a much more complex and expensive technique.

   Several well-designed clinical trials have been conducted, which confirm the efficacy of cFOBT. The Minnesota clinical trial showed a significant reduction in deaths by CRC of 20% with annual screening and of 17% with screening twice a year [22]. In 2007, a Cochrane review showed a 15% reduction in mortality [23].

   There is little scientific evidence regarding iFOBT, but some published studies show a higher sensitivity regarding cFOBT, which is proven by comparative studies [24].

2. *Flexible sigmoidoscopy*: This is a simple technique that allows visualization of the mucosa of the large intestine until it reaches 60 cm, that is, it does not allow examination of the proximal colon. If any lesion is demonstrated, the study is complemented with a full colonoscopy.

Several studies confirming the benefits of sigmoidoscopy as a screening test have been published. In 1998, a prospective study was published that included 25,000 men aged 40–70 years old, which showed a reduction in the incidence of CRC in any location of 48%, and a reduction in death risk of 44% [25]. Another study confirmed a reduction in mortality by CRC of up to 31% after performing one single flexible sigmoidoscopy in patients aged 55–64 years old [26].

3. *Colonoscopy*: This is the most sensitive and specific screening test, allowing visualization of the entire large intestine and biopsies or resections of lesions demonstrated. The patient must be prepared prior to the procedure, and often it is performed under sedation. The complication rate is higher than with flexible sigmoidoscopy.

Although there are no randomized clinical trials assessing its efficacy in terms of mortality, the evidence based on indirect studies shows its usefulness in the detection of CRC at the initial stages and in reducing incidence.

There is a marked tendency to consider colonoscopy as the screening test of choice. Up to 50% of patients with proximal advanced adenoma do not present distal lesions, so the use of sigmoidoscopy in these cases would not be effective [27]. Okamoto et al. [28] have shown a high prevalence of localized advanced neoplasia at the level of the proximal colon in elderly compared with young patients (younger than 50 years old), so they concluded that colonoscopy would be the right screening test in this group of patients.

Colonoscopies may also assume an advantage regarding other noninvasive tests, such as FOBT. There are ongoing studies on the superiority of colonoscopy as a screening test.

Screening Recommendations

The probability of developing CRC divides subjects into

1. *Medium risk*: Individuals 50 years old or older without additional risk factors
2. *High risk*: This group includes patients diagnosed with adenomatous polyps or inflammatory disease (Crohn and/or ulcerative colitis), people belonging to families with familial aggregation of cancer, people with personal and/or family history of CRC, and people with family history of familial adenomatous polyps or hereditary nonpolyposis CRC.

The Council of the European Union currently recommends FOBTs in men and women aged 50–74 years old every 2 years as a screening test for middle-risk individuals [3].

Different national scientific societies, such as the Spanish Society of Gastroenterology, recommend a screening of colorectal cancer in middle-risk patients aged older than 50 years by using the following tests:

- FOBT once a year
- Flexible sigmoidoscopy every 5 years
- Colonoscopy every 10 years

According to the guidelines of American scientific societies, besides the previously mentioned tests, other possible screening diagnostic methods include FOBT combined with flexible sigmoidoscopy every 5 years, or a double-contrast barium enema every 5 years [16]. However, there is currently no scientific evidence available enabling us to determine the best strategy for CRC screening. In high-risk individuals, it is recommended to conduct surveillance at an earlier age, with less time between timely screening tests (usually with a colonoscopy), always following the recommendations established in clinical practice guidelines.

Screening in Cervical Cancer

Introduction

Based on the information provided by the Spanish Network of Cancer Registries (REDECAN) [5], cervical cancer is the fourth most common cancer in women worldwide, representing 7.9% (527,500 new cases in 2012) of the total of malignant tumors in this gender. It is estimated that about 500,000 new cases of this cancer are diagnosed each year in the world, of which 83% occur in developing countries [29]. In Europe and Spain, it ranks 6th and 12th, respectively, Spain being one of the countries with lower incidence in the European Union.

The 5-year survival decreases based on the stage at which the disease is diagnosed, being over 90% for localized disease, 54% in cases of regional involvement, and 15% if there is remote involvement [20]. Thanks to the implementation of primary and secondary prevention strategies, mortality by cervical cancer has decreased in most developed countries.

Human papillomavirus (HPV) infection is the main risk factor for cervical cancer but is not sufficient on its own—that is, the development and evolution of this cancer require the presence of other risk cofactors (smoking, prolonged use of oral contraceptives, immunosuppression, etc.).

Screening and Diagnostic Methods

The natural history of cervical cancer is characterized by the presence of a long preclinical period, with precursor lesions that can be detected by cytology, and treatment of which prevents the occurrence of invasive cancer.

In the 1960s, exfoliative cervicovaginal cytology or the *Papanicolaou test* was introduced as the main diagnostic method. Screening allows for detection of both precursor lesions and invasive cancer, with the purpose of preventing its occurrence or diagnosing cancer in the early stages. Papanicolaou cytology is a simple procedure based on the morphological study of cervical cells scraped from different locations. The sample obtained is later examined under a microscope, and results are interpreted; the *Bethesda Classification System* provides a standardized terminology that, aside from classifying findings, also assesses the suitability of the sample [30].

According to published studies, the number of FNs is very high. Screening tests have a specificity of 98%; however, in low-prevalence populations, they have a sensitivity of about 50% [31]. In order to improve accuracy and minimize errors in sample gathering and handling and interpretation of results, new methods, such as liquid-based cytology and automated sample reading, have been developed. Although there are no randomized studies proving the efficacy of Papanicolaou cytology, observational, case, and control studies show a significant reduction in mortality that can exceed 70% in countries where screening has been massively applied [32].

The role of the high-risk human papillomavirus (HR-HPV) detection test as a screening method, or to complement cytology, has been analyzed in recent years. Published studies show that the HR-HPV test presents better sensitivity and reproducibility at the expense of a discreet reduction in specificity and positive predictive value, mainly in women aged under 30 years, due to the high frequency of temporary infections in this age group [33].

There is enough evidence from randomized studies to confirm an increased detection of high-grade intraepithelial lesions and a significant reduction in the incidence of cervical cancer with the HR-HPV test or as a co-test with cytology, compared with cytology alone [34–36].

Screening Recommendations

There is a general consensus about performing cytology as a screening method, although in the last decade, most scientific societies have been including HPV detection tests in their screening protocols.

In Spain, several scientific societies, such as the Spanish Society of Cervical Pathology and Colposcopy, recommend performing the first cytology at 25 years old or within 3 years after first intercourse, with a 3-year repeat cycle, after two annual examinations with normal results. One of the recommendations of the American Cancer Society is to reduce the age of onset for screening to 21 years old.

Screening in patients aged between 30 and 65 years can be carried out with one of the following diagnostic methods:

1. HPV test every 5 years
2. Cytology every 3 years
3. Screening using cytology as a co-test with HR-HPV testing every 5 years

Screenings should be discontinued at 65 years of age provided prior results within 10 years were appropriate and negative, and patients show no history of intraepithelial cervical neoplasia or cervical cancer treated during the previous 20 years.

There are specific subgroups of patients at a higher risk of developing this type of cancer (immunocompromised patients, subjects with history of condyloma acuminata, HPV infection, or sexually transmitted diseases) that require closer surveillance through timely screening tests, always following the recommendations established in clinical practice guidelines.

REFERENCES

1. Wilson JMG, Jungner G. *Principles and Practices of Screening for Disease.* Geneva, Switzerland: World Health Organization; 1968. Report No.: Public Health Papers No. 34. Available from: http://whqlibdoc.who.int/php/WHO_PHP_34.pdf
2. Cerdá Mota T, Ascunce Elizaga N. Implementation and Evaluation of Population Screening Programs. Madrid: EMISA, 2006.
3. Consejo de la Unión Europea. Recomendación del Consejo de 2 de diciembre de 2003 sobre el cribado del cáncer. *Diario Oficial de la Unión Europea.* 16–12–2003;L327:34–8.
4. Cabanes A, Pérez-Gómez B, Aragonés N, Pollán M, López-Abente G. *La situación del cáncer en España, 1975–2006.* Madrid: Instituto de Salud Carlos III; 2009 Jun.
5. Galceran J, Ameijide A, Carulla M et al. *Estimaciones de la incidencia y la supervivencia del cáncer en España y su situación en Europa.* Red española de registros decáncer (REDECAN), 2014 [consultado 11 Oct 2017]. Disponible en: http://redecan.org/es/page.cfm?id=196&title=estimaciones-de-la-incidencia-y-la-supervivencia-del-cancer-en-espana-y-su-situacion-en-europa
6. De Angelis R, Sant M, Coleman MP et al. Cancer survival in Europe 1999–2007 by country and age: Results of EUROCARE-5-a population-based study. *Lancet Oncol.* 2014;15:23–34.
7. Kearney AJ. Increasing our understanding of breast self-examination: Women talk about cancer, the health care system, and being women. *Qual Health Res.* 2006;16(6):802–20.
8. O'Driscoll D, Warren R, MacKay J, Britton P, Day NE. Screening with breast ultrasound in a population at moderate risk due to family history. *J Med Screen.* 2001;8(2):106–9.
9. Kuhl CK, Schmutzler RK, Leutner CC et al. Breast MR imaging screening in 192 women proved or suspected to be carriers of a breast cancer susceptibility gene: Preliminary results. *Radiology.* 2000 Apr; 215(1):267–79.
10. Shapiro S, Venet W, Strax P, Venet L, Roeser R. Ten- to fourteen-year effect of screening on breast cancer mortality. *J Natl Cancer Inst.* 1982 Aug;69(2):349–55.
11. Shapiro S. Periodic screening for breast cancer: The Health Insurance plan project and its sequelae. *J Natl Cancer Inst Monogr.* 1997;(22):27–30.
12. Baker LH. Breast Cancer Detection Demonstration Project: Five-year summary report. *Cancer J Clin.* 1982 Jul-Aug;32(4):194–225.
13. Tabár L, Vitak B, Chen HH et al. The Swedish Two-County Trial twenty years later. Updated mortality results and new insights from long-term follow-up. *Radiol Clin North Am.* 2000 Jul;38(4):625–51.
14. Bjurstam N, Björneld L, Warwick J et al. The Gothenburg Breast Screening Trial. *Cancer.* 2003 May 15;97(10):2387–96.
15. Andersson I, Janzon L. Reduced breast cancer mortality in women under age 50: Updated results from the Malmö Mammographic Screening Program. *J Natl Cancer Inst Monogr.* 1997;(22):63–7.
16. Castells X, Sala M, Ascunce N et al. *Descripción del cribado del cáncer en España: Proyecto DESCRIC.* Cataluña: Ministerio de Sanidad y consumo, 2007.
17. Burke W, Daly M, Garber J et al. Recommendations for follow-up care of individuals with an inherited predisposition to cancer. II. BRCA1 and BRCA2. Cancer Genetics Studies Consortium. *JAMA.* 1997 Mar 26;277(12):997–1003.
18. Fracheboud J, Groenewoud JH, Boer R et al. Seventy-five years is an appropriate upper age limit populationbased mammography screening. *Int J Cancer.* 2006;118:2020–25.
19. González JR, Moreno V, Fernández E, Izquierdo A, Borrás J, Gispert R. Grupo de Investigación sobre el Impacto del Cáncer en Cataluña. Probabilidad de desarrollar y morir por cáncer en Cataluña en el periodo 1998–2001. *Med Clin (Barc).* 2005;124:411–4.

20. Holland J, Frei E et al. *Cancer medicine.* 6th ed. Ontario: BC Decker; 2003.
21. López-Abente G, Ardanaz E, Torrella-Ramos A, Mateos A, Delgado-Sanz C, Chirlaque MD. Colorectal Cancer WorkingGroup. Changes in colorectal cancer incidence and mortality trends in Spain. *Ann Oncol.* 2010 May;21(Suppl 3):iii76–82.
22. Mandel JS, Church TR, Bond JH et al. The effect of fecal occult-blood screening on the incidence of colorectal cancer. *N Engl J Med.* 2000;343:1603–7.
23. Hewitson P, Glasziou P, Irwig L et al. Screening for colorectal cancer using the faecal occult blood test, Hemoccult. *Cochrane Database Syst Rev.* 2007;2007(1):CD001216.
24. Van Rossum LG, van Rijn AF, Laheij RJ et al. Random comparison of guaiac and immunochemical fecal occult blood tests for colorectal cancer in a screening population. *Gastroenterology.* 2008;135:82–90.
25. Kavanagh AM, Giovannucci EL, Fuchs CS, Colditz GA. Screening endoscopy and risk of colorectal cancer in United States men. *Cancer Causes Control.* 1998 Aug;9(4):455–62.
26. Atkin WS, Edwards R, Kralj-Hans I et al. Once-only flexible sigmoidoscopy screening in prevention of colorectal cancer: A multicentre randomised controlled trial. *Lancet.* 2010 May 8;375(9726):1624–33.
27. Imperiale TF, Wagner DR, Lin CY, Larkin GN, Rogge JD, Ransohoff DF. Risk of advanced proximal neoplasms in asymptomatic adults according to the distal colorectal findings. *N Engl J Med.* 2000;343:169–74.
28. Okamoto M, Shiratori Y, Yamaji Y et al. Relationship between age and site of colorectal cancer based on colonoscopy findings. *Gastrointest Endosc.* 2002 Apr;55(4):548–51.
29. Ferlay J, Steliarova-Foucher E, Lortet-Tieulent J et al. Cancer incidence and mortality patterns in Europe: Estimates for 40 countries in 2012. *Eur J Cancer.* 2013;49:1374–403.
30. Solomon D, Davey D, Kurman R et al. The 2001 Bethesda System: Terminology for reporting results of cervical cytology. *JAMA.* 2002;287:2120–9.
31. Agency for health care policy and research. *Evidence Report on Evaluation of Cervical Cytology.* Rockville: Agency for Health Care Policy and research; 1999:1–148.
32. Johannesson G, Geirsson G, Day N. The effect of mass screening in Iceland, 1965–74, on the incidence and mortality of cervical carcinoma. *Int J Cancer.* 1978 Apr 15;21(4):418–25.
33. Torné A del Pino M, Cusidó M et al. Guía de cribado del cáncer de cuello de útero en España 2014. *Rev Esp Patol.* 2014;47:1–43.
34. Bulkmans NW, Rozendaal L, Voorhorst FJ, Snijders PJ, Meijer CJ. Long-term protective effect of high-risk human papillomavirus testing in population-based cervical screening. *Br J Cancer.* 2005;92:1800–2.
35. Naucler P, Ryd W, Tornberg S et al. Human papillomavirus and Papanicolaou tests to screen for cervical cancer. *N Engl J Med.* 2007;357:1589–97.
36. Ronco G, Dillner J, Elfstrom KM et al. Efficacy of HPV-based screening for prevention of invasive cervical cancer: Follow-up of four European randomised controlled trials. *Lancet.* 2014;383:524–32.

5

Tumor Markers

Raquel Benlloch Rodríguez

Introduction

Tumor markers (TMs) are substances produced in response to a malignant tumor, which can be detected in blood, body fluids, or tissue qualitatively or quantitatively by laboratory testing. There is a wide variety of substances that can be classified as TMs, including glycoproteins (CA 15.3, prostate-specific antigen), hormones (corticotropin [ACTH], human chorionic gonadotropin hormone, calcitonin), enzymes (LDH, alkaline phosphatase), oncofetal antigens (carcinoembryonic antigen, α-fetoprotein), serum proteins (β_2-microglobulin), and genetic markers (HER2, P53).

TMs can be produced by the tumor itself, like the human chorionic gonadotropin (HCG) hormone in choriocarcinoma, or as a response of the body to the tumor lesion (acute phase proteins or immune system modulators) [1].

The first published reference dates back to 1846, when Bence Jones identified the first TM, a protein named after him that is found elevated in patients with multiple myeloma. The concept became more widespread from the mid-twentieth century onward, with the discovery of the human chorionic gonadotropin (HCG) hormone in 1927, the α-fetoprotein (AFP) in 1963, and the carcinoembryonic antigen (CEA) in 1965 [2]. Many hormones, enzymes, and other proteins were identified thereafter, which, in malignant conditions, altered their concentration in body fluids.

It must be taken into account that these TMs are not specific to neoplasms; significant concentrations can be found in a great number of nontumor pathologies or physiological conditions. However, in most cases, elevated concentrations of a certain TM are indicative of the presence of a tumor. In order to optimize their use and differentiate a benign from a malignant pathology, three strategies can be used [1]:

1. *Serum concentration of the TM*: The higher the concentration of the TM, the more likely that elevation is due to a tumoral process. In the absence of neoplasm, elevations are usually moderate. For example, in smokers or patients with liver or kidney failure, CEA may be slightly increased (2.5–5 ng/mL), but larger concentrations (>10 ng/mL) indicate a high probability of the presence of a tumor.
2. *Rule out the existence of benign processes*: It is necessary to know if the person shows any physiological or pathological condition that may alter the marker's concentration. Liver or renal failure, among others, can cause an increase in TM values.
3. *Evolution monitoring of the marker*: The progressive elevation, in time, of a TM with a higher interval than the TM's half-life is highly indicative of a neoplastic disease.

For proper clinical applicability of TMs, it is fundamental to consider their sensitivity and specificity from an epidemiological perspective. Sensitivity is the percentage of people who are tumor-marker positive and have cancer, and specificity is the percentage of people who are tumor-marker negative and do not have cancer. The perfect TM would be one that could be detected in the earlier stages of the disease (100% sensitivity) and that could only be detected in patients with that type of cancer (100% specificity) [1]. Validated TMs must have reproducible and repeatable results and must be determined through minimally invasive tests.

Tumor Marker Applications

In 1978, Herberman [3] established five potential applications of a TM: early detection, help in cancer diagnosis, tumor location, prognosis, and monitoring of cancer evolution. More recently, in 1994, George [4] highlighted four of these applications: early diagnosis, diagnosis, prognosis, and monitoring of the neoplastic disease.

Most TMs are insensitive in the initial stages of the disease, so, to date, it is not a useful instrument for early diagnosis of cancer in most cases; however, they may be helpful to select high-risk patients (e.g., with elevated AFP to conduct more specific supplementary tests. To date, as a screening method, failure to detect any TMs has proven to be a survival benefit in randomized clinical trials.

In most cases, the determination of TMs in isolation does not constitute enough evidence to prove the existence of a tumoral process. Elevated TMs with suspected malignant tumor support the diagnosis, but their negativity does not exclude it.

Main TM applications in clinical practice are to help in the diagnosis, to determine the potential origin and extension of the tumor, to point to the histological type, to serve as an early detection marker of a potential relapse and as a prognostic marker of the disease, to help control the evolution of the disease, and to monitor treatment responses. Furthermore, TMs are also starting to be used as risk markers, that is, as predictive markers of future diseases [5–7].

Recently, the identification of biomarkers has focused on the selection of patients who will benefit from a certain therapy, thus avoiding the side effects and costs derived from a nonoptimal treatment. It also tries to identify subsets of high- and low-risk patients who will benefit from the administration—or not—of adjuvant treatments.

Main Tumor Markers and Their Applicability

Main TMs used in daily clinical practice are presented in the following sections.

Carcinoembryonic Antigen

This is a high-molecular-weight oncofetal glycoprotein, with normal values below 2.5 ng/mL in nonsmokers and below 5 ng/mL in smokers. Levels above 10 ng/mL are highly indicative of a neoplastic process [8]. It may be elevated in malignant and benign pathologies, or even in patients without an apparent disease, and the probability of malignancy increases directly with CEA concentration.

It is frequently associated with tumors in the gastrointestinal tract, mainly increasing in colorectal cancer (CRC). Its values may also be increased in advanced epithelial carcinomas of other origins, such as breast, pancreatic and stomach cancer, melanoma, lymphoma, liver, medullary thyroid, and head and neck cancer. Elevated levels of CEA may be objectified in patients who smoke or who have nononcological diseases, such as intestinal inflammatory disease, gastric ulcer, pancreatitis, or hepatic diseases.

The proportion of subjects with CRC and elevated CEA increases based on the stage of the disease. Less than 25% of patients with localized disease show high levels of CEA; however, this percentage increases up to 75% in patients with disseminated disease [8].

CEA determination is not a useful method for early diagnosis of cancer. It has a fundamental role in patients treated with healing intention during disease follow-up, and early detection of relapses sometimes is the first indication of the presence of a recurrence. Likewise, it is a marker of great interest to assess responses to treatment and as a prognostic parameter.

Carbohydrate Antigen 19.9

This glycoprotein synthesized in several epithelia is typically elevated in patients with pancreas tumors. Its values may be increased both in other tumoral processes, such as bile duct, liver or esophageal cancer, or mucinous ovarian neoplasms, and in benign pathologies (pancreatitis, liver diseases, cholangitis), although in this case the elevation is less pronounced. The marker is elevated in 80%–90% of patients with pancreatic cancer, and in 60%–70% of patients with bile duct cancer [8].

Values below 40 U/mL are considered normal for both sexes, and there are no differences between smokers and nonsmokers. Values greater than 1000 U/mL are highly indicative of malignancy and predict the presence of metastatic disease [9].

Carbohydrate antigen (CA) 19.9 is not a useful tool for early diagnosis of cancer. Its main clinical indications are to monitor responses to treatment and as a prognostic factor, since preoperative values greater than 1000 U/mL or maintenance of high levels after surgery are associated with a worse prognosis.

Carbohydrate Antigen 125

CA 125 is a high-molecular-weight glycoprotein expressed on the surface of the cells of the celomic (mesothelium of the pleura and peritoneum, myocardium, pericardium) and müllerian epithelium (fallopian tube, endocervix, and vaginal fundus). CA 125 is the quintessential serum marker in ovarian epithelial carcinoma, although there are other neoplasias, such as endometrial, breast, lung, pancreatic and liver cancer, and melanoma that may increase its values.

Some benign pathologies associated with elevated CA 125 include endometriosis, liver diseases, ascites, cirrhosis, pleural or pericardial effusion, sarcoidosis, and tuberculosis, as well as pregnancy or menstruation.

In general, levels lower than 35 U/mL are considered normal. It is found elevated in 80% of patients with epithelial ovarian cancer, although this number decreases to 50% in the initial stage, so it is not a useful marker for early diagnosis [2]. In recent years, TM sensitivity in ovarian cancer has improved with the inclusion of the human epididymis protein 4 (HE4), which is found elevated in over 70% in the initial stages [10]. When combining the determination of CA 125 and HE4, the sensitivity and specificity of the diagnosis increase, facilitating distinguishing between malignant and benign diseases.

Currently, CA 125 is more useful to monitor responses to treatment and follow-up patients after full remission to detect relapses, and it also acts as a prognostic factor.

Carbohydrate Antigen 15.3

CA 15.3 is a high-molecular-weight glycoprotein, with normal values below 35 U/mL. It is the marker of choice for breast cancer, although it may be elevated in ovarian, lung, and prostate cancers, and in the case of benign breast or ovarian pathologies, liver diseases or kidney failure, as well as in pregnancy or lactation.

This marker is not usually elevated in the initial stages of the disease, so it is not considered useful for breast cancer screening. It rises in 20%–50% of patients with breast cancer, said elevation being more frequent in the advanced stages, when it reaches a sensitivity over 70% [11].

The determination of CA 15.3 is significant for prognosis, to monitor treatments, and combined with CEA determination, to follow up patients after treatment for early detection of relapses.

Prostate-Specific Antigen

Prostate-specific antigen (PSA) is a glycoprotein produced by the prostate epithelium. Of the total PSA detectable in serum, nearly 15% is present as free PSA, whereas the remaining PSA is bound to α-1-antichymotrypsin [2]. It is the tumor marker of choice in patients with prostate cancer, although it can also be elevated in benign prostate pathologies, such as prostatic hypertrophy, prostatitis, or prostate trauma.

Plasma PSA normal levels are below 4 ng/mL, although this value may be modified by factors like age. When PSA values are between 4 and 10 ng/mL, the specificity for malignant pathology is low, so determining speed and free PSA may be useful to plan the next steps. A PSA increase of speed over 0.75 ng/mL in 1 year, as well as free PSA values below 25%, are predictive of cancer [12] or a neoplastic process [13]. This marker is elevated in serum in more than 75% of patients with prostate cancer, and there is a correlation between PSA serum levels and the tumor stage.

PSA determination as a screening method is controversial. There is currently no evidence that decreasing mortality is a benefit, but it does increase the number of diagnoses in the early stage. Although for the time being it is not recommended to conduct a massive population screening, certain scientific societies recommend using PSA as a screening method in males over 50 years old and selected groups [8].

The main clinical applications of PSA, as with most TMs, lie in the assessment of treatment efficacy, patient follow-up for the early diagnosis of relapses, and as a prognostic factor, since low levels of PSA prior to surgery have been associated with better survival.

Alpha-Fetoprotein

AFP is an oncofetal glycoprotein equivalent to albumin, which in normal conditions is synthesized in the fetal liver, the yolk sac, and amniotic fluid [1]. Synthesis begins in the fetus, later decreasing and becoming virtually undetectable in adults. Values of up to 10 ng/mL may be considered normal.

This is the marker of choice in patients with hepatocarcinoma and nonseminomatous germ cell tumors, although it can also be elevated with other neoplasias (pancreatic, bile duct, and stomach cancer), benign processes such as liver diseases (hepatitis, cirrhosis), or physiological processes such as pregnancy.

In primary liver cancer, AFP is elevated in 80% of patients, with greater than 1000 ng/mL in 40% of cases [8]. There are no recommendations to determine this marker as a screening method, but most scientific societies suggest determination of AFP and abdominal ultrasound as screening methods in high-risk groups (patients with liver cirrhosis secondary to hepatitis B or C viruses). In patients with hepatocarcinoma, an AFP value greater than 400 ng/mL at diagnosis, or persistent high levels of AFP after surgical resection are associated with a worse prognosis [11]. AFP determination is useful for posttreatment monitoring and follow-up of the disease evolution.

In patients with nonseminomatous germ cell tumors, AFP plays a highly important role, being elevated in over 80% of cases. The elevation of this TM in the initial stages is poor, so it is not useful as a screening method. Its determination, together with the human chorionic gonadotropin hormone, is crucial to assess posttreatment efficacy and later patient follow-up. AFP values greater than 10,000 at diagnosis, or persistent high levels after treatment are associated with a worse prognosis [8].

Beta-Subunit of the Human Chorionic Gonadotropin (β-HCG) Hormone

The β-subunit of the human chorionic gonadotropin (β-HCG) hormone is a glycoprotein hormone made up of two subunits, α and β, expressed in placenta under normal conditions. The β-HCG is found elevated in germ cell tumors and gestational trophoblastic disease, as well as in other conditions, including pregnancy, marijuana consumption, and hypogonadism. Values below 5 mIU/mL are considered normal [8].

It is not useful as a screening method. Levels of β-HCG greater than 50,000 mIU/mL at diagnosis, and/or the persistence of value increase after treatment are associated with a worse prognosis. Its determination, together with AFP's, is essential for patient follow-up and to assess treatment efficacy [11].

Other Tumor Markers

Within the management of oncological patients, there are other TMs, the use of which is more restricted to certain situations. The antigen associated with squamous cell carcinoma (SCC) can be determined in patients with epidermoid tumors (predominantly lung and cervix) or neuron-specific enolase (NSE) in case of neuroectodermal tumors (such as small-cell undifferentiated carcinoma of the lung). Also, β_2-microglobulin, successfully used as a prognostic marker of multiple myeloma and Hodgkin disease, and as an early indicator of relapse in non-Hodgkin lymphoma [14], thyroglobulin for medullary thyroid carcinoma, or chromogranin A for neuroendocrine tumors should be noted.

New Era of Biomarkers

In recent years, changes in DNA and gene patterns produced by tumor cells have been studied to generate potential biomarkers. Thanks to a wider knowledge of the genetic and molecular biology of cancer, new biomarkers with significant diagnostic, prognostic, and predictive response values to new therapies have been identified, which have enabled optimization of the treatments administered and a change in the paradigm of oncological disease, preparing the way for "personalized medicine" in cancer. The incorporation of new biomarkers in daily clinical practice requires them to be validated, so current efforts are focused on conducting clinical trials that can justify their applicability.

In metastatic CRC, the determination of the *KRAS* gene mutational status as a predictive marker is essential prior to administering an antiepidermal growth factor receptor (anti-EGFR) treatment, since the benefit of these therapies is limited in patients with mutated *KRAS*. However, determining microsatellite instability (MI) in localized CRC is currently a consolidated prognostic marker, the presence of which gives a better prognosis. Genetic tests such as ColoPrint or Oncotype DX, as well as the determination of other biomarkers, including the *PTEN* or *BRAF* gene, are not yet being used as routine practice in this type of tumor [15].

In breast cancer, there are currently new, validated predictive markers of treatment response, such as determination of estrogen and progesterone receptors, which are crucial before recommending a hormone treatment, and determination of the HER2 oncogene, which is associated with more aggressive behavior (overexpressed in 20%–30% of breast cancers). The determination of HER2 is essential to indicate the administration of targeted therapies (like trastuzumab), but it is not useful as a prognostic marker in patients with early breast cancer [16].

However, the analysis of gene expression profiles (Oncotype DX) in breast cancer currently constitutes a very useful instrument, because it can predict both the risk of relapse and the benefit of chemotherapy in selected groups of patients [17].

New biomarkers predictive of response have been identified in nonmicrocytic lung cancer. There is sufficient scientific evidence in favor of determination of EGFR and rearrangements of the anaplastic lymphoma kinase (*ALK*) gene in patients with lung adenocarcinoma stage IV. EGFR mutations and *ALK* rearrangements are mutually exclusive. Other biomarkers of current interest, but which are not routine practice, include translocation of the *ROS* gene or alteration of the *MET* gene [18].

In gastrointestinal stromal tumors (GISTs), the determination of the Kit CD117 protein is routine practice, but of use only for diagnosis. The analysis of the c-Kit and PDGFRA gene mutations has a response-predictive value to treatment with targeted therapies (imatinib or sunitinib) as well as a prognostic value [19].

In melanoma, based on the results of published articles, experts recommend the determination of the *BRAF* gene mutational status, since it has implications for management. It is estimated to be mutated in 50% of cases and constitutes a prognostic and response-predictive marker to new targeted drugs (vemurafenib), which improve control and survival rates obtained with chemotherapy [20].

Determination of the HER2 oncogene, as with breast cancer, is also routine practice in advanced stages of gastric cancer. Its overexpression is associated with a worse prognosis [21]. Furthermore, as mentioned before, it has a response-predictive marker to targeted therapies (like trastuzumab).

A lot of biomarkers with diagnostic value, predictive response to targeted therapies, and/or with prognostic value have been included in lymphoproliferative syndromes. CD20, BCL2, CD79, CD5, CD23, or CD30 are some markers used in routine practice.

It is recommended to conduct routine analysis of germline mutations of the *BRCA1* and *BRCA2* genes in all women with high-grade, nonmucinous epithelial ovarian cancer. The presence of mutations in said genes is associated with a better prognosis. Studies published in recent years have shown increased sensitivity to poly(ADP-ribose) polymerase (PARP) enzyme inhibitor drugs, currently constituting a validated biomarker for the use of olaparib. New biomarkers have been recommended, such as the determination of p53 gene mutations, which may be used as early markers of treatment response [22].

Finally, for central nervous system tumors, several biomarkers have been identified and included in daily clinical practice. The determination of isocitrate dehydrogenase (*IDH1/2*) gene mutations has a clear diagnostic value and is associated with a favorable prognosis. The analysis of 1p/19q codeletion is also very helpful for diagnosis, since it is often found in oligodendroglial tumors, enabling a differential diagnosis with other neoplasias. Furthermore, it may serve as a response-predictive marker because the presence of codeletion is associated with more favorable responses after first-line chemotherapy and radiotherapy treatments. The determination of enzyme O^6-methylguanine-DNA-methyltransferase (MGMT) gene promoter methylation constitutes another new biomarker characteristic of this type of tumor; hypermethylation of said gene has a favorable prognostic value and is predictive of response to alkylating agents (temozolomide) [23].

REFERENCES

1. Hermida Lazcano I, Sanchez Tejero E, Cristina NS et al. Marcadores tumorales. *Rev Clín Med Fam.* 2016;9(1):31–42.
2. Martín Suárez A et al. Utilidad clínica de los marcadores tumorales séricos. *Aten Primaria.* 2003;32(4):227–39.
3. Herberman RB. Immunodiagnosis and its applicability for cancer screening. *Antibiotics Chemother.* 1978;22:59–66.
4. George SL. Statistical considerations and modeling of clinical utility of tumor markers. *Hematol/Oncol. Clin North Am.* 1994;8:457–70.
5. Duffy MJ. Tumor markers in clinical practice: a review focusing on common solid cancers. *Med Princ Pract.* 2013;22(1):4–11.
6. Senra A, Quintela D. Los marcadores diagnósticos y pronósticos del cáncer de mama. *Rev Senología Y Patol Mam.* 1999;12(3):121–32
7. Díaz Rubio E, García Conde J. *Oncología clínica básica.* Primera edición. Madrid: ARAN, 2000.
8. Perkins GL, Slater ED, Sanders GK, Prichard JG. Serum Tumor Markers. *Am Fam Physician.* 2003; 68(6):1075–82.
9. Steinberg W. The clinical utility of the CA 19-9 tumor-associated antigen. *Am J Gastroenterol.* 1990;85:350–5.
10. Escudero JM, Auge JM, Filella X, Torne A, Pahisa J, Molina R. Comparison of serum human epididymis protein 4 with cancer antigen 125 as a tumor marker in patients with malignant and nonmalignant diseases. *Clin Chem.* 2011;57(11):1534–44.
11. Ocaña Pérez E, Aceituno Azaustre MI. Utilidad clínica delos marcadores tumorales. *Revista Médica de Jaén.* 2014;4: 2–12
12. Carter HB, Pearson JD, Metter EJ et al. Longitudinal evaluation of prostate-specific antigen levels in men with and without prostate disease. *JAMA.* 1992;267:2215–20.
13. Catalona WJ, Partin AW, Slawin KM et al. Use of the percentage of free prostate-specific antigen to enhance differentiation of prostate cancer from benign prostatic disease: A prospective multicenter clinical trial. *JAMA.* 1998;279:1542–7.
14. Lacosta Esclapez P, Ramos Trujillo MF, Ugarte López N. *Diccionario de términos oncológicos para los no oncólogos. primera edición.* Madrid: Didot, 2018.
15. Navarro S, Pérez-Segura P, Ramón Y, Cajal S et al. Recomendación para la determinación de biomarcadores en el carcinoma colorrectal. Consenso Nacional de la Sociedad Espanola de Anatomía Patológica y de la Sociedad Espanola de Oncología Médica. *Rev Esp Patol.* 2012;45(3):130–144.
16. Heinz-Josef L. *Biomarkers in Oncology.* 1 ed. New York: Springer, 2013.
17. Austillo de la Vega H, Ruiz García E, Muñoz González D et al. Biomarcadores del cáncer de mama vs fi rmas genómicas: Hacia la búsqueda de una terapia personalizada. *Rev Mex Mastol* 2014;4(1):9–17.
18. López Ríos F, De Castro J, Concha Á et al. Actualización de las recomendaciones para la determinación de biomarcadores en el carcinoma de pulmón avanzado de célula no pequena. Consenso Nacional de la Sociedad Española de Anatomía Patológica y de la Sociedad Española de Oncología Médica. *Rev Esp Patol.* 2015;48(2):80–9.
19. González-Cámpora R, Ramos Asensio R, Vallejo Benítez A et al. Tumores del estroma gastrointestinal: Breve actualización y consenso de la SEAP-SEOM sobre diagnóstico patológico y molecular. *Rev Esp Patol.* 2017;50(2):89–99.

20. Rodríguez Peralto JR, Espinosa E, Ríos-Martin JJ et al. Recomendaciones para la determinación de biomarcadores en el melanoma metastásico. Consenso Nacional de la Sociedad Española de Anatomía Patológica y de la Sociedad Española de Oncología Médica. *Rev Esp Patol*. 2014;47(1):9–21.

21. Grávalos C, Jimeno A. HER2 in gastric cancer: A new prognostic factor and a novel therapeutic target. *Ann Oncol*. 2008;9:1523–9.

22. Oaknin A, Guarch R, Barretina P et al. Recomendaciones para la determinación de biomarcadores en cáncer de ovario epitelial. Consenso nacional de la Sociedad Española de Anatomía Patológica y de la Sociedad Española de Oncología Médica. *Rev Esp Patol*. 2018;51(2):84–96.

23. Manrique Guzmán S. Biomarcadores en gliomas de alto grado: Revisión sistemática. *Gac Med Mex*. 2016;152:87–93.

6

The Psychological Approach: The Healing Power of Image and Comprehensive Assistance to Cancer Patients

Carmen Yélamos

Disease and oncological treatments sometimes bring changes in physical appearance, which can alter the psychic and emotional balance of the person with the disease. Studies show how dissatisfaction with body image is related to low self-esteem, poor self-image, problems in gender identity, interpersonal anxiety, sexual problems, and depressive disorders. Patients with cancer can develop alterations in their body image temporarily or permanently caused by the disease itself (the presence of the tumor, associated weight loss, and so on) as well as by treatments (whether surgery, chemotherapy, radiotherapy, or hormone therapy) and their side effects that can impact on their appearance and body integrity. We should refer not only to alterations in appearance (e.g., hair loss, scarring, swelling, or weight loss), but also to sensory changes (e.g., pain or numbness) and functional impairment (e.g., dysphagia, dysarthria, impotence).

In this chapter, we analyze the psychological approach to alterations of body image in cancer patients in order to highlight strategies of prevention, evaluation, and psychological intervention empirically supported to treat these difficulties. We focus exclusively on the adult population, since the psychological approach in children and adolescents differs significantly from that in adults.

Theoretical Models of Body Image and Cancer

Several theoretical models address the problem of body image developed specifically for the oncology population. White proposes a cognitive-behavioral model based on that developed by Cash for patients with eating disorders, highlighting the subjective nature of the body image concept and the importance of considering the patient's perspective regardless of whether the changes suffered are perceived by others or not. It is expected that changes in appearance produce negative emotional reactions, especially if body image is an aspect valued by the patient, and there is a discrepancy with their ideals of beauty or physical appearance.

Fingeret conceptualizes concerns about the body image of cancer patients along a continuum, distinguishing normal and extreme levels of concern about body image and the behaviors that these concerns generate. For example, patients with mild to moderate difficulties can participate in social situations, despite feeling a certain degree of discomfort depending on the level of difficulty perceived; patients with extreme concerns would avoid

social situations almost completely and would tend to isolation because of the suffering they cause. This model postulates that many patients tend to minimize the difficulties of body image due to shame, fear, or guilt. Within this framework, concerns about body image are not necessarily considered pathological, but in most cases, they are normative experience.

Recently, new theoretical models have been developed, focusing on specific pathologies such as head and neck cancer or breast cancer. Rhoten addresses alterations in body image and dysfunction as a consequence of surgery in the adjustment of patients with head and neck cancer. Fingeret proposes a model focused on breast reconstruction after cancer, taking into account the pathology, the type of surgery and reconstruction, and the complications that can influence the body image of the patients.

Evaluation and Psychological Intervention in Cancer Patients

Studies conducted with long-term breast cancer survivors show that between 15% and 30% of the worries they experience are related to their body image [2]. Adequate and early detection of the alterations that concern cancer patients would increase the number of them who can benefit from psychological care programs as well as other available psychosocial support resources. Early intervention would allow the patient to be equipped with strategies of coping and of adaptation to the change and would improve the patient's approach to the problem or its symptomatology, enhancing adherence to the medical treatment and therefore quality of life.

In this sense, programs and preventive interventions based on emotional support and psychological counseling are recommended to increase the patient's abilities in the face of unwanted changes and favor their adaptation, through acceptance and integration to a new body image. Programs like Look Good Feel Better, Recover Your Smile, among others, facilitate access to necessary resources so patients can find solutions that minimize the limitations that the disease entails and transform them into factors of improvement while enhancing coping resources.

In addition to preventive and supportive interventions, some patients present a problem that is important enough to require a specific psychological evaluation and intervention. White [19] argues that there is a disorder in body image in the oncological population when a clear discrepancy is observed between the objective or perceived physical appearance of a part of the body, attribute, or bodily function and the mental representation (scheme) that the subject has of the attribute.

Frequently, we observe how the patient with cancer perceives himself or herself as a sick person and idealizes the rest of society, with sentiments such as "healthy people have everything," "people realize that I am sick with cancer," "my appearance is responsible for my problems with people and at work," "if my partner sees me bald and without chest, he will not like me and he will reject me"—thoughts that generate feelings of sadness, shame, dissatisfaction, and disgust, and can lead to behaviors of avoidance, camouflage, realization of extreme diets, and so on.

The psychological evaluation of body image in cancer patients should always include perceptual, emotional, cognitive, and behavioral aspects. Different evaluation instruments are available, but almost none of them is specifically designed for cancer patients. One of the most complicated issues in body image research concerns evaluation. The published works on the subject often use different instruments, so it can be difficult to generalize results.

The most specific scales used in oncological patients are the Body Image Scale (BIS), the Body Image Subscale (part of the breast cancer supplementary module BR23 of the QLQ-C30 scale), Sexual Functioning Subscale (part of the module complementary to BR23 breast cancer of the QLQ-C30 scale), FACT-B (Functional Assessment of Cancer Therapy-Breast) questionnaire, and the Rosenberg Self-Esteem Scale.

Regarding intervention aimed at increasing tolerance and facilitating adaptation to changes, Fernández proposes to focus on five objectives:

1. Facilitate the acceptance of loss or bodily harm, which entails a process of elaboration of mourning in which the identification and adequate expression of feelings is fundamental. *Strategies*: Information, participation in the decision-making process, emotional expression.
2. Promote support and family and social integration. *Strategies*: Identify and enhance contact with people who favor support or participation in groups of mutual support.
3. Promote the implementation of strategies and effective coping resources that minimize the impact of physical change. *Strategies*: Rehabilitation, reconstructive techniques, health education, use of prosthesis or other resources, promotion of skills development, operator techniques (planning and combining programs and establishing reinforcement programs and graded goal planning to favor a sense of achievement and control and making the new learning become automatic).
4. Facilitate the development of a new body image (accepting and integrating the changes in a new mental representation). *Strategies*: Techniques of cognitive restructuring, systematic desensitization, use of humor, contact with patient survivors, group dynamics.
5. Enhance self-esteem and the feeling of personal worth. *Strategies*: Cognitive techniques for the modification of beliefs, establishment of goals and achievable goals, development of self-reinforcing skills.

The therapeutic modality that has been shown to be most effective in the treatment of body image disorders in oncological patients has been cognitive-behavioral. The main components and the most used techniques are the following:

- Relaxation and breathing for the management of anxiety symptoms.
- Cognitive restructuring that allows work with the most negative and irrational thoughts. It seems more appropriate to do this before they present.
- Exposure to areas of physical appearance that cause discomfort by visualizing those areas or areas of the body that create discomfort. It can be applied in imagination, in front of the mirror, and through virtual reality. This technique can prevent ritual behaviors such as repeated checking, excessive grooming, camouflage, and so on.
- Designing positive experiences and pleasure with the body, sensory exercises, pleasurable activities, fulfilled toward oneself and one's own body, and so on.
- Prevention of relapses: Identification of risk situations and training in coping strategies.
- Motivation: Psychological treatment cannot change the patient's external aspect, but it can help the patient accept the body and live better in a more satisfactory way.
- Information about body image: How it is constructed; its alterations; physical appearance; the impact of thoughts, emotions, and perception of the body; the role of avoidance; and the rituals and behaviors that maintain a negative body image.
- Agreement on the therapeutic objectives: Psychological treatment is aimed at the patient learning new patterns of thought, emotion, and behavior.

In general, there are few studies on standardized psychological interventions aimed at the treatment of body image alterations in patients with cancer. The majority of studies focus on patients with breast cancer and cancer of the head and neck, so it is necessary to create a model of psychological intervention based on evidence to improve body image in cancer patients.

The Healing Power of Image

The interest in studies on body image and aesthetic care in patients with cancer is growing. We must not forget that the human being is primarily visual. The image has a universal value that positions, locates, and distinguishes us. We are biologically programmed to perceive the world in this way, and as a consequence, an aesthetic model is imposed that generates great social pressure, especially to certain strata of the population such as women, adolescents, and young people. Undoubtedly, the concern for body image also transcends the world of health and disease, both physical and mental [1,2].

Body Image and Self-Esteem

Classically, body image has been defined as the representation of the body that each individual constructs in his or her mind.

It is a complex construct that includes the perception we have of the whole body and each of its parts; its movement and limitations; the subjective experience of attitudes, thoughts, feelings, and valuations that we make and feel; and the way we behave derived from the cognitions and feelings that we experience [3]. It is, therefore, a concept that refers to the way in which each one of us perceives, imagines, feels, and acts with respect to his or her own body [4].

The body image that each individual has is a subjective experience, and there does not have to be a correct correlation with reality; that is, body image is not necessarily correlated with the actual physical appearance, since the thoughts, attitudes, and valuations that the individual makes of his or her own body are key. Basically, it is much more important how we see our body from within than what we see from the outside [5].

Self-esteem is a concept clearly related to body image. It is an attitude or feeling, positive or negative, toward oneself, based on the evaluation of one's own characteristics, and includes feelings of satisfaction with oneself [6]. Both terms—body image and self-esteem—are part of the self-concept.

Image and Society: Beauty Ideal

The body image is built evolutionarily. Adolescence is the key period in which the body is lived as a source of identity, self-concept, and self-esteem in which self-awareness develops on one's physical image, which may lead to greater or lesser dissatisfaction with the body.

A key element to consider in the formation of body image is the sociocultural context. The aesthetic ideal is determined by culture and has the ability to elicit different perceptions and opinions of people based on their physical characteristics (beauty is good, idealization of thinness, stigmatization of fatness, etc.). In this sense, the environment exerts great pressure and continually shows, mainly through advertising, that to succeed in society, it is essential to respond to an established canon of beauty. Therefore, the concept of beauty that manages society ends up directly affecting the ways people perceive their bodies [2].

On the other hand, and together with the two previous factors, the family environment and the social group exert an important influence, although finally, the eagerness to reach a certain physical stereotype will depend on the value that each one of us gives to the physical [7], so that we must forget the important role that personal characteristics will play in the construction of this concept. Thus, internalization, which refers to the degree to which ideals at the physical level are accepted, also influences personal assessment [6].

In Western society, one-third of women and a quarter of men have body dissatisfaction [8]. But this dissatisfaction and concern for the body become a disorder (i.e., a significant malaise) in 4% of women and in less than 1% of men [9].

Body Image, Self-Esteem, and Cancer

Cancer and cancer treatments greatly affect the person and his or her physical appearance. The body image of the cancer patient is clearly affected both by the consequences of surgery (loss of a part of the body or of a function, scars, asymmetry, etc.) and by the side effects of adjuvant treatments (chemotherapy,

radiotherapy, or treatment hormones that can cause alopecia, increase or decrease in body weight, skin lesions in the irradiated area, fatigue, etc.). These changes in the patient's self-image represent a new source of stress as well as impact on their self-esteem, and therefore their self-concept, finally altering the quality of life.

The oncological patient must face not only a serious illness associated with suffering, pain, and sometimes death, but must also adapt to changes in his or her image in a society where physical appearance acquires great importance. Some of these changes will be observable for others (such as tumors that affect the head and neck area, alopecia, etc.), which undoubtedly will influence adaptation to the disease process and treatment. The patient's ability to accept and adapt to these changes, and the possible stigma they generate, will directly affect their emotional state, as well as their personal, family, social, and work functioning. This situation will be especially significant in those patients who base their self-concept on their attributes or physical qualities.

The variables that influence the change in body image of cancer patients are as follows [10]:

- *The type of physical change experienced, the location and the degree of associated disability.* The literature shows greater emotional burden when the tumor affects the head and neck area, not only because of the loss of function (such as communication ability through speech) but also because of the important role of the face in social interaction, communication, and emotional expression [11]. The psychological morbidity is greater in the face of the loss of a bodily function. In these cases, the concern for the physical aspect comes to occupy a secondary position [12].

There is evidence that radical surgical treatments (whether they are followed by reconstruction or not) present greater psychological and adaptive problems than conservative surgical treatments [13].

Finally, the patients with greater risk of developing psychological and social problems are those with greater deformity and physical dysfunction [14,15].

- *Reaction of the environment and perceived social support.* The acceptance and support of family and friends play a key role in facilitating acceptance of the new body image. Shame and fear of rejection by people in the patient's environment can lead to avoidance of social relationships and isolation [10].

- *Availability and access to the necessary resources* (prostheses, handkerchiefs, caps, wigs, etc.), appropriate and adapted to the needs of each patient. Learning new forms of personal care, and attention or access to surgical reconstruction methods will facilitate a patient in facing in a more adaptive way the needs derived from the disease and treatments.

- *Characteristics of the personality.* The concept of a resilient personality with protective features and personal well-being enhancements (such as optimism, flexibility, locus of internal control) has been related to less emotional intensity in the face of changes in physical appearance and to the ability to mobilize and optimize existing resources in order to accept the change and overcome the limitations entailed [16,17].

- *The value or meaning* that the person makes of the physical alteration suffered. The important thing is not always the objective change but the meaning attributed to it. This assessment is mediated by the beliefs that the individual has about his or her body image, the person's coping skills, and the individual's personality [18].

In the case of oncological patients, we should not forget that—unlike what happens with other alterations of the body image—it is not about imagined defects or slight anomalies, but in most cases, we have an objective deformity, asymmetry, real losses of physical functions, and disability. It can be said that the "abnormal" or excessive aspect is not the response of the patient, but the situation that must be faced.

White [19] points out the presence of a disorder in the body image in the oncological population when there is a marked discrepancy between the objective or perceived physical appearance of a part of the body, attribute, or bodily function and the mental representation (schema) that the subject has of that attribute. For White, this discrepancy (due to its association with dysfunctional assumptions about the appearance and about oneself, and with the personal meaning that the subject gives to these changes) causes the appearance of negative emotional responses and compensatory behaviors, which interfere significantly with occupational and social functioning, with normal routine, and with interpersonal relationships.

In general, we can say that when the concern for body image and the dissatisfaction with physical appearance invade a patient's thoughts with intensity and frequency and generate discomfort in the same, interfering negatively with their daily lives, we can talk about body image disorder. These disorders are not very frequent in cancer patients, but difficulties or problems of body image as a result of cancer and its treatment are very common.

Comprehensive Assistance to Cancer Patients

Attention in oncological disease is currently immersed in an important paradigm shift, in which the focus has shifted from a disease-centered to a patient-centered approach; attention is increasingly being paid to psychosocial aspects, to the improvement of the quality of life, to the coverage of the needs and rights of patients, to their empowerment, and to comorbidities and survival [20].

There are increasing numbers of patients who show care and attention for all aspects that are affected by their disease, including their appearance and body image, during and after the oncological process. The physical changes that occur as a result of the disease or treatments can be associated with a deterioration in the perception of body image and are often accompanied by great personal dissatisfaction, a decrease in self-esteem, and avoidance of social relationships, placing the person in a situation of great psychological and emotional vulnerability.

Therefore, the care of cancer patients has a special relevance and should be considered in oncology centers and services with a holistic approach, given its epidemiological importance and its psychosocial connotations. Even today there are still many unmet needs that are in practice only addressed by those cancer centers that can offer comprehensive, multi-, and interdisciplinary cancer care to their patients.

Comprehensive and Multidisciplinary Care for Cancer Patients

Multidisciplinary care units in oncology are dedicated to the treatment and specific care of cancer patients. These units incorporate the criterion of interaction and synergies between the different resources of medical and radiotherapy oncology, as well as that of other specialties, organized into care networks aimed at guaranteeing quality, safe, and efficient care for oncological patients. To this end, they include coordination with primary care services, as well as with other nonspecific specialized units and services (such as Rehabilitation and Physiotherapy Unit, Nutrition and Dietetics, and Plastic, Aesthetic and Reconstructive Surgery) as well as with home services and palliative care units.

The multidisciplinary units represent the alliance of all health professionals involved in the treatment of patients with a tumoral pathology, whose performance is guided by their willingness to agree on clinical decisions based on scientific evidence and to coordinate the provision of care in all stages of the process, encouraging patients to take an active part.

Criteria of Quality of Care

The disposition of these resources within the multidisciplinary care units is an indicator of the quality of the unit, service, or center. In oncology, teamwork and interdisciplinarity are especially important because no specialty can meet all the requirements necessary for the comprehensive management of cancer patients; therefore, the coordination of different specialties is necessary.

Having support services for rehabilitation and physiotherapy, nutrition and dietetics, aesthetic medicine, as well as psychological and social care, and having referral protocols to these services are indicators of quality in multidisciplinary care.

In this way, multidisciplinary care is the hallmark of quality cancer care, and its key element is the tumor committee. Any hospital that offers oncological treatment must have tumor committees that evaluate decisions prior to treatment and establish a global intervention and follow-up plan for the patient.

Concept of Multidisciplinarity

Multidisciplinarity refers to something encompassing several disciplines, with the concept of several specialists and professional categories cooperating and working together for the same patient and to achieve the best results. The fundamental characteristics that distinguish the interdisciplinary team are the persistence of a work methodology, coordination and cooperation among the members of the team, and the existence of common objectives.

The multidisciplinary team in oncology is composed of a group of professionals from different disciplines that come together to work toward the best therapeutic results for the patient, using a common methodology and sharing the same care project and minimum care objectives. A specialist is usually the person responsible or coordinator of the multidisciplinary unit [21].

Integral Vision

The formation of coordinated interdisciplinary teams will lead to the treatment of the oncological patient with a comprehensive vision of the disease and the patient, thus facilitating the approach and prevention of the different aspects that can cause physical, psychological, and social disorders that aggravate the prognosis, thus favoring the patient's best adaptation to the disease and treatment. This good coordination will provide the patient with a referral specialist and the security of the existence of a common thread among the various professionals involved in the healing process.

These units, therefore, facilitate identifying and treating in a personalized and comprehensive way not only the patient's illness but also the possible repercussions that oncologic processes produce in the people who suffer them and the impact on their quality of life (e.g., on the perception of their own body image), contributing in this way to offering the best oncological care.

Undoubtedly, multidisciplinary care units have important advantages for patient, health professionals, and the social environment alike. They produce better results in terms of survival and the reduction of waiting time between diagnosis and treatment initiation, and contribute positively to patient and clinician satisfaction, both at the level of coordination and in professional cooperation [22,23].

The Needs of Cancer Patients

The need for comprehensive, systematic, and continuous management of patients with cancer requires a care network based on close collaboration between the different services and areas dedicated to providing the best care for patients with cancer, as well as other social and health resources. It is therefore necessary that the care centers offer a wide range of care and support modalities that allow guaranteeing and offering the best care to patients undergoing oncological treatment.

This is a need and request that patients with cancer voice more frequently. Patients are increasingly active, calling on public administrations at national, regional, and local levels; medical societies; patient associations; the media; and the pharmaceutical and biotechnology sectors to undertake the necessary actions to address the key needs of people living with cancer. Of these, the need for multidisciplinary assistance by qualified professionals in reference services and the increase of information and patient support services are usually their main requests and demands.

Until relatively recently, the points of view and the preferences of the patients were considered to be of little relevance, and often requests for information or additional attention were not met. Currently, it is noted that the problems of communicating information about the disease and treatment are the most frequent cause of patient dissatisfaction [24,25], which is why knowing and meeting the needs of cancer patients has become a priority.

The greater interest in knowing the preferences of patients in relation to the options of clinical management of the disease is a central element in relation to the participation of the patient in the care plan and in making informed and shared decisions [26]. Without a doubt, it is essential that health professionals, in addition to offering the best therapeutic alternatives available for each case, can assess the needs, preferences, and values expressed by patients; if patients have been able to express these in any way, the doctor is interested to know them before being able to make decisions regarding the therapeutic plan [27].

During the evolution of the disease, patients present complex physical and psychological needs that must be treated appropriately. Even when the patient is in complete remission or "cured," quality of life surveys reveal the presence of physical symptoms and psychosocial discomfort that alter and condition their existence. Physical needs are usually the type of unmet needs most demanded by patients, followed by economic and employment problems, communication and information needs with specialists, problems with the care and attention system, psychological and emotional problems, support and social resources, concerns related to the experience of having lived through cancer, problems of body image, and existential/spiritual needs [28].

Therefore, improvements in survival should not be the only objective to define the failure or success of a specific oncological therapy. Unless the natural history of cancer changes substantially, the patient will end up suffering the consequences of a progressive and incurable disease. Quality of life is also important and very necessary to contemplate in the overall therapeutic plan for cancer [29,30].

Conclusions

Alteration of body image is a critical psychosocial problem for patients with oncological diseases, since cancer and treatments frequently produce significant changes in the appearance and functioning of the body. The knowledge of the psychological impact is essential to offer better psycho-oncological interventions that constitute an essential component in the biopsychosocial support of the cancer patient.

There are many references in the literature that show the negative consequences derived from changes in the physical appearance of cancer patients and their repercussion in their psychological adjustment, self-esteem, sexuality, and therefore, quality of life. Body image disorders are not very frequent; however, in the future more attention should be paid to these needs of cancer patients, given that they can produce great dissatisfaction and should be specifically analyzed in groups of women, adolescents, and young people because of the greater risk and vulnerability to develop psychological alterations.

The human being is composed of different dimensions—physical, psychological, social, spiritual, ethical, interpersonal, emotional, and aesthetic—hence, it is important to provide comprehensive and global therapeutic care to each person, and therefore to the patient with cancer, in all its complex multidimensionality. No single discipline or professional can provide this care or meet the different needs of the patient, so teamwork is one of the fundamental pillars in the care of the oncological patient. Coverage and support by all professionals involved in the therapeutic relationship and help to the patient with cancer are needed in order to ensure the best possible care.

REFERENCES

1. Haimouitz D, Lansky LM, O'Reilly P. Fluctuations in body satisfaction across situations. *Int J Eating Disord.* 1993;13(1):77–84.

2. Killen DJ, Taylo CB, Hayward C, Haydel FH, Wilson D, Hammer L. Weight concerns influence the development of eating disorders: A 4-year prospective study. *J Consult Clin Psychol.* 1996;64:936–940.

3. Raich RM. ¿Qué es la imagen corporal? En: Raich RM, ed. *Imagen corporal. Conocer y valorar el propio cuerpo.* Madrid: Ed. Pirámide, 2000:17–26.

4. Rosen JC. The nature of body dysmorphic disorder and treatment with cognitive behavior therapy. *Cognitive and Behavioral Practice.* 1995;2:143–166.

5. Cash TF. *The Body Image Work Book. An 8–Step Program for Learning to Like Your Looks.* Oakland. New Harbinge, 1997.

6. Rosenberg M. *Society and the Adolescent Self Image.* Princeton, NJ: Princeton University Press, 1965.

7. Rajagopalan J, Shejwal B. Influence of sociocultural pressures on body image dissatisfaction. *Psychol Stud.* 2014;59(4):357–64.

8. Grant JR, Cash TF. Cognitive-behavioral body image therapy:comparative efficacy of groups and modest-contact treatments. *Behav Ther.* 1995;26:69–84.

9. Rosen JC, Reiter J, Orosan P. Cognitive-behavioral body image therapy forbody dysmorphic disorder. *J Consult Clin Psychol.* 1995; 63:263–269.

10. Fernández AI. Alteraciones psicológicas asociadas a los cambios en la apariencia física en los pacientes oncológicos. *Psicooncología.* 2004;1(2–3):169–80.

11. Rhoten BA, Murphy B, Ridner SH. Body image in patients with head and neck cancer: A review of the literature. *Oral Oncol.* 2013;49(8):753–60.

12. Die Trill M, Die Trill J, Die Goyanes A. Tumores de cabeza y cuello. En: Die Trill M, ed. *Manual de Psico-oncología.* Madrid: Editorial Ades, 2003:145–63.

13. Yurek D, Farrar W, Andersen BL. Breast cancer surgery: Comparing surgical groups and determining individual differences in postoperative sexuality and body change stress. *J Consult Clin Psychol* 2000;68(4):697–709.

14. Gamba A, Romano M, Grosso I. Psychosocial adjustment of patients surgically treated for head and neck cancer. *Head Neck.* 1992;14:218–23.

15. Langius A, Bjrvell H, Lind M. Functional status and coping in patients with oral and pharyngeal cancer before and after surgery. *Head Neck.* 1994;16:559–68.

16. Cobaza S, Maddi S, Kahn S. Hardiness and Health. A prospective study: Clarification of the resistance personality. *J Pers Soc Psychol.* 1993;65(1):35–47.

17. Abend TA, Williamson GM. Feeling attractive in the wake of breast cancer: Optimism matters, and so do interpersonal relationships. *Pers Soc Psychol B.* 2002;28(4):427–36.

18. Raich RM. ¿Por qué hay personas que sufren el trastorno de la imagen corporal? Desarrollo del trastorno de la imagen corporal. En: Raich RM, ed. *Imagen corporal. Conocer y valorar el propio cuerpo.* Madrid: Ediciones Pirámide, 2000: 67–93.

19. White CA. Body I Image dimensions and cancer: A heuristic cognitive behavioural model. *Psychooncology.* 2000;9:183–92.

20. European Partnership Action Against Cancer Consensus G, Borras JM, Albreht T et al. Policy statement on multidisciplinary cancer care. *Eur J Cancer.* 2014;50(3):475–480.

21. Unidades asistenciales del área del cáncer. Estándares y recomendaciones de calidad y seguridad. Informes, estudios e investigación. *Ministerio de Sanidad, ServiciosSociales e Igualdad,* 2013. [fecha de consulta: 4 noviembre 2017]. Disponibleen: http://www.mscbs.gob.es/organizacion/sns/planCalidadSNS/docs/Cancer_EyR.pdf.

22. CanNET National Support and Evaluation Service – Siggins Miller 2008. *Managed Clinical Networks – a literature review,* Cancer Australia, p.56. Canberra:ACT, 2008.

23. National Support and Evaluation Service - Siggins Miller. *Managed Clinical Networks - A Literature Review. CanNET Cancer Service Networks National Demonstration Program.* Canberra: Cancer Australia, 2008.

24. Coulter A. Patient information and shared decision-making in cancer care. *Br J Cancer.* 2003;89:S15–S16.

25. Grol R, Wensing M, Mainz J, Jung HP, Ferreira P, Hearnshaw H et al. Patients in Europe evaluate general practice care: An international comparison. *Br J Gen Pract.* 2000;50:882–887.

26. Kraetschmer N, Sharpe N, Urowitz S, Deber RB. How does trust affect patient preferences for participation in decision making? *Health Expect.* 2004;7(4):317–26.

27. Blank T, Graves K, Sepucha K, LlewellynThomas H. Understanding treatment decision making: Contexts, commonalities, complexities, and Challenges. *Ann Behav Med.* 2006;32(3):211–7.

28. Burg MA, Adorno G, López EDS, Loerzel V, Stein K, Wallace C, Sharma DKB. Current unmet needs of cancer survivors: Analysis of open-ended responses to the American Cancer Society Study of Cancer Survivors II. *Cancer.* 2015;121:623–630.

29. Arraras JL, Martínez M, Manterota A, Laínez N. La evaluación de la calidad de vida del pacienteoncológico. *El Grupo de Calidad de Vida de la EORTC Psicooncología.* 2004;1(1):87–98.

30. Aaronson NK. Assessment of quality of life benefits from adjuvant therapies in breast cancer. *Recent Results Cancer Res.* 1993;127:201–10.

7

The Role of the Family

Ana Isabel Cobo Cuenca

Cancer, like other diseases, requires great adaptation efforts. Not only does it affect the person who has it, but it also causes a great emotional burden in the family environment. When a family member has cancer, family dynamics become destabilized. Family emotional responses and the degree to which family dynamics are destabilized will depend on the following:

1. Cancer (type of cancer, location, phase in which it is located, degree of disability)
2. Who is the relative who is sick (spouse, parent, child, sibling, grandparent) and role played within the family
3. Health beliefs held by the family
4. Previous experiences of illness (e.g., it is not the same to have a history of family members who died from cancer, family members who were cured of cancer, or family members who had the same or different types of cancer)
5. Family type (functional or dysfunctional)

The family, and especially the main caregiver, plays an important role in the life of the cancer patient, since family members are usually in charge of basic care, hygiene, food, medication administration, emotional support, transportation to health centers, and communication with the health team.

Family members, besides being the main caregivers, tend to empathize too much with the patient's pain and discomfort. In different studies, it has been observed how family members may have higher levels of anxiety than patients themselves. In addition, they may have other symptoms such as pain, insomnia, and fatigue.

The care of health professionals has to be directed not only to the cancer patient, but also to the family.

Psychological interventions in the family, as in the person with cancer, will be performed according to which period of the process they are in:

1. The moment of diagnosis
2. During the curative treatment
3. In the survival period
4. During palliative care

At the beginning, it is convenient to make a family evaluation, with the objectives to be able to meet the family, identify the competencies (knowledge, skills, and attitudes) that are required to take care of the cancer patient, know the coping strategies usually used, know the aids needed, and be able to identify family crises that may arise (caregiver claudication).

It is generally considered that cohesion, good communication, and intrafamilial affection are the most important family aspects required to achieve greatest adaptation to the disease.

Effective communication improves family cohesion, the expression of emotions among family members, and the solution of conflicts that may appear, and also reinforces new changing roles and improves family support and functioning.

A fundamental area in the family is the relationship of a couple, in which communication, marital adjustment, and the form of conflict resolution become very important in times of crisis (as, in this case, having a relative with cancer).

To determine the family functioning, there are different questionnaires:

1. APGAR Familiar [1] is an easy-to-use questionnaire, which explores family functioning from the patient's perspective. It consists of five questions with three answer options; the higher the score, the better is the family functioning.
2. Family Relationship Index (FRI) [2] is a self-filled questionnaire that measures interpersonal relationships between family members. It consists of 12 items with two yes or no answer options in three subscales (cohesion, conflicts, and expressiveness). Cohesion is understood as the degree to which the members are united and help each other; conflicts refer to the way in which conflicts in the family are freely expressed; and expressiveness refers to the way they share their feelings.
3. Self-report Family Inventory (SFI) [3] is a self-filled questionnaire with 36 items that values the competence and style of the family. It has five subscales: health-competition, conflict, cohesion, leadership, and emotional expressiveness.

The scales that can be used to know family communication are among others:

1. The Family Communication Scale (FCS) is a validated scale of ten items with five response options. This assigns value to family communication, with different family members and at different stages of the life cycle, and considers family communication as the transmission of ideas, feelings, and knowledge.

2. The Parent-Adolescent Communication Scale (PAC) is a 20-item questionnaire that measures parents' communication with teenagers.

Family Interventions

Galindo Vázquez et al. [4], after a review of the literature, concludes that the interventions that help the most and have more evidence are as follows:

1. Informative/psychoeducational interventions, which are aimed at providing the caregiver with training to be able to effectively carry out care for the cancer patient, management instruction and care of ostomies and catheters, and teaching of diets appropriate to the pathology and treatment.
2. Interventions for the couple/family, which are aimed at improving communication within the family, facilitating the relationship of couple and conflict resolution. Cognitive behavioral therapy, psychoeducational techniques, and activation control techniques are usually employed.
3. Therapeutic orientation directed to the caregivers themselves, improving or facilitating skills to attend their own physical and emotional health, self-confidence, self-efficacy, quality of life, and support systems.

Interventions can be done face to face, by telephone, or online, although they are usually done in person. They can be individual, with the whole family, or as a group with other families.

There are numerous studies that report that group techniques tend to be much more effective than individual techniques, since they foster interpersonal relationships; improve empathy, self-esteem, and feelings of self-efficacy; and favor emotional relief. They tend to have a psychoeducational character and often teach multiple techniques for coping with stress, decreased activation, sensory focusing techniques, communication skills, skin care, and so on. Often they act as self-help groups, favoring communication between the members of the groups.

Communication with the Family

The correct communication of the diagnosis and of the evolution of the disease in the family will affect the adaptation of the process, both in the patient and in the rest of the members of the family nucleus.

The moment of communicating the diagnosis to the family is usually unpleasant for the patient, causing anxiety and fear through not knowing what to communicate and how to communicate it. Generally, when communicating the diagnosis to children, siblings, or parents, doctors usually rely on the couple. If it is not known how to do this, it is important that health professionals be asked.

To adapt the information, the following must be taken into account:

1. Location where the information is to be imparted: it is not suitable for communication of the diagnosis to take place either in the street or in places where you cannot facilitate expression of emotions, such as in an open space with people outside the family (e.g., bars).
2. The information must be gradual, clear, real, and with an appropriate language to the family to whom it is addressed, taking into account the age, the cultural level, and the resources the family has to face crisis situations.
3. Time should be provided so that emotions or doubts and questions about the process can be expressed.

It is common that when there are children, they are not given due attention, leaving them out of the disease process and trying to protect them, which makes the disease seem taboo within the family environment.

Leaving children out of the process is often counterproductive, as children often realize that something is not working well in the family. They usually score high on anxiety, since they usually anticipate and magnify situations. Also, for the rest of the family, both the sick and others, trying to keep the disease hidden, so that children do not know, is a great effort. It is important not to leave children out of the cancer process.

When talking with the family, you have to choose the right time and place, so there are no interruptions. The disease should be explained with vocabulary appropriate for the child's age. The information has to be close to reality, but it must be given gradually, respecting the needs and rhythm of the child. We must explain that nobody is to blame and that it is not contagious. Children's reactions are very different and must be respected. You can use stories or pictograms appropriate to the ages of the children to inform them.

The age and maturity of the child must be taken into account:

1. *Early childhood (0–24 months)*: Although they do not understand the meaning of disease, they are able to perceive that something is wrong. They usually have changes in sleep, food, and crying.
2. *Preschool stage (2–6 years)*: They can interpret the disease in a magical way, even thinking that it is a consequence of some behavior they have had or that it is contagious.
3. *School stage (6–9 years)*: They usually worry about their safety and that of the family. They may have more interest in knowing about the disease.
4. *Preadolescent stage (9–12 years)*: They have a greater capacity to understand the complexity of the disease and often demand more information.
5. *Teen stage (12–18 years old)*: At this stage, they already understand the disease as a long process. Adolescence is a time of life crises. Sometimes, teenagers hide their feelings, expressing little concern or indifference to the family, even if this is not true, and they have a high sensitivity.

Normally, to know if the child needs psychological intervention, it should be taken into account that it is normal to be sad, and this does not mean that the child has a problem. Normally, children's moods manifest through behavior. Changes in behavior, a drop in school performance, isolation, or changes in game playing can tell us if something is wrong for the child. It is important that the school is aware of the occurrence of the disease in the child's environment so that problems can be detected and alleviated.

Key Points

- Cancer has a great impact on the person and family that suffer from it.
- Psychological intervention is aimed at improving adaptation to the disease, preventing and treating psychopathological problems.
- The psychological intervention will depend on the stage of the disease.
- The psychological intervention is also aimed at the family.
- It is important to know how the family functions to facilitate the adaptation of the family and to prevent crisis situations.
- It is important that there is a multidisciplinary team (doctors, psychologists, nurses, physiotherapists) that treats both people with cancer and their families.

REFERENCE

1. Smilkstein G. The family APGAR: A proposal for a family function test and its uses by physicians. *J Fam Pract.* 1978;6:1231–1239.
2. Kissane DW, Bloch S, McKenzie M, McDowall AC, Nitzan R. Family grief therapy: A preliminary account of a new model to promote healthy family functioning during palliative care and bereavement. Psycho-Oncology: *J Psychol, Soc Behav Cancer,* 1998;7(1):14–25.
3. Beavers WR, Hampson RB, Hulgus YF. Commentary: *The Beavers systems approach to family assessment.* 1985.
4. Galindo Vázquez O, Rojas Castillo E, Ascencio Huertas L et al. Guía de Práctica clínica para la Atención Psico-Oncológica del cuidador primario informal de pacientes con cáncer. *Psicooncología.* 2015;12(1):87–104.

BIBLIOGRAPHY

Cortés-Funes F, Bueno JP, Narváez A, García-Valverde A, Guerrero-Gutiérrez L. Funcionamiento familiar y adaptación psicológica en oncología. *Psicooncología.* 2012;9(2–3):335–54.

Cruzado Rodríguez JA. *Manual de psicooncología. Tratamientos Psicológicos en pacientes con cáncer.* Madrid: Pirámide; 2013.

Hawrylak MF, Maíllo LH, García IM. Comunicación intra-familiar y cáncer de mama. *Psicooncologia.* 2018;15(1):13.

Osborne RH, Elsworth GR, Sprangers MA, Oort FJ, Hopper JL. The value of the Hospital Anxiety and Depression Scale (HADS) for comparing women with early onset breast cancer with population-based reference women. *Qual Life Res.* 2004; 13(1):191–206.

Rodríguez Vega B, Ortiz Villalobos A, Palao Tarrero A, Avedillo C, Sánchez-Cabezudo A, Chinchilla C. Síntomas de ansiedad y depresión en un grupo de pacientes oncológicos y en sus cuidadores. *The European Journal of Psychiatry (Edición en Español)*, 2002;16(1):27–38.

Visser A, Huizinga GA, van der Graaf WT, Hoekstra HJ, Hoekstra-Weebers JE. The impact of parental cancer on children and the family: A review of the literature. *Cancer Treat Rev.* 2004;30(8):683–94.

8

The Oncological Patient Environment: Legal Framework and Ethics

Rosa María Rodríguez Arias

Introduction

Thanks to new studies, research, and breakthrough treatments, the survival rate for cancer has significantly increased. This encouraging fact has also led to frequent consequences for patients, some of them aesthetic. In order to cope with these sequelae and improve patients' quality of life, aesthetic medicine for oncological patients has developed. If every patient has to be treated with respect based on truthful, simple, and transparent information, this is even more critical for patients who have undergone a serious disease and desire to return to social and labor life in the best circumstances. For this reason, it is fundamental to offer to the oncological patient adequate information and appropriate informed consent.

Information Consent

In the last century, the doctor-patient relationship moved from a vertical, paternalistic relation, in which the aphorism was "all for the patient, but without the patient," to a relationship in which the patient is more informed. This change occurred due to the greater complexity of the medical profession itself (with an increase in invasive diagnostic methods and high-risk therapies) and to significant social changes (the rise of the Internet and medical information being searched for on the web, increased legal protection, and communication of patients' rights). Whatever the reason, patients' individuality has been promoted, and they, with the maximum amount of information possible, must make their own decisions about medical acts and take full responsibility for them.

This shift toward a more formal, or standardized, informed consent should not be interpreted as a break in the relationship of trust between doctor and patient. On the contrary, the legal and ethical regulation of informed consent should be seen as a renewal of this trust in the search of equality. The doctor will increase the quality of his or her performance by informing the patient about the treatment (benefits, alternatives, adverse events, and risks), and in case of failure, the patient will need to make a decision only about possible future treatment.

This historical evolution has led to the corresponding legal evolution. The modern doctrine of informed consent was born in the early twentieth century in the Anglo-Saxon world, which highlighted individual inviolability and that every human being has the right to decide for his or her own body. After the Second World War, the "Nuremberg Code" [International Court of Nuremberg of 1947] represents a good reference: The voluntary consent of the human subject is absolutely essential. This means that the person involved should have legal capacity to give consent; should be so situated as to be able to exercise free power of choice, without the intervention of any element of force, fraud, deceit, duress, overreaching, or other ulterior form of constraint or coercion; and should have sufficient knowledge and comprehension of the elements of the subject matter involved, as to enable him or her to make an understanding and enlightened decision. This latter element requires that, before the acceptance of an affirmative decision by the subject of an experiment, there should be made known to him or her the nature, duration, and purpose of the experiment; the method and means by which it is to be conducted; all inconveniences and hazards reasonably to be expected; and the effects upon health or person, which may possibly come from participation in the experiment. The duty and responsibility for ascertaining the quality of the consent rests upon each individual who initiates, directs, or engages in the experiment. It is a personal duty and responsibility that may not be delegated to another with impunity.

More recently, the Convention for the Protection of Human Rights and Dignity of the Human Being with regard to the Application of Biology and Medicine: Convention on Human Rights and Biomedicine (signed in Oviedo, Spain, in 1997) devotes Chapter II, Articles 5 to 9, to Informed Consent. Article 5 has special relevance for the definition on Informed Consent: "An intervention in the health field may only be carried out after the person concerned has given free and informed consent to it. This person shall beforehand be given appropriate information as to the purpose and nature of the intervention as well as on its consequences and risks. The person concerned may freely withdraw consent at any time."

Informed consent is also referenced in the Charter of Fundamental Rights of the European Union (2000/C 364/01): Article 3 (Right to the integrity of the person) states, "In the fields of medicine and biology, the following must be respected in particular: the free and informed consent of the person concerned, according to the procedures laid down by law."

The European Committee for Standardization (CEN) has developed a European standard (EN) for aesthetic medicine, EN16844. CEN 403 "Aesthetic medicine services—non-surgical medical treatments" in which Informed Consent is regulated in section 4.3, starting with the definition "Consent is an ongoing process extending from the time of first contact until the day of the aesthetic-medical treatment; the majority of this process should be completed prior to booking." In the second paragraph of the same section, informed consent content is detailed:

4.3.2 The process shall include the following:

a. A clear explanation of the limitations of the aesthetic-medical treatment and alternative treatments that may be available (including those not offered by the practitioner).
b. A clear explanation of the implications of the aesthetic-medical treatment, including a clear explanation of the recovery time, duration of recommended absence from work and follow up plans.
c. The practitioner shall ensure that the patient clearly understands the risks involved with the planned treatment. The frequently occurring and the rare, but serious, complications should be fully explained and understood. A personal low rate of complication shall not be used to entice patient to undertake aesthetic-medical treatment.

If data are available, personal risks should be stated in natural numbers and in relation to a number of treated patients, for example 1 out of 200 patients suffer from this side effect rather than 0.5% of all patients.

d. The discussion shall include an explanation, in clear and understandable terms, of the practitioner's expectations of outcome and the relation between the outcome of the treatment with those of alternative treatments.
e. Written information shall be given as additional material and shall not take the place of an informed discussion. Practitioners should keep a record of both the discussions and of the information given to the patient. Both parties shall sign the informed consent form.
f. The practitioner shall ensure that the patient is informed of the limitation, implications and potential complications of the aesthetic-medical treatment before booking it.
g. Until the initial consent process is complete (the time at which the patient fully understands the limitation, implications and potential complications of the aesthetic-medical treatment) all monies, except for any previously declared non-refundable deposit, shall remain refundable.
h. No patient shall undergo an aesthetic-medical treatment without completion of the consent process.
i. Aesthetic-medical treatments for patients under the age of 18 years should be exceptional and linked to a documented medical assessment of the risks and benefits (health, social consequences). In those cases where it is clinically or psychologically necessary, the consent form shall be available in a legal form of words appropriate to the patient and/or their parents or guardians prior to the aesthetic-medical treatment. Parental or guardian written agreement is mandatory.

j. The consent forms should be legible, understandable and signed by both parties.
k. The patient's consent shall be performed in a language both parties can understand and agree on.

In Spain, Law 41/2002, regulating patient autonomy, specifically standardizes informed consent throughout Chapter IV on Respecting the Autonomy of the Patient. Before this chapter, Article 3 gives a rather appropriate definition of what can be understood as informed consent as "the free, voluntary and conscious conformity of a patient, manifested in the full use of his faculties after receiving the adequate information, in order for an action that affects his health to take place."

At a more general level, the International Code of Medical Ethics, adopted by the 3rd General Assembly of the World Medical Association in the UK in 1949 and last amended at the 57th General Assembly of the AMM, in South Africa in 2006, does not specifically mention informed consent (contrary to some local medical codes of practice, such as the Spanish) but does allude to the autonomy of the patient by stating: "the physician must respect the right of the competent patient to accept or reject a treatment."

Conclusions

Delivering complete information to patients regarding the treatment they will undergo is fundamental. When it comes to oncological patients, the information should not be limited to the treatment and usual side effects but should include the most frequent risks and complications, based on their medical background, and potential implications that those antecedents may lead to.

BIBLIOGRAPHY

Charter of the fundamental rights of the European Union. (2000/C364/01)
Código de deontología médica. Guía de ética médica de 2011. Consejo General de Colegios Oficiales de Médicos de España.
Convention for the protection of Human Rights and Dignity of the Human Being with regard to the Application of Biology and Medicine: Convention on Human Rights and Biomedicine. Oviedo, 04/04/1997.
EN16844. CEN 403 'Aesthetic medicine services - Non-surgical medical treatments' European Standard by CEN/CENELEC. June, 2017.
Galan Cáceres JC. *Medicina y responsabilidad legal. Medicina y Derecho, dos Mundos en Convergencia*. España: Editorial Follas Novas, 2014.
International Code of Medical Ethics. 1949.
Ley 44/2003 de 21 de noviembre de Ordenación de las Profesiones Sanitarias.
Ley española Ley 41/2002, de 14 de noviembre, básica reguladora de la autonomía del paciente y de derechos y obligaciones en materia de información y documentación clínica.
Nuremberg Code, International Court of Nuremberg, 1947.
Romeo Casabona CM. El consentimiento informado en la relación entre el médico y el paciente. en *Problemas prácticos del consentimiento informado*. Barcelona: Publicación de la Fundación Víctor Grífols i Lucas, 2002.

9

Radiotherapy: The Prevention of Secondary Effects, Radiodermatitis, and Long-Term Toxicity

Eglee Montilla de Somaza

Introduction

Shortly after radiation was introduced as a therapeutic modality at the beginning of the twentieth century, the effects of x-rays on the skin were recognized as one of the main dose-limiting toxicities. Despite these historical advances in our understanding of radiation therapy (RT) and its effects on normal tissue, radiation dermatitis continues to be one of the most common side effects of modern RT [1].

The combination of radiation therapy and systemic therapy, such as chemotherapy, can exacerbate skin reactions, leading to severe xerosis, inflammation, thinning of the skin, and necrosis of the upper dermis and epidermis [2].

These findings, although rarely fatal, can result in significant morbidity, cosmetic disfigurement, and psychological distress. These reactions can lead to the interruption of therapy, which could be detrimental to the outcome of cancer treatment [1,3].

Predisposing Factors

There are factors that predispose to radiodermatitis related to the characteristics of the patient, the categories of the radiation treatment technique, and the type of chemotherapy used [4].

With regard to the patient, large volumes of irradiation produce radiation dermatitis, especially in patients with large breasts, large body mass index, black skin color, or those who are postmenopausal [5].

In relation to treatment, new techniques such as three-dimensional (3D) conformal and intensity modulated radiation therapy (IMRT) have a markedly improved lower rate of radiodermatitis, hyperpigmentation, edema, and desquamation. Studies have shown that irradiation doses, the time the treatment lasts, and whether it is fractionated or standard, are important. In fact, the data suggest that hypofraction presages improvements in the rates of dermatitis, pruritus, hyperpigmentation, and breast pain in the acute context [5].

Radiation therapy and the combined radiotherapy and chemotherapy protocols have improved the prognosis and long-term survival of many malignancies. Therefore, patients and treating physicians are increasingly forced to control the acute skin reactions associated with these treatments. Radiation therapy causes a variety of acute skin reactions, commonly defined as acute radiodermatitis, that occur in the first 6 months from the start of treatment and range from mild erythema and dry desquamation to severe confluent wet desquamation. A study conducted by Barkham in the United Kingdom in 2014, cited in Berger et al. [2,3], revealed that 52% of radiotherapy centers reported having observed dry desquamation associated with radiotherapy. It has also been reported that acute radiodermatitis occurs in 90% of patients treated with breast cancer and head and neck cancer. In fact, any patient with head and neck cancer or breast cancer who receives RT and chemotherapy or systemic therapy may have some risk of developing these reactions [2,5].

Acute damage occurs directly from the initial radiation dose when the first batch of basal cells is destroyed, although acute side effects become apparent on average 2–3 weeks after the start of therapy. The remaining cells become cornified and, therefore, break off faster than healthy skin. This process disrupts the balance between normal cell production in the basal layer and cell destruction on the surface of the skin and will appear as long as the treatment continues. Skin barrier dysfunction manifests as dryness, peeling skin, or scaling, such as folliculitis (rash), xerosis, pruritus, and hyperpigmentation. The skin becomes more sensitive to allergens and ultraviolet radiation, making it prone to infection. The main function of supporting skin care is to maintain the integrity of the epidermal barrier [5].

Protection of the Skin in the Cancer Patient

Before starting treatment with radiotherapy, it is necessary to reinforce the skin so that it is in the best conditions to face the usual treatments. Adequate nutrition and micronutrition are important; the cleaning and hydration and photoprotection are no less important. Aggressive treatments such as peeling and dermabrasion should be avoided [6].

The primary function of skin care products is to provide exogenous support that maintains the intactness of the epidermal barrier. Skin hydration relieves symptoms associated with dry skin and reduces the aggravation associated with the itching that leads to secondary infections. This hydration must be with ingredients, without perfumes, and without alcohol and must be manufactured in sterile conditions [6].

During the treatment, it is recommended patients use neutral soaps of neutral or nonalkaline pH, without perfume colors or preservatives, so they produce a variation of the physiological pH of the skin, avoiding an imbalance that causes alteration or elimination of the hydrolipidic film, the transformation of the corneum stratum of the skin, the modification of the structure of the keratin, or the alteration of the bacterial flora that is at physiological pH and that prevents the proliferation of pathogens, so that these could then develop and lead to infections [7].

The usual hygiene during and after the radiation with washing and the use of deodorant are labeled as "recommended for practice" by the Oncology Nursing Society's Putting Evidence into Practice [4,5].

Bolderston et al. [1] reported that if wet desquamation occurs, it should include several types of dressings and antimicrobials (the most common is Flamazine or silver sulfadiazine and Fucidin). The objective is the management of wet desquamation (when the dermis is exposed with loss of serous fluid) to minimize trauma, protect the skin, promote healing, and prevent infection from occurring [1].

Dreno et al. [8] recommend that general measures should be continued to avoid further deterioration of topical barrier treatments, taking care not to apply occlusive creams. The role of emollients is to protect the epidermal barrier. The topical application of humectants or emollients joins the water with the stratum corneum, providing partial hydration of the surface. This will improve the function of the epidermal barrier and reduce the itching, scaling, redness, and cracks associated with xerosis, and will prevent secondary infections by scratching, induced by radiation. Therefore, skin care with moisturizers, cleansers, and low irritation makeup is effective to improve the skin's hydration and control or conceal some skin reactions [8].

Several experts [9–11] have proven that patients receiving calendula in ointment have significantly fewer cases of grade 2 major dermatitis and greater pain relief.

It is believed that hyaluronic acid accelerates the healing process by stimulating fibroblasts and fibrin formation. Some authors recommend the use of hyaluronic acid in topical cream in the management of grade 2 and 3 skin toxicity in the absence of infection [9].

After oncological treatment, adverse effects persist for several weeks after radiotherapy. Women had greater concerns about dry skin and skin irritation once cancer therapy had been completed. There is a very high prevalence (81%) of xerosis grade 1 or 2 in the total study population [12,13].

Multiple prospective randomized trials have established that topical corticosteroids are effective in decreasing radiation dermatitis in patients with breast cancer [11,12,14]. Kole et al. [5] evaluated the effect of mometasone furoate for the prevention of radiation dermatitis. These results have been validated in two larger recent studies that tested the efficacy of mometasone furoate. The preventive effect of betamethasone on radiation dermatitis has been observed in both conventional and hypofractionated radiation environments. Some nonsteroidal agents have shown promise. Silver sulfadiazine cream 3 days per week during RT and for 1 week after showed a reduction of the dermatitis rates compared to a control group without intervention [5].

An open observational study, conducted in four radiotherapy centers, suggests that following a proper routine for skin care could delay the onset of early skin reactions. This is the first study found in the literature that presents a complete protocol of skin care specific to the oncological patient that includes thermal water, cleanser, emollient, cream to heal wounds, and sunscreen.

Although the study was prospective, the design was limited by the absence of a control group. However, this study provides additional support for the use of an appropriate skin care protocol in the treatment of skin reactions due to radiotherapy [4].

Included in the usual care to prevent radiodermatitis is nonpharmacological care. The guidelines include local hygiene, reduction of exposure and friction of the irradiated area, use of suitable clothing (preferably cotton), and avoidance of contact with extreme temperatures and pruritus in the irradiated area. Direct exposure to the sun should be avoided; use sunscreen with a sun protection factor (SPF) of at least 15. Apply hypoallergenic moisturizing creams without perfumes or preservatives. The natural oil-based emulsion containing allantoin seems to have similar effects for managing skin toxicity compared with aqueous cream up to week 5; however, it becomes significantly less effective at later weeks into the radiation treatment and beyond treatment completion (week 6 and beyond). Avoid the use of acne products that have alcohol or retinoids [14–16].

Long-Term Toxicity of Radiation Therapy

Chronic changes are a unique subset of adverse reactions from the long-term toxicity of radiation therapy. Chronic radiation dermatitis is a late skin toxicity that develops after a period of latency that can vary between 2 and 10 years after exposure to radiation therapy; one of the most common causes is the exposure of the irradiated area to the sun. The condition can develop in patients who have only experienced minimal acute radiation dermatitis and, therefore, can develop into almost normal-looking skin. Chronic radiation dermatitis is unlikely to repair itself and may remain indefinitely. The defining characteristics of long-term toxicity are thin and vulnerable skin, with telangectasias, hyper- or hypopigmentation, fibrosis, atrophy, and sometimes, the development of cutaneous malignancies. Postinflammatory depigmentation is common and, depending on the type of skin of the patient and the severity of the reaction, can resolve slowly or worsen over time. The skin may become xerotic, scaly, and hyperkeratotic. With severe skin lesion, there may be permanent loss of nail and skin appendages, absence of hair follicles and sebaceous glands with resultant alopecia, and absent or reduced sweating [16]. When the skin and subcutaneous tissue develop fibrosis, there may be a limited range of motion, contractures, and pain. Fibrosis occurs more frequently in patients with breast cancer who were previously treated with a combination of surgical intervention and RT. These patients may experience pain, retraction, and induration of the skin, restricted movements of the arms and neck, lymphedema, necrosis, and ulcerations of the skin. Radiation-induced fibrosis is limited to the region treated with RT, and a biopsy should be obtained to confirm fibrosis [16].

Recommended Ingredients for Prevention of Radiodermatitis

In general, a galenic formula must be composed of individual or combined elements that include nutrients and regenerators such as Rosa Mosqueta oil, almond oil, olive oil, karite butter, grape seed oil, amino acids, jojoba oil, vitamins E or K, aqueous extracts of plants, allantoin, pentoxifylline, sucralfate, copper and zinc sulfate, hyaluronic acid, and urea [17].

Ferreira et al. [15], in a paper on topical interventions to prevent acute dermatitis by radiation, analyze descriptively the characteristics of 13 studies to evaluate the use of trolamine, aloe vera, allantoin, olive oil, Liambai liquid, sucralfate, octasulfate Na-sucrose, hyaluronic acid, and dexpanthenol as active ingredients to prevent radiation dermatitis [7,15]. Additionally, there are studies on topical melatonin and radiodermatitis that show significantly less radiation dermatitis compared to in patients who received placebo. In Tresguerras et al. [18], nonpharmacological topical controls were routinely used in care, such as in aqueous creams, mild soaps, thermal water gel, ointments, and emulsions, the latter being the most recommended for these patients [6].

The period of topical application is another important factor. The preferable application of the product was during the night, allowing the product to remain on the skin for a longer period [7].

Chang et al. [14] investigated the effects of an oil-based natural emulsion containing allantoin versus an aqueous cream, to prevent and control radiation-induced skin reactions. In general, aqueous cream seems to be a more preferred option.

Kodiyan et al. [19] demonstrated that use of topical sucralfate showed a significant improvement in radiodermatitis.

Conclusions

For the oncological patient, the cutaneous effects related to the treatment during and after radiotherapy constitute in many occasions a great inconvenience. Although radiotherapy is an essential treatment for the patient's improvement and to treat cancer, it alters the function of the cutaneous barrier, causing a reaction, shortly after the start of treatment, which affects the quality of life of the patient. Skin reactions can cause physical discomfort with clinical symptoms, alterations in body image, and emotional stress that in some cases may even cause delays in treatment and/or reductions in the overall dose planned and administered, which may compromise the results of the treatment [1,10,17].

During treatment, several factors can affect the skin's toxicity characteristics in terms of intensity, duration, and recovery time. Some of them are related to the characteristics of RT, such as the total dose, the fractionation, the radiation energy, and the volume of the treated regions. The addition of standard chemotherapy and/or biological agents can systematically increase the toxicity profile [5].

Although there are recommendations for the pharmaceutical treatment of skin reactions, there are no recommendations for the choice or use of specific products for skin care affected by the toxicity of RT.

The treatment for radiodermatitis must be seen from the point of view of prophylaxis prior to treatment, during the application of the same, and after the end. Currently, there are no specific guidelines for skin care during or after RT; however, work on ingredients recommended and not recommended in galenic forms has shown the ideal components of galenic forms in the light of current knowledge and their impact on the cosmetic concerns of the cancer patient.

REFERENCES

1. Bolderston A, Cashell A, McQuestion M et al. A Canadian survey of the management of radiation-induced skin reactions. *J Med Imaging Radiat Sci.*, 2018;49(2):1–9. https://doi.org/10.1016/j.jmir.2018.01.003. In Press.
2. Bensadoun RJ, Humbert P, Krutman J et al. Daily baseline skin care in the prevention, treatment, and supportive care of skin toxicity in oncology patients: Recommendations from a multinational expert panel. *Cancer Manag Res.* 2013;5:401–8.
3. Biswal SG, and Mehta RD. Cutaneous adverse reactions of chemotherapy in cancer patients: A clinicoepidemiological study. *Indian J Dermatol.* 2018;63(1):41–6.
4. Chan RJ, Larsen E, and Chan P. Re-examining the evidence in radiation dermatitis management literature: An overview and a critical appraisal of systematic reviews. *Int J Radiat Oncol Biol Phys.* 2012;84(3):e357–62.
5. Kole AJ, Kole L, and Moran MS. Acute radiation dermatitis in breast cancer patients: Challenges and solutions. *Breast Cancer – Targets Therapy* 2017;9(5):313–23.
6. Berger A, Regueiro C, Hija T et al. Interest of supportive and barrier protective skin care products in the daily prevention and treatment of cutaneous toxicity during radiotherapy for breast cancer. *Breast Cancer (Auckl).* 2018;12:1178223417752772.
7. Fernández Martín ME. Introducción a la Estética Oncológica. *Primer Curso de Introducción a la Estética Oncológica GEMEON.* Abril 2018.
8. Dreno B, Bensadoun RJ, Humbert P et al. Algorithm for dermocosmetic use in the management of cutaneous side-effects associated with targeted therapy in oncology. *J Eur Acad Dermatol Venereol.* 2013;27(9):1071–80.
9. Feight D, Baney T, Bruce S, and McQuestion M. Putting evidence into practice. *Clin J Oncol Nurs.* 2011;15(5):481–92.
10. Bolderston A, Lloyd NS, Wong RK, Holden L, and Robb-Blenderman L; Supportive Care Guidelines Group of Cancer Care Ontario Program in Evidence-Based Care. The prevention and management of acute skin reactions related to radiation therapy: A clinical practice guideline support care cancer. 2006;14(8):802–17.
11. Chan RJ, Webster J, Chung B, Marquart L, Ahmed M, and Garantziotis S. Prevention and treatment of acute radiation-induced skin reactions: A systematic review and meta-analysis of randomized controlled trials. *BMC Cancer.* 2014;14:53.
12. Butcher K, and Willianson K. Management of erythema and skin preservation; advice for patients receiving radical radiotherapy to the breast: A systematic literature review. *J Radiother Pract.* 2012;11:44–54.
13. Dalenc F, Ribet V, Rossi AB et al. Efficacy of a global supportive skin care programme with hydrotherapy after non-metastatic breast cancer treatment: A randomised, controlled study. *Eur J Cancer Care (Engl).* 2018;27(1).
14. Chan RJ, Mann J, Tripcony L et al. Natural oil-based emulsion containing allantoin versus aqueous cream for managing radiation-induced skin reactions in patients with cancer: A phase 3, double-blind, randomized, controlledtrial. *Int J Radiat Oncol Biol Phys.* 2014;90(4):756–64.
15. Ferreira EB, Vasques CI, Gadia R et al. Topical interventions to prevent acute radiation dermatitis in head and neck cancer patients: A systematic review. *Support Care Cancer.* 2017;25(3):1001–11.

16. Cancer.Net, American Society of Clinical Oncology (ASCO). 2005–2018 https://www.cancer.net/es/. Reacciones en la piel por la terapia dirigida y la inmunoterapia.
17. Montilla Somaza E. Criterios que debe reunir un cosmético para uso en paciente oncológico. *Trabajo fin de experto para el máster en calidad de vida y cuidados estéticos del paciente oncológico.* Universidad de Alcala. 2018.
18. Tresguerres A. Prevención de la radiodermitis con melatonina tópica. *Master en calidad de vida y cuidados médico estéticos.* I edición. Universidad de Alcala. 2017.
19. Kodiyan J, and Amber KT. A review of the use of topical calendula in the prevention and treatment of radiotherapy-induced skin reactions antioxidants (Basel). 2015;4(2):293–303.

10

Prevention and Treatment of Dermatological Secondary Effects of Cancer Therapy

Sheila K. Mota Antigua

Introduction

Cancer therapies, such as chemotherapy, radiotherapy (RT), targeted therapies, hormone therapy, and recently immunotherapy, have managed to increase the survival of patients diagnosed with this disease, being increasingly specific and effective, thus achieving an increase in life expectancy and, in some cases, turning cancer into a chronic pathology [1]. Despite these great advances, antineoplastic treatments present a series of dermatological adverse effects (DAEs) [2], considerably affecting quality of life (QoL), self-esteem, social life, work life, and relationships [3], and are also an impediment to proper fulfillment and adherence to treatment to such an extent that it is sometimes necessary to interrupt treatment, with a negative impact on the evolution and prognosis of the disease [4]. Several studies have shown that DAEs can have a negative impact on the QoL of cancer patients, while others have emphasized the psychological effects, such as depression, anxiety, and vulnerability. Identifying and developing prevention plans and individual treatment according to what each patient needs is essential to improve the QoL of this group and its subsequent sequelae [3].

DAEs can be addressed in three stages. The first stage corresponds to the *preventive stage*, which begins at the moment at which the treatment to which the patient will be submitted is decided. At this point, we can begin to put into practice nonpharmacological measures that allow care and preparation of the skin to face future aggressive treatment, with the purpose of avoiding alterations occurring at all (and if they occur, of their being as nonaggressive as possible). The second stage corresponds to the *treatment and maintenance stage*, where nonpharmacological and pharmacological therapies will be used, if necessary, to alleviate the adverse effects that may occur during antineoplastic treatment. Finally, in the third stage, the *repair stage*, efforts will be focused on returning the skin to vitality and normalcy.

Adverse/Expected Dermatological Effects of Cancer Therapies

The DAEs of cancer treatments are very frequent and represent a real burden for cancer patients, which is why these manifestations are known as "expected effects of treatment." In order to be able to help cancer patients in terms of counseling, prevention,

and treatment of DAEs, it is necessary that professionals who are in direct contact with these patients learn to recognize these symptoms, their origin, and their impact (both physical and psychological), to prevent them as far as possible, and finally to treat them, so that the negative impact on the QoL of those affected is minimized and treatment interruptions avoided [2].

Among the most common symptoms and signs are alopecia and modifications of hair, eyebrows and body hair, acneiform eruptions, toxic erythema due to chemotherapy, acute radiodermatitis and chronic radiodermatitis caused by radiation therapy, skin fissures, hyperkeratosis, hypersensitivity, photosensitivity, changes in pigmentation, mucositis (which can affect all mucous membranes), nail changes, cutaneous xerosis, and induced cutaneous tumors [2].

The cells of the skin are affected due to the nonspecificity of the treatments, which attack not only the tumor cells but also those of rapid proliferation, causing an imbalance of the stratum corneum with subsequent alteration of the barrier function of the skin [2].

Prevention and Treatment of Dermatological Adverse Effects

DAEs, according to various studies, can be prevented and treated with nonpharmacological measures, such as dermocosmetic guidelines; depending on the degree of involvement and if the dermocosmetics have not been sufficient to slow them down, physicians will use additional pharmacological measures. Skin dermocosmetic care is defined, according to experts, as personal hygiene, which includes cleaning, hydration, and photoprotection of the skin, using nonpharmacological or cosmetic products. For its use to be suitable in oncological patients, these products must have been tested in patients with dermatological diseases and have demonstrated a good tolerance profile [5]. It has been proven that the good choice of a cosmetic can delay or even prevent the appearance of a DAE related to antineoplastic treatments, while inappropriate use can make them worse [5].

Objective of Dermocosmetic Therapy

The objective of dermocosmetic therapy should be to maintain intact the barrier function of the skin through the application of preventive and maintenance measures during antineoplastic treatment, with nonpharmacological and cosmetic products. The intention is to prevent and manage more effectively cutaneous toxicity and improve the patient's QoL, avoiding dose changes or interruptions due to DAEs, which in many cases can become incapacitating [4–6].

In order for a dermocosmetic to be safe in an oncological patient, it must comply with a series of criteria in its composition—both active ingredients and excipients and additives—as well as in its form of manufacture, to ensure that it will not be harmful to the cancer patient with an altered skin barrier.

The criteria that a dermocosmetic must comply with for use in oncological patients are the following [7]:

- Hypoallergenic
- Formulations with a high percentage of natural ingredients of high purity
- No irritants
- No preservatives
- pH greater than 5.5
- Cleaners must be Syndet (synthetic detergent)
- Emollients should be synthetic, with vegetable oils
- Natural gellants of the xanthan gum type
- No AHAs (alphahydroxy acids)
- No alcohol
- No hormonal disruptors
- No parabens
- No perfumes
- Dermatologically tested on skins with altered barrier function

Knowing the necessary requirements so that a dermocosmetic can be prescribed to an oncological patient, we advance to the next step, which is to recognize the dermatological needs that the patient is going to present, in order to cover each patient with a specific dermocosmetic treatment that helps to prevent the appearance of DAEs. Within the dermocosmetic needs could be listed facial and body hygiene, facial and body hydration, photo protection, care of the oral mucosa, care of the vaginal mucosa, care of the nails, care of the scalp, corrective makeup, and repair creams (Table 10.1).

TABLE 10.1

Dermocosmetic Pillars for the Prevention and Treatment of Dermatological Adverse Effects of Antineoplastic Therapies

Fundamental since the beginning of therapies	Hygiene
	Hydration
	High sun protection
Other pillars for prevention and treatment	Care of the oral mucosa
	Genital mucosa care
	Nail care
	Scalp care
	Skin repair
	Camouflage makeup

Description, Prevention, and Treatment of the Most Common Dermatological Adverse Effects

Alopecia and/or Alterations in Hair

This can manifest as loss of hair on head and body, in its entirety, gradually, or in sections, or a reduction in density, as well as alterations in the quality and quantity of hair. It is usually transient, but with the use of certain molecules such as taxanes (Paclitaxel, docetaxel), it can be permanent. It begins at 2–3 weeks of treatment with a maximum point at 2 months. It usually represents the main burden of the disease. Recovery occurs from 3 to 6 months after cessation of therapies [2,8].

Induction Molecules

Chemotherapy: Taxanes, etoposide, cyclophosphamides, doxorubicin, Adriamycin, among others. Less frequently: vinblastine, vincristine, bleomycin, fluorouracil, cytarabine, methotrexate. Normally without alopecia: carboplatin, capecitabine, cisplatin.

Targeted therapies: Inhibitors of EGF (cetuximab, erlotinib, gefitinib, etc.). Inhibitors of RAF (sorafenib, etc.).

Interferon-α and interferon-β.

Anti-CTLA-4 antibodies (ipilimumab).

Hormone therapy: Antiestrogens (tamoxifen), antagonists of the estrogen receptor (fulvestrant), anti-aromatases (anastrozole, letrozole) [2,8].

Some therapies can cause hypertrichosis and trichomegaly, a rare adverse effect that can develop 2–5 months after starting treatment with targeted therapies, which may persist for the duration of the treatment. For trichomegaly, it is recommended to cut the eyelashes to avoid corneal irritation; for hypertrichosis, laser hair removal is recommended once the oncological treatment is finished and the skin has recovered all its vitality [9].

Prevention

- Use of a cooling cap (DigniCap) to reduce the frequency and intensity of hair loss during chemotherapy is approved by the U.S. Food and Drug Administration (FDA) for use in patients with solid tumors. This works through the contraction of the blood vessels of the scalp, which reduces the amount of chemotherapy that reaches the hair follicle cells. The low temperature also decreases the activity of the follicles, reducing the speed of cell division, which makes them less affected by the chemotherapy. This method does not guarantee efficacy with all chemotherapeutic agents and is contraindicated in certain types of cancers, in pediatric patients, and in some chemotherapy regimens [10,11]. Several studies have shown its effectiveness in preventing a little more than 50% of hair loss, but they admit that more long-term studies are necessary to obtain information about the possible adverse effects (the currently known ones being headache, nausea, and dizziness) [12–15].

General Recommendations

- Use hair prostheses, handkerchiefs, or turbans. If a capillary prosthesis is used, leave the scalp free at least 6–8 hours a day.
- Do not use dyes with ammonia or paraphenylenediamine (PPD), only nonpermanent, natural dyes.
- Use pencils and shadows to disguise loss of eyebrows and eyelashes.
- Use delicate scalp shampoos.
- May use 2% or 5% Minoxidil to prevent chemotherapy-induced alopecia (CIA), but its efficacy has been shown to be lower than scalp cooling [9,11].

Ungual Alterations

Modifications in the nails include fragility, appearance of stretch marks, color alterations, roughness, painful inflammation of the periungual tissue, pigmented areas, pain, and fissures. These are observed in 10%–15% of patients; they appear after the first 2 weeks of treatment, and there is a risk of superinfection [2,8,16].

Induction Molecules

Chemotherapy: taxanes more frequent, paclitaxel, docetaxel, among others. Targeted therapies, less frequent: inhibitors of mTOR, inhibitors of EGF [2,8].

Prevention

- Use products for care of the nail, such as hardeners, liquid bandages, among others
- Use wide footwear
- Adequate hygiene with antiseptics

Treatment

- Antibiotic creams (nystatin, mupirocin) and oral tetracyclines to prevent and treat superinfections
- Topical corticosteroids to treat inflammation
- Electrocautery for granulomas [5,6,9]

General Recommendations

- Avoid using traditional nail varnishes:
  - Use hypoallergenic nail polish
- Cut the nails with caution to avoid injuries that can trigger infections
- Do not use false nails:
  - Use protective gloves, preferably made of cotton, to reduce the risk of infection [17]

Acneiform or Papulopustular Rash

This is a localized eruption on the face, trunk, and other areas rich in sebaceous glands, with papules and pustules associated with pain, itching, and discomfort. They are not comedogenic lesions and differ from acne due to their clinical and histopathological differences [9]. They affect more than 70% of patients treated with monoclonal antibodies and tyrosine kinase inhibitors. The impact on QoL is important and can be very disabling. This appears progressively at the beginning of treatment [2,5,8]. Its appearance is considered as a marker of efficacy of the treatment, and it disappears 4 weeks after the end of treatment, although it may leave sequelae such as postinflammatory hyperpigmentation, telangiectasias, and erythema.

According to the National Cancer Institute Common Terminology for Adverse Events (CTCAE) version 4.0, papulopustular eruptions are divided into five grades (Table 10.2) [9].

Induction Molecules

Targeted therapies: erlotinib, gefitinib, cetuximab, etc. [2,9].

Prevention

- Hygiene and intense hydration of the skin
- Photoprotection
- Some authors also recommend the use of prophylactic treatment, which should be initiated at the same time as the antineoplastic treatment, consisting of oral tetracyclines 100 mg twice daily, combined with low-potency topical corticosteroids, twice daily, on the face and trunk, between 6 and 8 weeks [9].

Treatment

The treatment of acneiform eruptions will be done according to the degree of severity at which the patient presents. Grade 1 can be treated successfully with Syndet-type cleansers, antiseptic soaps, and topical antibiotics (clindamycin 1%, erythromycin 3%, twice a day for 4 weeks), low-potency topical corticosteroids, twice a day, as well as the use of nonocclusive makeup to camouflage the lesions and scars, which should then be removed with nonirritating, nonalcoholic, hypoallergenic makeup removers. If there was no improvement and progress to grade 2, grade 1 measures would

TABLE 10.2

Grades of the Papulopustular Rash Reaction due to Epidermal Growth Factor Receptor Inhibitor

Grade 1	Papules and/or pustules covering less than 10% of the body surface area (BSA) with or without symptoms of pruritus or tenderness.
Grade 2	Papules and/or pustules covering 10%–30% of the BSA with or without symptoms of pruritus or tenderness; with psychosocial impact.
Grade 3	Papules and/or pustules covering greater than 30% of the BSA with or without symptoms of pruritus or tenderness; limiting self-care activities of daily living, associated with local superinfection with oral antibiotics indicated.
Grade 4	Covering any percentage of the BSA with or without symptoms of pruritus or tenderness; associated with extensive superinfection with intravenous antibiotics indicating life-threatening consequences.
Grade 5	Death.

Source: Adapted from Lupu I et al. *J Med Life*. 2015;8(Special Issue):57–61.

be used, and doxycycline 200 mg per day for 4–6 weeks would be added. If after 2 weeks, the patient has been refractory to treatment, we would face grade 3, in which the dose of the antineoplastic should be adjusted, allowing improvement to a degree 2, and oral corticosteroids should be administered (prednisone 0.5 mg/kg). If the progression continues, some authors have described the use of isotretinoin 20–30 mg/day as beneficial, with the aggravating factor that it worsens xerosis, for which moisturizers can be prescribed, and antihistamines for pruritus. If none of the measures described earlier provides good results, the dose reduction, interruption, or discontinuation of chemotherapy should be considered [9]. Acne products containing benzoyl peroxide, and topical retinoids such as tretinoin, adapalene, and tazarotene, should be avoided because they are very irritating, although there are studies that mention efficacy—albeit limited—against the rash [5,18]. The use of creams with 0.1% vitamin K1, twice a day, has shown evidence of improvement [18].

General Recommendations

- Use photoprotection
- Avoid the sun
- Avoid hot showers
- Use corrective makeup

Cutaneous Fissures

These are fissures of varying depth, due to cutaneous dryness, more frequently occurring in fingertips and heels. They are usually painful and can interfere with the patient's daily life. It is possible that they superinfect. They appear after several weeks of treatment [2].

Induction Molecules

Targeted therapies of the epidermal growth factor (EGF) receptor and mitogen-activated protein kinase kinase (MEK) (cetuximab, erlotinib, gefitinib, cobimetinib, etc.) and less frequently some chemotherapy [2,8].

Prevention

- Apply emollient and keratolytic cream daily in case of associated hyperkeratosis
- Avoid hot and prolonged baths
- Use antiseptic products [2]

Treatment

- Emollient creams
- Master formulas based on propylene glycol and salicylic acid
- Hydrocolloid dressings, prepared based on copper sulfate, zinc sulfate, and sucralfate
- Topical corticosteroids, provided there is no associated bacterial infection

- Liquid cyanoacrylate [2,9]

General Recommendations

- Use cotton gloves

Photosensibility

Greater sensitivity to sun exposure can result in serious skin burns. Hypersensitivity to light or photoallergy often affects both skin that has been exposed and skin that has not [2,8].

Induction Molecules

Chemotherapeutics (fluoracil, capecitabine, vinblastine, etc.) and targeted therapies (vandetanib, vemurafenib, etc.) [2,5,8]

Prevention and Treatment

- Photoprotection with very high protection factor

General Recommendations

- Avoid sun exposure
- Use wide-brimmed hats
- Use appropriate clothing

Hyperpigmentation

Increased coloration of the skin and mucous membranes can occur, especially in photoexposed areas. The hyperpigmentation of the skin and mucous membranes can be partial or generalized. The time of appearance is variable, depending on each patient and the sun exposure. It usually disappears with the cessation of treatment [2,8].

Induction Molecules

Chemotherapeutics: Capecitabine, 5-fluorouracil, liposomal doxorubicin, among others [2,8].

Prevention

- Use photoprotection with a very high protective factor
- Avoid sun exposure
- Use corrective makeup for sensitive skin

Treatment

If the hyperpigmentation does not disappear after finishing the treatment, when the skin is fully recovered, depigmenting creams can be initiated, as well as light therapies.

General Recommendations

- Wear wide-brimmed hats
- Wear loose clothing that protects as much skin as possible

Mucositis

Mucositis can affect the digestive tract from the mouth to the anus. It may consist of erythema or complete necrosis of the mucosa.; it appears from the first days after the first treatment cycle. Its clinical repercussions are very important, because it can significantly alter the nutritional status of the patient, making it difficult to eat, making it necessary to modify or interrupt treatment, if the mucositis is severe [2,8].

Induction Molecules

Chemotherapy and radiation therapy; occurs less with targeted therapies (inhibitors of EGF, inhibitors of ErB, inhibitors of mTOR).

Prevention and Treatment

According to the scientific literature, the best methods of treatment and/or prevention of oral mucositis are laser therapies, cryotherapy, antimicrobial and antifungal agents, royal jelly, *Lactobacillus brevis* lozenges (lactobacillus with anti-inflammatory activity), zinc supplements, chlorhexidine and palifermin (a growth factor) human keratinocyte (KGF) produced by recombinant DNA technology in *Escherichia coli*, prepared oral glutamine 30 gr/day divided in three doses, and preparations based on hyaluronic acid as barrier products [6,17,19,20].

General Recommendations

- Soft diet
- Good oral hygiene
- Systemic analgesics
- Increased fluid intake
- Avoidance of hot, acidic, or spicy foods

Radiodermatitis

Radiodermatitis is the damage to superficial cells and blood vessels of the skin by the direct action of RT. Cutaneous exposure to ionizing radiation can cause some alterations of a reversible nature (hair removal, erythema, pruritus, burning sensation, pain, desquamation, suppression of sebaceous glands, abnormalities of pigmentation) and some that are irreversible (acute and chronic radiodermatitis, induced neoplasms by radiation as basal cell carcinoma and squamous cell carcinoma) [5,16]. Acute radiodermatitis appears after the second week, with a feeling of tightness; hyperpigmentation, desquamation, painful blisters, and ulcers may appear and usually disappear after 2–3 months after the completion of RT [2,8], while chronic radiodermatitis appears after 90 days or more after the end of RT, causing scarring, hyperpigmentation, loss of skin adnexa, and epidermal and dermal atrophy [2,8].

Prevention

- Apply emollient moisturizers

Treatment

- Use repairers, such as rosehip oil, dexpanthenol, omega-3, omega-6, allantoin, *Centella asiatica*, calendula, niacinamide, vitamin F, among others
- Use syndet cleaners
- Apply emollient moisturizing dermocosmetics such as aloe vera, hyaluronic acid, urea, and so on, suitable for patients with altered skin
- Use topical anti-inflammatories such as α-bisabolol, vitamin E, calendula, shea butter, among others
- Use photoprotection

Depending on the severity, it may be necessary to use treatments such as follows:

- Corticosteroids, due to their anti-inflammatory effect as a vasoconstrictor and inhibitor of leukocyte chemotaxis. Studies have not shown a statistically significant efficacy in their use in prevention of the disease [16].
- Sucralfate in dressings, although its effectiveness has not been demonstrated.
- Antibiotics in cream, when there is risk of infection.

General Recommendations

- Avoid sun exposure in the treated areas
- Use natural fabric clothes, such as cotton
- Avoid baths with very chlorinated water
- Do not use any cream 4 hours before exposure to ionizing radiation
- Avoid shaving or any other depilatory method

Hand-Foot Syndrome

Palmoplantar erythrodysesthesia manifests with tingling, swelling, and redness in the hands and/or feet. It can be one of the most severe side effects. It is most commonly associated with capecitabine and 5-fluorouracil derivatives. The early recognition of this DAE is very important, since it can progress rapidly to higher degrees of toxicity, with debilitating consequences [5]. It appears after two to three cycles of treatment and usually disappears 2–4 weeks after the end of treatment. It worsens without dermocosmetic treatment [2,8].

Induction Molecules

Chemotherapy (capecitabine, doxorubicin, etc.) and targeted therapies (sunitinib and sorafenib) [2,8].

Prevention

- Use extreme hydration with nourishing and repairing creams
- Avoid sun exposure

Treatment

The use of urea-based hydrating creams and salicylic acid-based ointments [5] as well as repairing emollients for hands and feet have been shown to be effective [6].

General Recommendations

- Use comfortable shoes
- Avoid irritating products
- Avoid activities that generate force or friction
- Use cold water jets on wrists and ankles:
    - Pay special attention to superficial cuts and chafing, in case of infection

Xerosis

Exaggerated dryness of the skin can be accompanied by desquamation, inflammation, pain, and pruritus. This is an adverse effect that affects more than 35% of patients. It can produce fissures and be superinfected with *Staphylococcus aureus* or with herpes simplex virus. It appears after the first month of treatment but improves with dermocosmetic treatment [2,8].

Induction Molecules

Chemotherapy, targeted therapies (erlotinib, gefitinib, cetuximab), and hormone therapy [2,8].

Prevention

- Use syndet cleansers
- Apply moisturizers and repairers
- Use photoprotection

Treatment

- Moisturizing creams based on emollients such as urea at 5%–10% are recommended; some studies also recommend the use of moisturizers with niacinamide [5]. These allow the hydrolipidic mantle of the stratum corneum to be reconstructed and thus avoid the loss of transepidermal water; they also provide natural hydration factors with a protective function [17].
- The use of antiseptics is also recommended to prevent infections.
- Antihistamines are indicated to improve pruritus.
- Low-potency topical corticosteroids can be used if eczema appears.
- Topical or oral antibiotics can be used in cases of superinfection [9].

General Recommendations

- Use clothes made of natural fabrics, such as cotton
- Shower with warm water:
    - Avoid scratching to minimize the risks of infection

Induced Cutaneous Tumors

Antineoplastic therapies can induce the appearance of secondary skin tumors, with a higher risk in this group than in the general population. It is not a very frequent situation, but melanomas, induced nevi, epidermoid carcinomas, basal cell carcinomas, keratoacanthomas, papillomas, among others, could be developed [2].

Induction Molecules

Targeted therapies, inhibitors of RAF proteins (vemurafenib, dabrafenib, sorafenib, etc.), and some chemotherapeutics [2].

Prevention

- Periodic dermatological monitoring throughout life, especially if the patient suffered from cancer in childhood
- Continuous use of broad-spectrum sun protection

Treatment

- Complete excision with safety margins

After neoplastic therapies, efforts will be aimed at repairing skin that has been injured with the objectives of normalizing the patient's appearance, thus improving acceptance of the patient's self-image, improving recovery of social and interpersonal relationships, providing greater self-confidence, improving self-esteem, and in general improving QoL [1]. To achieve these objectives, we can use dermocosmetic and corrective makeup products and minimally invasive medical-aesthetic procedures, especially those designed to deeply hydrate the skin, to improve hyperpigmentation and telangiectasias that had appeared, and to recover the quality of the hair. Treatments with thermal waters are also indicated for their soothing, repairing, anti-irritant, antioxidant, healing, antipruritic, and decongestant properties [1].

Conclusions

The DAEs of antineoplastic therapies cause a significant impact on the lives of this group of patients, physically, emotionally, and psychosocially, negatively affecting the QoL of the patient and the treatment, since sometimes it will be necessary to reduce the dose or interrupt the therapy; that is why we must put more emphasis on prevention and treatment of DAEs, involving the different health professionals who will be in contact with these patients during the evolution of their disease.

To reduce these DAEs, it is also necessary to educate patients (and not only health professionals), through general care courses and workshops, dermocosmetic and corrective makeup, which allows them to improve their appearance and self-esteem, resulting in an improvement in the QoL and adherence to antineoplastic therapies.

The dermocosmetic care of the oncological patient is an indispensable strategy for the management and prevention of the DAEs. As it has been observed, the prevention of the same and the treatment is done initially with non-pharmacological products, postponing the use of drug for progression to more severe degrees. The non-use of dermocosmetic products, in cases such as xerosis, hand-foot syndrome, and hyperpigmentation increases the progression of these DAEs.

More studies are needed to test the dermocosmetic products in populations with damaged and sensitive skin.

Registered guidelines for prevention and treatment of these DAEs should be implemented.

REFERENCES

1. Prieto, L. "La importancia de la dermocosmética para los pacientes oncológicos". *Master en calidad de vida y cuidados médico estético del paciente oncológico*. La Roche Posay, Madrid, España. Julio 2017.

2. Sibaud V, Delord JP, Robert C. *"Dermatología de los tratamientos contra el cáncer. Guía práctica"*. Toulouse: Editions Privat, 2015.

3. Charalambous A. "Living with the Effects of Cutaneous Toxicities Induced by Treatment". *Asia-Pacific Journal of Oncology Nursing*. July-September 2017;4(3):220–3.

4. Hernández A, Zarzuelo A, Sánchez A. "Cuidados de la piel del paciente oncológico". *Farma Journal*. 2017;2(2):127–37.

5. Bensadoun RJ, Humbert P, Krutmann J, Luger T, Triller R, Rougier A. "Daily baseline skin care in the prevention, treatment, and supportive care of skin toxicity in oncology patients: Recommendations from a multinational expert panel". *Cancer Management and Research*. 2013;27:401–8.

6. Dreno B, Bensadoun RJ, Humbert P et al. "Algorithm for dermocosmetic use in the management of cutaneous side-effects associated with targeted therapy in Oncology". *J Eur Acad Dermatol Venereol*. 2013;27:1071–80.

7. Mota Antigua SK, Almonte Medina GM. "Dermocosmética para paciente Oncológico". *XI Jornadas de medicina estética de la AMECLM*. Toledo, España, 2018.

8. Seskimo Group. Grupo español para el cuidado de la piel en oncología. "La importancia del cuidado de tu piel". La Roche Posay.

9. Lupu I, Voiculescu VM, Bacalbasa N et al. "Cutaneous adverse reactions specific to epidermal growth factor receptor inhibitors". *J Med Life*. 2015;8(Special Issue):57–61.

10. U.S. Food & Drug Administration. Silver Spring, MD: FDA 2017. Last updated 03/28/2018. News and events (2–3 screens). https://www.fda.gov/NewsEvents/Newsroom/PressAnnouncements/ucm565599.htm

11. Shin H, Jo SJ, Kim DH, Kwon O, Myung SK. "Efficacy of interventions for prevention of chemotherapy – induced Alopecia: A systematuc review and meta-analysis". *Int J Cancer*. 2015; 136:E442–454.

12. Nagia J, Wang T, Osborne C et al. "Effect of a Scalp Cooling Device on Alopecia in Women Undergoing Chemotherapy for Breast Cancer: The Scalp Randomoized Clinical Trial. *JAMA*. 2017;317(6):596–605.

13. Cigler T, Isseroff D, Fiederlein B, Schneider S, Chuang E, Vahdat L. "Efficacy of Scalp Cooling in Preventing Chemotherapy Induced Alopecia in Breast Cancer Patients receiving adjuvant docetaxel, and cyclophosphamide chemotherapy." *Clin Breast Cancer*. 2015;15(5):332–4.

14. Rugo HS, Klein P, Melin SA et al. "Association Between Use of a Scalp Cooling Device and Alopecia After Chemotherapy for Breast Cancer. *JAMA*. 2017;317(6):606–14.

15. Vasconcelos I, Wiesske A, Schoenegg W. "Scalp cooling successfully prevents alopecia in breast cancer patients undergoing anthracycline/taxane based chemotherapy". *Breast*. 2018;40:1–3.

16. Barco D, Puig L, Vilarrasa E, López-Ferrer A, Ruiz V. "La Piel del paciente oncológico". *Farmacia Profesional*. 2009;23(6):52–5.

17. Bonet R, Garrote A. "Cuidados dermatológicos del paciente oncológico". *Farmacia Profesional*. 2016;30(2):12–4.

18. Kozuki T, "Skin problems and EGFR-tyrosine kinase inhibitor". *Jpn J Clin Oncol*. 2016;46(4):291–8.

19. Daugelaite G, Uzkuraityte K, Jagelaviciene E, Filipauskas A. "Prevention and treatment of chemotherapy and radiotherapy induced oral Mucositis". *Medicina (Kaunas)*. 2019 Jan 22;55(2).

20. Sayles C, Hickerson SC, Bhat RR, Hall J, Garey KW, Trivedi MV. "Oral glutamine in preventing treatment-related Mucositis in adult patients with cancer: A systematic review". *Nutr Clin Pract*. 2016;31(2):171–9.

11

Prevention and Treatment of Adverse Effects of Antineoplastic Therapy and of Delayed-Onset Side Effects: Prevention and Treatment of Hair Loss

Emma Iglesias Candal

Hair loss associated with antineoplastic therapies is one of the most shocking aspects of treatment for oncological patients, but the impact is commonly underestimated by physicians. Hair loss makes the disease visible for everyone, and this fact can create discomfort and insecurity in the patient. Additionally, it negatively impacts on body image, sexuality, and self-esteem. The influence of these different reasons means that up to 8% of patients decide to refuse chemotherapy if there is a risk of hair loss [1–3].

Of all the antineoplastic therapies, chemotherapy presents the greatest risk of associated alopecia, with an average of 60%–70%. However, the incidence and posttreatment recovery are conditioned by the type of drugs used, administration intervals, duration of treatment, age of the patient, and previous condition of hair: with antimicrotubule agents, alopecia is reported with more than 80% incidence; with alkylators, around 60%; with antimetabolites, the range is very wide (10%–50%). The combination of different agents is associated with a higher incidence compared to monotherapy; for example, the combination of anthracycline, cyclophosphamide, and doxorubicin has a 98% risk of complete alopecia [4–6].

Chemotherapy-induced alopecia (CIA) is a common and stressful adverse effect for cancer patients who undergo chemotherapy. When it occurs, it usually begins 1–3 weeks after the first cycle of chemotherapy and gets worse with the following cycles [7,8]. Fortunately, in most cases, there is usually a spontaneous recovery of lost hair after about 3–6 months from the end of chemotherapy treatment. However, a not insignificant percentage of patients suffer from definitive alopecia, and many suffer changes in their hair related to color, texture, and speed of hair growth for a long time after the end of treatment [9–11].

The first attempts to reduce the adverse effects of chemotherapy on hair were carried out in the 1970s. The idea was to reduce cytostatic exposure of the hair follicles through mechanical methods like the use of tourniquets or by the use of cold with ice caps. These first attempts had no success [12,13]. After these, there were different pharmacological methods to reduce CIA; the use of minoxidil in topical application was shown to be ineffective in prevention but can reduce the time to complete hair regrowth [14–16]; the use of vitamins like D_3 had shown preventive effect in hair loss in animal models, but not in humans [17,18].

More recently, the technique of scalp cooling has shown promising results in the prevention of hair loss in patients who received chemotherapy. The mechanism of action of cold therapy has been explained through two theories: first, by vasoconstriction, which generates less blood flow in the follicles during the infusion of chemotherapy and therefore interrupts the arrival of cytotoxic agents to the hair follicle; and second, by reducing biochemical activity, the follicles are presented with less cold biochemical activity that makes them less susceptible to damage by chemotherapeutic agents [19,20]. However, despite its promising success rate, there are few hospitals offering this procedure [19].

DigniCap scalp cooling system was the first system of scalp cooling to obtain U.S. Food and Drug Administration (FDA) approval (in 2015) for use in stages I and II breast cancer patients receiving chemotherapy that may cause significant alopecia. Since then, the Paxman Scalp Cooling System has been FDA approved for the same application, and DigniCap was approved for prevention of alopecia in patients receiving chemotherapy for other solid tumors [19,21–23] (Figure 11.1).

The scalp cooling systems consist of a refrigerator unit and a control unit; depending on the type of system, one or two cooling caps are connected, the second option allowing two patients to be treated at the same time. The cap consists of two layers: the inner layer is made of silicone, and its smooth surface allows snug fitting and optimal contact between the cap and the patient's scalp. The canals in the silicone cap are divided into two separate circuits, one for the forehead and one for the back of the head. Liquid coolant is pumped through the tubes, which run to the cap. The outer cap is made of neoprene that functions as an insulator. The system allows a gradual reduction from room temperature to the desired temperature. Deviations from the set temperature are detected and adjusted by the system (Figure 11.2).

Scalp temperature can be controlled with an accuracy of ±2°C. Scalp cooling is usually initiated 30 minutes before the administration of chemotherapy and is maintained at 5°C throughout the session and after chemotherapy. The duration of postchemotherapy cooling time differed according to the chemotherapy regimen used [19].

The most common reason for discontinuing scalp cooling was intolerable side effects. The side effects reported in scientific articles were headaches, cold sensation in the scalp, and vomiting [19,23].

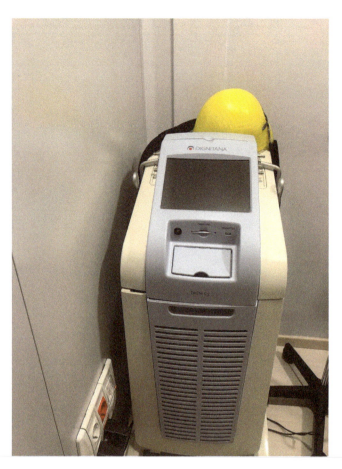

FIGURE 11.1 DigniCap system (by courtesy of Dr. Victoria Zamorano, clinician, Roman Oncology Clinic).

One concern about using scalp cooling to prevent CIA is the possibility of an increased risk of developing scalp metastasis due to decreased chemotherapeutic drug perfusion in the scalp caused by reduced blood flow. However, recent reviews and meta-analyses have found that scalp cooling did not increase the incidence of scalp metastasis [19,23–25].

Several types of biological therapies, especially immunotherapies, are being used or developed for cancer treatment. Many of these therapies are associated with dermatological complications; there may be change in the appearance of the hair (curly, brittle, depigmented hair). Alopecia is much more moderate than with conventional chemotherapy [26,27].

In the case of radiotherapy, it is important to remember that the hair follicles are radiosensitive, especially when they are in the anagen phase [28]. Radiation damage can be observed as early as the fourth day of treatment. It produces anagenic effluvium (loss of dystrophic hairs) due to damage in the cellular mitosis activity of the matrix cells. This is followed by a telogenic effluvium due to the premature passage from the late anagen to the catagen phase. Alopecia associated with loss of sebaceous and sweat glands in irradiated sites is a dose-dependent phenomenon that can be temporary or irreversible but is generally limited to the area of application [28–30].

If more than 1000 cGy was administered (as a total dose), alopecia is observed in the area. The doses used for the treatment of intracranial malignancies are usually high and produce definitive destruction of the hair follicles. There is consensus to affirm that the integral dose of about 5000–6000 cGy, fractionated in a daily dose of 200 to 500 cGy, produces permanent alopecia. However, it is important to consider variables such as radiotherapy modality, sites to radiate, radiant focus distance to skin, among others. Cases of temporary alopecia have been reported after radiological or angiographic studies of the skull and neck for diagnostic purposes [28,31].

There have been trials with some prevention measures: the use of tempol, vitamin D_3, and prostaglandins E2. It is believed that they would have a protective effect against radiotherapy-induced alopecia. However, there are still no totally effective methods to prevent alopecia by radiation [29,32]. In all patients, it is very important to ensure strict photoprotection of the hairless area by means of caps, handkerchiefs, and/or sunscreen products. In cases of permanent alopecia, reconstructive surgery or hair transplantation may be used in selected patients.

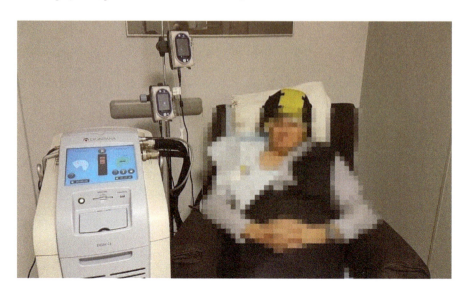

FIGURE 11.2 DigniCap system in use with a male patient receiving chemotherapy for prostate cancer (by courtesy of Dr. Victoria Zamorano, clinician, Roman Oncology Clinic).

We must continue to study alternatives for the prevention of hair loss associated with antineoplastic treatments. Although it has been downplayed by many oncologists and medical professionals, it has serious psychological consequences for patients who have it.

REFERENCES

1. Rosman S. Cancer and stigma: Experience of patients with chemotherapy-induced alopecia. *Patient Educ Couns.* 2004; 52: 333–9.
2. Helms RL, ÓHea EL, Corso M. Body image issues in women with breast cáncer. *Psychol Health Med.* 2008; 13: 313–25.
3. Lemieux J, Manunsell E, Provencher L. Chemotherapy induced alopecia and effects on quality of life among women with breast cáncer. *Psychooncology.* 2008; 17: 317–28.
4. Trueb RM. Chemotherapy-induced alopecia. *Curr Opin Support Palliat Care* 2010; 4(4): 281–4.
5. Breed W, van der Hurk CJG, Peerboms M. Presentation, impact and prevention of chemotherapy-induced hairloss. *Experts Rev Dermatol.* 2011; 6 (1): 109–25.
6. Paus R, Haslam IS, Sharov AA, Botchkarev VA. Pathobiology of chemotherapy-induced hair loss. *Lancet Oncol.* 2013; 14(2): e50–59.
7. Rossi A, Fortuna MC, Caro G, Pranteda G, Garelli V, Pompili U, Carlesimo M. Chemotherapy-induced alopecia management: Clinical experience and practical advice. *J Cosmet Dermatol.* 2017; 16 (4): 537–41.
8. Roe H. Chemotherapy induced alopecia: Advice and support for hair loss. *Br J Nurs.* 2011; 20(10): S4–11.
9. Kim IR, Cho J, Choi EK et al. Perception, attitudes, preparedness an experience of chemotherapy-induced alopecia, among breast cancer patients, a qualitative study. *Asia Pac J of Cancer Prev* 2012; 13(14), 1383–8.
10. Batchelor D. Hair and cancer chemotherapy: Consequences and nursing care – A literature study. *Eur J Cancer Care.* 2001:10: 47–63.
11. Wang H, Lu Z, Au JL. Protection against chemotherapy-induced alopecia. *Pharm Res.* 2006; 23: 2505–14.
12. Hyoseung S, Seon JJ, Do HK, Ohsang K, Seung KM. Efficacy of interventions for prevention of chemotherapy induced alopecia: A systematic review and meta-analysis. *Int J Cancer.* 2015; 136: E442– 54.
13. Maxwell MB. Scalp tourniquets for chemotherapy-induced alopecia. *Am J Nurs.* 1980, 80: 900–3.
14. Rodriguez R, Machiavelli M, Leone B et al. Minoxidil s a prophylaxis of doxorubicin-induced alopecia. *Ann Oncol.* 1994;5: 769–70.
15. Duvic M, Lemak NA, Valero V et al. A randomized trial of minoxidil in chemotherapy-induced alopecia. *J Am Acad Dermatol.* 1996; 35: 74–8.
16. Granai CO, Frederickson H, Gajewski W et al. The use of minoxidil to attempt to prevent alopecia during chemotherapy for gynecologic malignancies. *Eur J Gynaecol Oncol.* 1991; 12: 129–32.
17. Jimenez JJ, Joaquin J, Yunis AA. Protection from chemotherapy-induced alopecia 1,25 Dihydroxyvitamin D3. *Cancer Res.* 1992; 52 (18): 5123–5.
18. Jimenez JJ, Yuniss AA. Vitamin D3 and chemotherapy induced alopecia. *Nutrition.* 1996; 12 (6): 448–9.
19. Saad M, Chong FLT, Bustam AZ, Ho GF, Malik RA, Ishak WZW, Ee Phua VC, Yusof MM, Yan NY, Alip A. The efficacy ad tolerability of scalp cooling in preventin chemotherapy-induced alopecia in patients with breast cáncer receiving anthracycline and taxane-based chemotherapy in an Asian setting. *Indian J Cancer.* 2018; 55(2) 157–61.
20. Kato MS, Imai R, Kobayashi T. Evaluation of DigniCap system for the prevention of chemotherapy-induced hair loss in breast cancer patient. *Breast.* 2011;20:S80.
21. Rugo HS, Voigt J. Scalp hypothermia for preventing alopecia during chemotherapy. A systematic review and meta-analysis of randomized controlled trials. *Clin Breast Cancer.* 2017;18(1). pii: S1526-8209(16)30543-2.
22. Auvinen PK, Mähönen UA, Soininen KM et al. The effectiveness of a scalp cooling cap in preventing chemotherapy-induced alopecia. *Tumori.* 2010;96:271–5.
23. Food and Drug Administration. Medical devices, general and plastic surgery devices; classification of the scalp cooling system to reduce the Likekihood of chemotherapy-induced Alopecia. *Federal Registe* 2016; 81: 7452–4.
24. Cigler T, Isseroff D, Fiederlein B et al. Efficacy of scalp cooling in preventing chemotherapy-induced alopecia in breast cancer patients receiving adjuvant Docetaxel and cyclophosphamide chemotherapy. *Clin Breast Cancer.* 2015;15:332–4.
25. Christodoulou C, Klouvas G, Efstathiou E et al. Effectiveness of the MSC cold cap system in the prevention of chemotherapy-induced alopecia. *Oncology.* 2002;62:97–102.
26. Belum VR, Marulanda K, Ensslin C et al. Alopecia in patients treated with molecurlaly targeted anticancer therapies. *Ann Oncol.* 2015; 26 (12): 2496–502.
27. Lacouture ME. Mechanisms of cutaneous toxicites to EGFR inhibitors. *Nat Rev Cancer.* 2006; 6 (10): 803–12.
28. Paus R, Cotsarelis G. The biology of hair follicles. *New Engl J Med* 1999;341:491–7
29. Ward JF. DNA damage produced by ionizing radiation in mammalian cells: Identities, mechanisms of formation and reparability. *Prog Nucleic Acid Res Mol Biol.* 1988; 35: 95–125.
30. Wen CS, Lin SM, Chen Y, Chen JC, Wang YH, Tseng SH. Radiation-induced temporary alopecia after embolization of cerebral arteriovenous malformations. *Clin Neurosurg.* 2003;105:215–7.
31. Deng Z, Lei X, Zhang X et al. mTOR signaling promotes stem cell activation via counterbalancing BMP mediated suppression during hair regeneration. *J Mol Cell Biol* 2015;7:62–72.
32. Greco V, Chen T, Rendl M et al. A two-step mechanism for stem cell activation during hair regeneration. *Cell Stem Cell.* 2009;4:155–69.

12

Melatonin for Prevention and Treatment of Complications Associated with Chemotherapy and Radiotherapy: Implications for Cancer Stem Cell Differentiation

Germaine Escames, Ana Guerra-Librero, Dario Acuña-Castroviejo, Javier Florido, Laura Martinez-Ruiz, Cesar Rodríguez-Santana, Beatriz I Fernandez-Gil, and Iryna Russanova

Introduction

Drug resistance and relapse are the principal limitations of clinical oncology for many patients. Following the failure of conventional treatments, drug resistance can be an extremely demoralizing experience. It has therefore become crucial to find new therapeutic targets and drugs to enhance the cytotoxic effects of conventional treatments without potentiating or offsetting their adverse effects.

For decades, scientists have been attempting to determine how cancers progress in order to develop more effective and accurate therapeutic strategies. One target of research has been cancer stem cells (CSCs), which, like normal stem cells, have a self-renewal capacity [1]. Studies carried out over the last 10 years have greatly advanced our understanding of the molecular pathogenesis of cancer. CSCs have been demonstrated to be the basis of resistance to conventional treatments, resulting in tumor recurrence and poor prognoses. In this context, the development of novel CSC eradication techniques to inhibit tumor recurrence is regarded as a major challenge in the field of cancer treatment. Novel compounds specifically designed to eliminate CSCs or to affect their microenvironment, combined with conventional chemo- and radiotherapy, can lead to tumor bulk shrinkage and, subsequently, ablate resistance and relapse [2].

Cancer Stem Cells: Special Features

CSCs, caused by oncogenic processes, initiate the formation of tumors and metastases [2,3]. CSCs: (i) initiate malignant tumors and promote neoplastic proliferation [4]; (ii) recreate the heterogeneous phenotype of the originating tumor through asymmetric cell division [5]; (iii) have a capacity for self-reconstruction via symmetric cell division [5]; (iv) are generally slow or nondividing cells and thus are relatively resistant to radio- and chemotherapy [6]; and (v), unlike the bulk tumor population, express a distinct repertoire of biomarkers, which can be used for CSC definition and isolation [7] (Figure 12.1).

The phenotypic diversity of tumor cells and their metastases derive from CSCs [8]. A CSC is assumed to fully regenerate the tumor from which it has been extracted [9,10]. However, like physiological tissues, cancers are composed of heterogeneous cell populations [11] that exhibit different morphological and functional phenotypes [11,12]. The tumor itself consists of at least two subpopulations: (i) a small population of CSCs and (ii) a mass population of non-self-renewing cancer cells. The self-renewing properties of these CSCs are thus the true driving force behind tumor growth. Additional testing of this model has shown that the selective removal of CSCs can stop tumor growth [13]. In fact, in the presence of CSCs that can reactivate tumor growth, conventional treatments, such as chemo- and radiotherapy, which only affect differentiated cells, are ineffective.

Origin of Cancer Stem Cells

CSCs, also known as tumor-initiating cells (TICs), like normal tissue stem cells (TSCs), have a proliferation, differentiation, and self-renewal capacity [14–16]. Although CSCs are widely believed to play a critical role in cancer initiation, metastasis, and relapse, their origin remains unclear [17] and is the subject of much debate. Many researchers have not yet determined whether CSCs are directly descended from mutated stem cells or more mature cells that take on the properties of stem cells during tumorigenesis [18,19].

Response of Cancer Stem Cells to Radio- and Chemotherapy

The prognosis for patients diagnosed with recurrent or metastatic diseases is poor [20]. In these cases, apart from treatment with antibodies, chemotherapy remains the only systemic treatment option, which, where possible, is combined with surgery and radiation. Clinically, the use of radiation and high doses of chemotherapy often results in a good initial tumor response. However, recurrences in patients who do not respond to subsequent treatment are frequent, and the presence of CSCs could be the cause. In recent years, researchers have, for the first time, investigated the therapeutic resistance of CSCs [21,22]. In this research, cell surface markers were used to identify and purify CSCs from tumors. The CSC fraction was found to be enriched

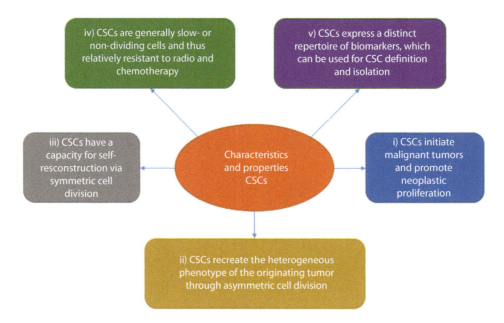

FIGURE 12.1   Characteristics of cancer stem cells.

in the tumor samples and cultures of cancer cells following treatment with radiation or chemotherapeutic drugs. Therefore, it was demonstrated that CSCs are particularly resistant to radio- and chemotherapy and, consequently, contribute to treatment failure. Thus, CSCs may represent a new target for therapeutic treatment [22–25]. Chemo- and radioresistance of CSCs have been investigated in numerous experimental models. In acute leukemia, CSCs show increased resistance to the chemotherapeutic drug daunorubicin [26]. CSCs from glioblastoma are also resistant to radiation and chemotherapy [23,27], which is in line with the resistance to chemotherapy observed in glioblastoma stem cells isolated from tumor xenografts [28,29]. Although the mechanisms underlying this resistance remain unclear, some studies have demonstrated that stem cells derived from brain tumors render apoptosis-related proteins resistant by altering their expression. A strong response to DNA damage and increased repair capacity are also responsible for this resistance. In addition, there is evidence of resistance associated with CSCs in other cancers such as breast cancer [30]. Similarly, CSCs derived from pancreatic tissue are highly resistant to chemotherapy [31], as well as those isolated from human hepatocellular carcinoma (HCC) cells, and colon cancer [32].

The mechanisms underlying this resistance have not been fully elucidated. Despite their ability to form certain types of tumors reported in several studies [33], little is known about the role of CSCs in tumoral chemo- and radioresistance. However, according to previous studies, clinical observations, and experimental evidence, it seems that increased resistance, potential recurrences, and metastases could be due to the resistance of CSCs to therapy.

Role of Oxidative Stress in Cancer Stem Cells

Reactive oxygen species (ROS) are powerful signaling molecules involved in the regulation of a variety of biological processes. Cancer cells have higher levels of ROS than their normal counterparts, which is partly due to their enhanced metabolism and mitochondrial dysfunction. However, the decrease in ROS generation in cancer cells increases tumor resistance to radio- and chemotherapy [34]. Thus, higher levels of ROS in cancer cells may provide a unique opportunity for their elimination by elevating ROS to highly toxic intracellular levels. This can activate various ROS-induced cell death pathways, inhibit cancer cell resistance to chemotherapy, and promote cell differentiation. These outcomes can be achieved through the use of agents to increase ROS generation or to inhibit antioxidant defenses or a combination of both [35].

Melatonin Cancer Treatment

Melatonin (*N*-acetyl-5-methoxytryptamine; aMT), a derivative of serotonin (5-hydroxytryptamine), was initially isolated from bovine pineal tissue [36]. For a number of years after its discovery by Lerner in 1958, melatonin, which regulates circadian and circannual rhythms, was considered to be produced exclusively in the pineal gland [37]. Following the identification of melatonin synthesis in the pineal gland, melatonin-related enzymes were found to be present in the retina and cerebellum [38,39] and were subsequently identified in many other peripheral tissues and organs [37]. Melatonin is also found in a very wide and diverse range of biological systems, ranging from single cells to highly complex human organisms [40]. Chronobiologists have traditionally regarded melatonin as a hormone that only regulates circadian day-night rhythms and seasonal biorhythms [41]. However, melatonin also performs functions that enable organisms to be protected against environmental changes. In addition, depending, for the most part, on its cellular redox state and inflammatory status, melatonin genomically regulates the expression of genes such as glutathione peroxidase (GPx), glutathione reductase (GRd), superoxide dismutase (SOD), inducible nitric oxide synthase (iNOS), and cytokines [42]. It is also a chemotoxicity-reducing agent, a putative anti-aging substance, and an anticancer agent, as well as an essential regulator of mitochondrial function.

Synthesis and Metabolism of Melatonin

The synthesis of melatonin begins with the hydroxylation of tryptophan to 5-hydroxy-tryptophan (5HTP) by tryptophan-5-hydroxylase (TPOH). This product is subsequently decarboxylated to 5-hydroxy-L-tryptamine (serotonin or 5-HT) under the catalytic action of aromatic amino acid decarboxylase (AADC). Serotonin is then acetylated to *N*-acetylserotonin by arylalkylamine *N*-acetyltransferase (AANAT). Finally, *N*-acetylserotonin is methylated to melatonin by hydroxyindole-O-methyl transferase (HIOMT), now known as *N*-acetyl-serotonin methyltransferase (ASMT) [43], which is a melatonin synthesis rate-limiting enzyme inhibited by light [44]. Therefore, melatonin concentrations in serum, mainly originating from the pineal gland, follow a circadian pattern.

In mammals, melatonin is metabolized either in the liver or directly at its site of production. Circulating melatonin in the liver is first hydroxylated by cytochrome P-450 monooxygenases and then conjugated with sulfate to form 6-sulfatoxymelatonin, which is excreted in the urine [45]. The three main metabolic pathways of melatonin (indolic, kynuric, and P450-dependent) involve both enzymatic and nonenzymatic reactions caused by free radicals [46]. Melatonin, which scavenges these free radicals, produces metabolites such as N^1-acetyl-N^2-formyl-5-methoxykynuramine (AFMK) and N^1-acetyl-5-methoxykynuramine (AMK), which also protect against oxidative stress.

Mechanism of Action of Melatonin

Melatonin can pass through the cellular, mitochondrial, and nuclear membranes and perform multiple functions in several cellular compartments. Studies of its distribution in different organelles have revealed that more melatonin accumulates in the cell's nucleus and mitochondria than in the cytosol [47].

Two groups of melatonin receptors have been identified and characterized: membrane receptors and nuclear receptors [48]. The membrane receptors, type 1 (MT1) and 2 (MT2), bind high-affinity melatonin [48] and, when activated, dissociate G proteins into α and $\beta\gamma$ dimmers, which interact with effector molecules involved in cellular signaling transmission [49]. Melatonin receptor type 3 (MT3), located in the cytosol of some cells, is not coupled to the G protein and exhibits low melatonin affinity [50]. Although melatonin interacts with a group of nuclear receptors to perform certain functions [51], its impact on mitochondria and its antioxidant effects are receptor independent.

Melatonin not only neutralizes and eliminates free radicals but also boosts cellular antioxidant enzyme production. Moreover, melatonin neutralizes free radicals in the mitochondria, which improves oxidative phosphorylation [52]. Unlike classical antioxidants, melatonin has no prooxidative activity, and the intermediates generated by its interaction with reactive species, such as AMK and AFMK, are also free radical scavengers. This reaction is referred to as a free radical scavenging cascade, which enables one melatonin molecule to potentially scavenge up to four or more reactive species [53].

Inflammasomes and inflammatory mediators are also targets of melatonin. The inflammasome complex contains proteins that regulate the release of interleukin-1β (IL-1β) and IL-18, as well as the activation of certain proapoptotic pathways [54]. Melatonin, an important antioxidant and widespread anti-inflammatory molecule, modulates both pro- and anti-inflammatory cytokines under different pathophysiological conditions. It is able to inhibit inflammasome following mitochondrial damage, leading to an attenuation of inflammatory cytokines.

Therefore, being an excellent antioxidant and anti-inflammatory molecule that protects cells against oxidative stress, melatonin can ameliorate and prevent damage caused by radiotherapy, as inflammatory responses and mitochondrial disruption after exposure to radiation are causes of chronic oxidative stress [54,55].

Mechanism of Melatonin Antitumor Action

Melatonin efficiently suppresses neoplastic growth in a variety of tumors and can be beneficial in the treatment of cancer patients. Numerous studies have shown that it has proven antiproliferative properties in a wide range of tumors [56–61], directly inhibits tumor cell proliferation and growth, and increases apoptotic cell death in several types of cancer cells while protecting normal cells against apoptosis. The possible mechanisms involved in melatonin oncostasis are its direct and indirect antioxidant impact, its regulation of metabolism, and its antiangiogenic and antimetastatic effects, as well as its capacity to reduce telomerase activity and to regulate the immune system. However, despite the involvement of virtually as many mechanisms as tumor types, the oncostatic impact of melatonin is difficult to explain. These mechanisms could be mere epiphenomena of an, as yet unknown, underlying fundamental mechanism caused by melatonin [50,62], whose oncostatic impact has not been analyzed in any clinical trials. Finally, its unexplored role in cancer treatments to reduce recurrence or resistance to oncotic therapies [63] highlights the importance of investigating the mechanisms involved in the oncostatic effects of melatonin and its ability to increase the cytotoxic impact of other tumor treatments.

Melatonin, Mitochondria, and Cancer Stem Cells

Given that mitochondria are well known to be the principal target of melatonin, some evidence points to (i) a direct relationship between oxidative stress in mitochondria and melatonin's potent antioxidant activity; (ii) the presence of a large amount of melatonin in these organelles; (iii) the existence of circadian/seasonal variations in mitochondrial structures and functions, suggesting that melatonin plays a physiological role in the modus operandi of mitochondria [64]; (iv) the major antiapoptotic impact of melatonin on normal cells given the mitochondrial origin of most apoptotic signals; and (v) the dependence of mitochondria on glutathione (GSH) uptake from the cytosol. Mitochondria also contain the antioxidant enzymes GPx and GRd which maintain the GSH redox cycle. This cycle is enhanced by melatonin, which also increases GSH content by stimulating its synthesis in the cytosol [65]. In addition, high levels of the indole have been identified in mitochondria as compared to other cellular compartments [64]. Thus, melatonin directly affects the physiological

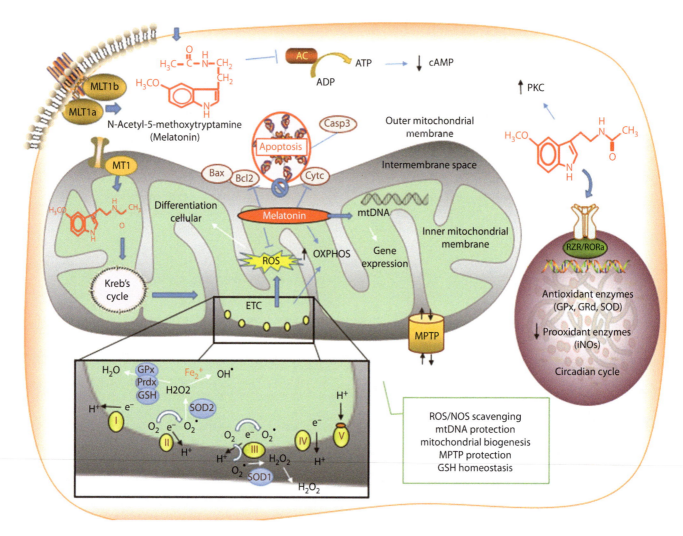

FIGURE 12.2 Melatonin's potential mechanisms in the cell. Melatonin interacts with cells in a receptor-dependent and receptor-independent manner. The MT1 (Mel 1a) and MT2 (Mel 1b) receptors on the cell membrane mediate a wide variety of mechanisms such as protein kinase C (PKC) activation and adenylate cyclase (AC) inhibition, which drives additional ATP production and a decrease in cyclic AMP (cAMP). Independently of the receptors, melatonin permeates cell membranes and scavenges reactive oxygen species (ROS) in the cell, cytoplasm, mitochondria, and nucleus. In the cytoplasm, melatonin maintains glutathione homeostasis and interacts with calmodulin and calreticulin proteins. Melatonin is also a ligand for nuclear retinoid related orphan nuclear hormone receptors (RZR/RORa), which regulate the expression of antioxidant enzymes, including glutathione peroxidase (GPx), glutathione reductase (GRd), and superoxide dismutase (SOD), and downregulate pro-oxidant enzymes, such as NOSs, particularly iNOS. Through interaction with the MT1 transporter, melatonin enters mitochondria, accumulates at high concentrations, directly scavenges ROS and reactive nitrogen species (RNS), stabilizes mitochondrial inner membranes, increases activity respiration (ETC), and plays an important role in cell differentiation. It also safeguards respiratory chain complexes and mtDNA against free radical damage, protects membrane permeability transition pores (MPTPs), and thus prevents cell apoptosis.

regulation and energy metabolism of mitochondria (Figure 12.2) and provides a novel homeostatic mechanism for regulating mitochondrial function.

Despite the known role played by mitochondria in stem cell differentiation, proliferation, and survival, the modus operandi of melatonin in cancer requires further research. Melatonin is well known to decrease cancer cell proliferation, self-renewal, and clonogenic capacity by reducing stem cell marker expression [66], although the mechanisms involved remain unclear. Considering its impact on mitochondrial physiology, it is also possible to hypothesize that melatonin affects stem cell mitochondria. Several studies have demonstrated that melatonin modulates the capacity of neuronal stem cells (NSCs) for their neuronal proliferation and differentiation in a time- and concentration-dependent manner [67–69]. Mendivil et al. have

reported that melatonin induces NSC differentiation in oligodendrocytes and mature neurons by enhancing mitochondrial respiration/membrane potential and by increasing mitochondrial mass-DNA complexes and ATP synthesis through an increase in mature neuron markers [69]. Other studies, which evaluated the effect of melatonin on hippocampal neurogenesis in adult mice, report an increase in new cell formation in the hippocampus [70]. According to the previously mentioned effect of melatonin on NSC proliferation, CSC differentiation and survival may be due to the role played by melatonin in mitochondrial dynamics, which requires further investigation in order to decipher the activities, specific molecular mechanisms, and possible targets of melatonin in cancer [69]. However, given that a number of relevant melatonin effects are triggered by targeting mitochondria, melatonin should be considered a pharmacological agent capable of modulating mitochondrial functions in cancer [56,61]. It is well known that the modulation of the mitochondrial respiratory chain by melatonin can disrupt the highly glycolytic bioenergetic pathway of cancer cells [71]. On the other hand, the depletion of ROS boosts CSC resistance to chemotherapy by decreasing toxic oxidized intermediates. Therefore, the restoration of normal ROS levels is associated with the loss of CSC-like properties and increased cisplatin sensitivity in HNSCC cells [72]. These findings point to the possibility that melatonin in CSCs acts as a mitochondrial agent that enhances oxygen consumption, generates ROS, and produces energy by maintaining and, in many cases, by increasing ATP production and mtDNA expression [73]. Inhibition of ROS-scavenging proteins such as SOD2 and catalase leads to an increase in ROS and, subsequently, in sensitivity to cisplatin [72].

Melatonin as an Adjuvant in the Treatment of Cancer

Melatonin has a number of properties that are not limited to an antitumor effect [74]. Melatonin has anxiolytic and antidepressant abilities that underline its possible application for depression and anxiety in cancer patients. Melatonin can be served as an effective adjuvant of chemotherapy and radiotherapy to increase the efficacy of treatment and decrease side effects. Taking melatonin as an adjuvant could effectively lower the threshold for chemotherapy or radiotherapy and protect normal tissues from being sensitized to the cytotoxicity of the therapies [55,74,75]. In most of the combination trials where melatonin was used in conjunction with therapeutic drugs, the presence of melatonin was found to prolong disease progression-free time and overall survival as well as improve patient suffering [76]. The concomitant administration of melatonin significantly reduces the frequency of thrombocytopenia, neurotoxicity, cardiotoxicity, stomatitis, and asthenia. Moreover, chemotherapy is better tolerated in patients treated with melatonin, and melatonin can enhance the immunological activities of patients [77].

Conclusions

Melatonin can provide an innovative adjuvant strategy in cancer by combining effects on the circadian rhythm with oncostatic and cytoprotective properties. As discussed, melatonin is effective in suppressing neoplastic growth in a variety of tumors. However, the mechanisms involved are not very clear. It is important to note that as mitochondria are regarded by the pharmaceutical industry as a potentially important drug delivery target, strategies based on mitochondrial damage prevention and mitochondrial function management may lead to the development of new cancer therapies [78,79].

Melatonin is an effective pharmacological tool in the treatment of mitochondria-related diseases. Unlike its impact on normal cancer cells, melatonin has a major effect on mitochondrial function in CSCs. This is due to the properties of melatonin, such as its ability to enter mitochondria, its regulation of redox state by increasing ROS levels, activating cell signaling pathways, and promoting cellular differentiation and mtDNA transcriptional capacity.

Besides these oncostatic properties, melatonin deserves to be considered in the treatment of cancer for two other reasons. First, because of its hypnotic-chronobiotic properties, melatonin use can allow the clinician to effectively address sleep disturbances, a major comorbidity in cancer. Indeed, as with many other diseases, evidence supports the hypothesis that metabolic rhythm attenuation and/or disruption contributes to the etiology of cancer. Second, because of melatonin's anxiolytic and antidepressant effects, it has a possible application in two other major comorbidities seen in cancer patients—that is, depression and anxiety.

Given these properties, melatonin can be regarded as a first-rate effective alternative therapeutic strategy in clinical trials [80].

Acknowledgments

We wish to thank Michael O'Shea for proofreading the chapter.

REFERENCES

1. Pakravan K, Amin Mahjoub M, Jahangiri B, Babashah S. Cancer stem cells: A quick walk through the concepts. In: Babashah S, ed. *Cancer Stem Cells: Emerging Concepts and Future Perspectives in Translational Oncology*. Cham, Switzerland: Springer, 2015: 3–12.
2. Medema JP. Cancer stem cells: The challenges ahead. *Nat Cell Biol*. 2013;15(4):338–44.
3. Valent P, Bonnet D, De Maria R et al. Cancer stem cell definitions and terminology: The devil is in the details. *Nat Rev Cancer England*; 2012;12(11):767–75.
4. Lobo NA, Shimono Y, Qian D, Clarke MF. The biology of cancer stem cells. *Annu Rev Cell Dev Biol*. 2007;23:675–99.
5. Morrison SJ, Kimble J. Asymmetric and symmetric stem-cell divisions in development and cancer. *Nature*. 2006;441(7097):1068–74.
6. Cortes-Dericks L, Carboni GL, Schmid RA, Karoubi G. Putative cancer stem cells in malignant pleural mesothelioma show resistance to cisplatin and pemetrexed. *Int J Oncol*. 2010;37(2):437–44.
7. Visvader JE, Lindeman GJ. Cancer stem cells in solid tumours: Accumulating evidence and unresolved questions. *Nat Rev Cancer*. 2008;8(10):755–68.
8. Baccelli I, Trumpp A. The evolving concept of cancer and metastasis stem cells. *J Cell Biol*. 2012;198(3):281–93.
9. Dalerba P, Cho RW, Clarke MF. Cancer stem cells: Models and concepts. *Annu Rev Med*. 2007;58:267–84.
10. Liu Y, Nenutil R, Appleyard M V et al. Lack of correlation of stem cell markers in breast cancer stem cells. *Br J Cancer*. 2014;110(8):2063–71.
11. Sun X, Yu Q. Intra-tumor heterogeneity of cancer cells and its implications for cancer treatment. *Acta Pharmacol Sin*. 2015;36(10):1219–27.
12. Hamburger AW, Salmon SE. Primary bioassay of human tumor stem cells. *Science (80-)*. 1977;197(4302):461–3.
13. Schatton T, Frank NY, Frank MH. Identification and targeting of cancer stem cells. *BioEssays*. 2009;31(10):1038–49.
14. Rawat N, Singh MK. Induced pluripotent stem cell: A headway in reprogramming with promising approach in regenerative biology. *Vet World*. 2017;10(6):640–9.

15. Reya T, Morrison SJ, Clarke MF, Weissman IL. Stem cells, cancer, and cancer stem cells. *Nature.* 2001;414(6859):105–11.
16. Weiner LP. Definitions and criteria for stem cells. *Methods Mol Biol.* 2008;438:3–8.
17. Bu Y, Cao D. The origin of cancer stem cells. *Front Biosci (Schol Ed).* 2012;4:819–30.
18. Regenbrecht CR, Lehrach H, Adjaye J. Stemming cancer: Functional genomics of cancer stem cells in solid tumors. *Stem Cell Rev.* 2008;4(4):319–28.
19. Rycaj K, Tang DG. Cell-of-origin of cancer versus cancer stem cells: Assays and interpretations. *Cancer Res.* 2015;75(19):4003–11.
20. Bozec A, Gros FX, Penault-Llorca F et al. Vertical VEGF targeting: A combination of ligand blockade with receptor tyrosine kinase inhibition. *Eur J Cancer.* 2008;44(13):1922–30.
21. Jia H, Li X, Gao H et al. High doses of nicotinamide prevent oxidative mitochondrial dysfunction in a cellular model and improve motor deficit in a Drosophila model of Parkinson's disease. *J Neurosci Res.* 2008;86(9):2083–90.
22. Krause M, Dubrovska A, Linge A, Baumann M. Cancer stem cells: Radioresistance, prediction of radiotherapy outcome and specific targets for combined treatments. *Adv Drug Deliv Rev.* 2017;109:63–73.
23. Bao S, Wu Q, McLendon RE et al. Glioma stem cells promote radioresistance by preferential activation of the DNA damage response. *Nature.* 2006;444(7120):756–60.
24. Kim JK, Jeon HY, Kim H. The molecular mechanisms underlying the therapeutic resistance of cancer stem cells. *Arch Pharm Res.* 2015;38(3):389–401.
25. Zhao J. Cancer stem cells and chemoresistance: The smartest survives the raid. *Pharmacol Ther.* 2016;160:145–58.
26. Morrison R, Schleicher SM, Sun Y et al. Targeting the mechanisms of resistance to chemotherapy and radiotherapy with the cancer stem cell hypothesis. *J Oncol.* 2011;2011:941876.
27. Ramirez YP, Weatherbee JL, Wheelhouse RT, Ross AH. Glioblastoma multiforme therapy and mechanisms of resistance. *Pharmaceuticals (Basel).* 2013;6(12):1475–506.
28. Eramo A, Ricci-Vitiani L, Zeuner A et al. Chemotherapy resistance of glioblastoma stem cells. *Cell Death Differ England.* 2006;13(7):1238–41.
29. Auffinger B, Spencer D, Pytel P, Ahmed AU, Lesniak MS. The role of glioma stem cells in chemotherapy resistance and glioblastoma multiforme recurrence. *Expert Rev Neurother.* 2015;15(7):741–52.
30. Kuo MT. Roles of multidrug resistance genes in breast cancer chemoresistance. *Adv Exp Med Biol.* 2007;608:23–30.
31. Whatcott CJ, Posner RG, Von Hoff DD, Han H. Desmoplasia and chemoresistance in pancreatic cancer. In: *Pancreatic Cancer and Tumor Microenvironment. Trivandrum (India): Transworld Research Network.* 2012.
32. Guo JF, Li K, Yu RL et al. Polygenic determinants of Parkinson's disease in a Chinese population. *Neurobiol Aging.* 2015;36(4):1765.e1-1765.e6.
33. Willers H, Azzoli CG, Santivasi WL, Xia F. Basic mechanisms of therapeutic resistance to radiation and chemotherapy in lung cancer. *Cancer J.* 2013;19(3):200–7.
34. Bigarella CL, Liang R, Ghaffari S. Stem cells and the impact of ROS signaling. *Development.* 2014;141(22):4206–18.
35. Galadari S, Rahman A, Pallichankandy S, Thayyullathil F. Reactive oxygen species and cancer paradox: To promote or to suppress? *Free Radic Biol Med.* 2017;104:144–64.
36. Lerner AB, Case JD, Heinzelman R V. Structure of melatonin. *J Am Chem Soc.* 1959;81(22):6084–5.
37. Acuña-Castroviejo D, Escames G, Venegas C et al. Extrapineal melatonin: Sources, regulation, and potential functions. *Cell Mol Life Sci.* 2014;71(16):2997–3025.
38. Cardinali DP, Rosner JM. Retinal Localization of the Hydroxyindole-O-methyl Transferase (HIOMT) in the Rat. *Endocrinology.* 1971;89(1):301–3.
39. Bubenik GA, Brown GM, Uhlir I, Grota LJ. Immunohistological localization of N-acetylindolealkylamines in pineal gland, retina and cerebellum. *Brain Res.* 1974;81(2):233–42.
40. Erren TC, Reiter RJ. Melatonin: A universal time messenger. *Neuro Endocrinol Lett.* 2015;36(3):187–92.
41. Bubenik GA, Smith PS, Schams D. The effect of orally administered melatonin on the seasonality of deer pelage exchange, antler development, LH, FSH, prolactin, testosterone, T3, T4, cortisol, and alkaline phosphatase. *J Pineal Res.* 1986;3(4):331–49.
42. Lopez A, Garcia JA, Escames G et al. Melatonin protects the mitochondria from oxidative damage reducing oxygen consumption, membrane potential, and superoxide anion production. *J Pineal Res.* 2009;46(2):188–98.
43. Axelrod J, Weissbach H. Enzymatic O-Methylation of N-Acetylserotonin to Melatonin. *Science.* 1960;131(3409):1312.
44. Wurtman RJ, Axelrod J, Phillips LS. Melatonin synthesis in the pineal gland: Control by light. *Science.* 1963;142(3595):1071–3.
45. Bojkowski CJ, Arendt J, Shih MC, Markey SP. Melatonin secretion in humans assessed by measuring its metabolite, 6–sulfatoxymelatonin. *Clin Chem.* 1987;33(8):1343–8.
46. Slominski A, Pisarchik A, Semak I, Sweatman T, Wortsman J. Characterization of the serotoninergic system in the C57BL/6 mouse skin. *Eur J Biochem.* 2003;270(16):3335–44.
47. Venegas C, Garcia JA, Escames G et al. Extrapineal melatonin: Analysis of its subcellular distribution and daily fluctuations. *J Pineal Res.* 2012;52(2):217–27.
48. Venegas C, García JA, Doerrier C et al. Analysis of the daily changes of melatonin receptors in the rat liver. *J Pineal Res.* 2013;54(3):313–21.
49. Dubocovich ML, Markowska M. Functional MT 1 and MT 2 melatonin receptors in mammals. *Endocrine.* 2005;27(2):101–10.
50. Reiter RJ, Tan DX, Galano A. Melatonin: Exceeding expectations. *Physiol.* 2014;29(5):325–33.
51. Acuña-Castroviejo D, Pablos MI, Menendez-Pelaez A, Reiter RJ. Melatonin receptors in purified cell nuclei of liver. *Res Commun Chem Pathol Pharmacol.* 1993;82(2):253–6.
52. Acuña-Castroviejo D, Carretero M, Doerrier C et al. Melatonin protects lung mitochondria from aging. *Age (Dordr).* 2012;34(3):681–92.
53. Tan D, Reiter RJ, Manchester LC et al. Chemical and physical properties and potential mechanisms: Melatonin as a broad spectrum antioxidant and free radical scavenger. *Curr Top Med Chem.* 2002;2(2):181–97.
54. Ortiz García F, Escames Rosa G, Doerrier Velasco C et al. Molecular basis of the radiotherapy-induced mucositis. Beneficial effects of melatonin. *Reports Pract Oncol Radiother.* 2013;18:S76.
55. Fernández-Gil B, Moneim AEA, Ortiz F et al. Melatonin protects rats from radiotherapy-induced small intestine toxicity. *PLOS ONE.* 2017;12:e0174474.

56. Fernandez-gil BI, Guerra-librero A, Shen Y et al. Melatonin enhances cisplatin and radiation cytotoxicity in head and neck squamous cell carcinoma by stimulating. *Oxid Med Cell Longev.* 2019;2019:1–12.

57. Blask DE, Sauer LA, Dauchy RT, Holowachuk EW, Ruhoff MS, Kopff HS. Melatonin inhibition of cancer growth *in vivo* involves suppression of tumor fatty acid metabolism via melatonin receptor-mediated signal transduction events. *Cancer Res.* 1999;59(18):4693–701.

58. Rodriguez C, Martín V, Herrera F et al. Mechanisms involved in the pro-apoptotic effect of melatonin in cancer cells. *Int J Mol Sci.* 2013;14(4):6597–613.

59. Hong Y, Won J, Lee Y, Lee S, Park K, Chang KT. Melatonin treatment induces interplay of apoptosis, autophagy, and senescence in human colorectal cancer cells. *J Pineal Res.* 2014;56(3):264–74.

60. Pariente R, Pariente JA, Rodriguez AB, Espino J. Melatonin sensitizes human cervical cancer HeLa cells to cisplatin-induced cytotoxicity and apoptosis: Effects on oxidative stress and DNA fragmentation. *J Pineal Res.* 2016;60(1):55–64.

61. Shen YQ, Guerra-Librero A, Fernandez-Gil BI et al. Combination of melatonin and rapamycin for head and neck cancer therapy: Suppression of AKT/mTOR pathway activation, and activation of mitophagy and apoptosis via mitochondrial function regulation. *J Pineal Res.* 2018;64(3):1–18.

62. Reiter RJ, Mayo JC, Tan DX, Sainz RM, Alatorre-Jimenez M, Qin L. Melatonin as an antioxidant: Under promises but over delivers. *J Pineal Res.* 2016;61(3):253–78.

63. Reiter RJ, Rosales-Corral SA, Tan DX et al. Melatonin, a full service anti-cancer agent: Inhibition of initiation, progression and metastasis. *Int J Mol Sci.* 2017;18(4).

64. Tan DX, Manchester LC, Qin L, Reiter RJ. Melatonin: A Mitochondrial Targeting Molecule Involving Mitochondrial Protection and Dynamics. *Int J Mol Sci.* 2016.

65. Acuna-Castroviejo D, Martin M, Macias M et al. Melatonin, mitochondria, and cellular bioenergetics. *J Pineal Res.* 2001;30(2):65–74.

66. Lee H, Lee HJ, Jung JH, Shin EA, Kim SH. Melatonin disturbs SUMOylation-mediated crosstalk between c-Myc and nestin via MT1 activation and promotes the sensitivity of paclitaxel in brain cancer stem cells. *J Pineal Res.* 2018;65(2):e12496.

67. Moriya T, Horie N, Mitome M, Shinohara K. Melatonin influences the proliferative and differentiative activity of neural stem cells. *J Pineal Res.* 2007;42(4):411–8.

68. Jenwitheesuk A, Boontem P, Wongchitrat P, Tocharus J, Mukda S, Govitrapong P. Melatonin regulates the aging mouse hippocampal homeostasis via the sirtuin1-FOXO1 pathway. *Excli J.* 2017;16:340–53.

69. Mendivil-Perez M, Soto-Mercado V, Guerra-Librero A et al. Melatonin enhances neural stem cell differentiation and engraftment by increasing mitochondrial function. *J Pineal Res.* 2017;63(2):1–18.

70. Liu J, Somera-Molina KC, Hudson RL, Dubocovich ML. Melatonin potentiates running wheel-induced neurogenesis in the dentate gyrus of adult C3H/HeN mice hippocampus. *J Pineal Res.* 2013;54(2):222–31.

71. Proietti S, Cucina A, Minini M, Bizzarri M. Melatonin, mitochondria, and the cancer cell. *Cell Mol Life Sci.* 2017;74(21):4015–25.

72. Chang CW, Chen YS, Chou SH et al. Distinct subpopulations of head and neck cancer cells with different levels of intracellular reactive oxygen species exhibit diverse stemness, proliferation, and chemosensitivity. *Cancer Res.* 2014;74(21):6291–305.

73. Bonnefont-Rousselot D, Collin F. Melatonin: Action as antioxidant and potential applications in human disease and aging. *Toxicology.* 2010;278(1):55–67.

74. Ortiz F, Acuña-castroviejo D, Doerrier C et al. Melatonin blunts the mitochondrial/NLRP3 connection and protects against radiation-induced oral mucositis. *J Pineal Res.* 2015;58:34–49.

75. Moneim AEA, Guerra-librero A, Florido J et al. Oral mucositis: Melatonin gel an effective new treatment. *Int J Mol Sci.* 2017;18:1–20.

76. Tahamtan R, Sc M, Monfared AS, Ph D, Tahamtani Y, Ph D. Radioprotective effect of melatonin on radiation-induced lung injury and lipid peroxidation in rats. *Cell J.* 2015;17(1):111–20.

77. Lissoni P, Chilelli M, Villa S, Cerizza L, Tancini G. Five years survival in metastatic non-small cell lung cancer patients treated with chemotherapy alone or chemotherapy and melatonin: A randomized trial. *J Pineal Res.* 2003;35(1):12–5.

78. Kumar A, Singh A. A review on mitochondrial restorative mechanism of antioxidants in Alzheimer's disease and other neurological conditions. *Front Pharmacol.* 2015;6:206.

79. Brown DA, Perry JB, Allen ME et al. Expert consensus document: Mitochondrial function as a therapeutic target in heart failure. *Nat Rev Cardiol.* 2017;14(4):238–50.

80. Andersen LP, Gogenur I, Rosenberg J, Reiter RJ. The Safety of Melatonin in Humans. *Clin Drug Investig.* 2016;36(3):169–75.

13

Chronic Antineoplastic Therapies and Their Impact on Quality of Life

Juana Deltell

Despite the advances in knowledge regarding the different types of cancer, mechanisms of carcinogenesis, new diagnostic methods, and new therapeutic systems, we still have not been able to find the cure for cancer. However, thanks to continuous care in medical oncology, cancer has become a real chronic disease for many [1]; this care will not cure cancer but seeks to improve patient survival, decrease symptoms, and increase intervals without signs of disease progression [2]. The term *chronic cancer* is defined as an active disease diagnosis—advanced or metastatic cancer that cannot be cured but can be controlled through continuous or cyclical long-term treatment [3] that will require frequent checkups to monitor its evolution and to adjust treatment and has similar needs to other chronic pathologies [4]. Some types of cancer may be included in this definition, such as ovarian cancer, chronic leukemia, some lymphomas, and even some types of cancer that have spread or metastasized in other parts of the body, such as breast or prostate cancer metastasis [5].

In the last decade, the different treatments have substantially changed, improving both their efficacy and safety compared with traditional cytotoxic drugs. We have new chemical therapies, molecular-targeted therapies, immunotherapy (biological response modifiers and vaccines), genic therapy, monoclonal antibodies, a new generation of immunoconjugates, and hormonal modulators.

Some of these may be administered as chronic or long-term treatments and can significantly increase patient survival, in which case they must be selected on an individual basis according to a series of variables: the patient's overall health status, the extension of the tumor, concomitant pathologies, treatments previously received and time interval since last administration, age, the patient's psychological and social characteristics, and so on. In this scenario, we cannot exclusively focus our attention on prolonging patients' lives: they must have a good quality of life. In recent years, health-related quality of life (HRQoL) is a concept that has been gradually but strongly introduced as an additional parameter to decide which treatment to administer to the patient. It is made by both objective and subjective factors (perceived by patients themselves), which explains its multiple individual particularities [6]; however, in order to minimize these and establish a common thread, specific standardized tests have been designed for its evaluation, such as the European Organisation for Research and Treatment of Cancer Quality of Life Questionnaire (EORTC QLQ C-30) or PROMs (patient-reported outcome measures), among others, which represent a simple way to assess physical and psychological disabilities

[7]. Studying HRQoL in this type of patient will enable us to accurately confirm the impact that these treatments have on it and discover their potential needs; however, there are still many tumors that do not include the study of HRQoL, even less in the case of long-term patients, so clearly there is a long way to go, and more research is needed to expand knowledge on the subject from different perspectives in order to better understand and help them. However, a few specific questionnaires are beginning to be developed, such as CCEQ (Chronic Cancer Experiences Questionnaire) [3], which have brought to light some of the needs (unmet or barely met) of patients who aspire to have a life as "normal" as possible; these needs are highly varied, but controlling the adverse effects of treatments, as well as decreasing the number of visits to the hospital and the feeling of uncertainty due to the evolution of the disease, are undoubtedly the most significant. However, we must note that based on patients' age, there are usually other needs that also occupy the top positions: in young patients, the priority is survival, and infertility is a great concern, while among the increasingly more abundant elderly population, the biggest concern is independence and preservation of cognitive functions [8].

Chronic treatments will be aimed at partial remission or control of the disease, but, as we have mentioned before, these do not lack adverse effects: some of these are significant because they may lead to fatal outcomes, the occurrence of comorbidities, and even treatment discontinuation due to dose-limiting toxicity [9]; others, although of low grade, significantly compromise patients' quality of life [10,11], such as, for instance, fatigue, which occurs in 82% of patients treated with tyrosine kinase inhibitors (TKIs) and is reported by patients as one of the adverse effects that, although not severe, conditions their HRQoL the most [12].

Due to the complexity of the disease, most patients usually receive combined treatments throughout the process (chemotherapy, surgery, radiotherapy, targeted therapies, immunotherapy, hormone therapy, cell therapy, etc.). The expression of symptoms of adverse effects and their involvement in HRQoL will change depending on the organ or system affected, as well as the development and evolution of the disease itself, and of course, on the vital characteristics and circumstances of each patient [13–15]. We should not forget that many of them already present with their own comorbidities prior to the cancer diagnosis, which will influence decision-making [16]. Several symptoms of adverse effects to consider that particularly compromise HRQoL are as follows: skin toxicity: rash, photosensitivity, hypersensitivity reactions, alopecia, hyper-/hypopigmentations, vitiligo, and so on; general symptoms: fatigue, fever, or pain (only 20% due to the different treatments; in most cases due to the tumor itself); at the digestive level: emesis, constipation, diarrhea, mucositis, and so on; liver and pancreatic toxicity; at the hematological level: anemia, coagulation alterations; neurological toxicity: motor and speech alterations, peripheral neuropathies, and so on; eye involvement: photophobia, dry eye, keratitis, and so on; genitourinary disorders; cardiac and pulmonary toxicity: arrhythmia, pericarditis, pneumonitis, and so on; endocrine alterations such as hyper-/hypothyroidism, and even autoimmune thyroiditis; gonadal and sexual dysfunction, among others. Due to this great variability, it is recommended that a physician know and perform a detailed follow-up on these effects, seeking their resolution as soon as possible in order to improve the treatment process and therefore patient survival and well-being, which in turn will improve HRQoL [16].

It is essential to integrate treatments into patients' daily routines because they may need them for the rest of their lives. Adherence to treatment is therefore an important point that will be conditioned by different factors: the presence of side effects of variable intensity; the need to take specific doses or medication that may negatively interact with dietary requirements or have restrictions in combination with the patient's usual medication prior to their oncological diagnosis [17]; and the administration route, because some patients need to have a catheter inserted that, although it reduces the amount of punctures and visits to the hospital, also generates discomfort and forces them to change part of their daily activities (mostly affecting young patients or those with an active work life) [18].

The administration regimen may be varied: some treatments are administered daily and permanently until there is a progression in the disease or an unacceptable toxicity occurs; others, on the contrary, will only be administered on specific days, with scheduled breaks between treatment cycles; and still others will be administered for a specific condition and then suspended, being resumed if there are changes in the evolution of the disease. Again, patients' lives are conditioned by the treatment because, in the case of having to alter the dose or suspend treatment, its efficacy might decrease along with their survival rate; or if the treatment interacts with their usual drugs, it may affect their prior comorbidities; and even if they modify their daily activities, their physical appearance, or sexual life, in some cases this leads them to discontinue the treatment, as often occurs in the case of males with prostate cancer undergoing antiandrogen therapy or women with breast cancer undergoing antiestrogen therapy [8]. To try to prevent this, it is key to customize the regimen, even using nonstandard posologies adapted to the clinical evolution of each patient [19].

As we have seen, the different treatments have many adverse effects, with patients increasingly demanding more care for their HRQoL; however, despite these patients needing specific care for the rest of their lives [8] because they are at a higher risk of the disease, no care models have yet been defined. Therefore, it is important to drive patient self-management abilities and lifestyle modifications (increased physical activity, healthy diet to prevent obesity, smoking cessation, decreased alcohol intake, etc.) without forgetting that, at the clinical level, it is necessary to keep the Hippocratic Oath, *primum non nocere* ("first, do no harm"), in mind by trying to minimize the morbidity/mortality associated

with the different treatments and prioritizing the preservation of basic global functions and the effective control of symptoms (even when these are of low grade), since it is critical to improve adherence to treatment or HRQoL of oncological patients. However, to know the real involvement of the different treatments, more studies are necessary that allow us to better understand their short-, middle-, and long-term alterations. Our final goal will be to achieve a therapeutic combination that allows a disease to be undetectable but always ensures the best HRQoL possible [20].

REFERENCES

1. Phillips JL, Currow DC. Cancer as a chronic disease. *Collegian*. [Internet]. 2010;17(2):47–50. Available from: http://dx.doi.org/10.1016/j.colegn.2010.04.007

2. Blasco Cordellat A. Los Cuidados Continuos (Terapia de Soporte y Cuidados Paliativos). In: Sociedad Española de Oncología Médica SEOM, ed. 2o Edición *Manual SEOM de Cuidados Continuos* [Internet]. Segunda: Sociedad Española de Oncología Médica SEOM, 2014: 477:(18–30). Available from: https://es.scribd.com/document/286417457/Manual-Seom-Cuidados-Continuos-2a-ed

3. Harley C, Pini S, Kenyon L, Daffu-O'Reilly A, Velikova G. Evaluating the experiences and support needs of people living with chronic cancer: Development and initial validation of the Chronic Cancer Experiences Questionnaire (CCEQ). *BMJ Support Palliat Care*. 2019 Mar;9(1):e15. Available from: http://spcare.bmj.com/lookup/doi/10.1136/bmjspcare-2015-001032

4. OMS (Organización Mundial de la Salud). Enfermedades crónicas [Internet]. OMS (Organización Mundial de la Salud). 2019 [cited 2019 Jan 18]. Available from: https://www.who.int/topics/chronic_diseases/es/

5. American Cancer Society. Managing Cancer as a Chronic Illness [Internet]. 2019. Available from: https://www.cancer.org/treatment/survivorship-during-and-after-treatment/when-cancer-doesnt-go-away.html

6. Higginson IJ. Measuring quality of life: Using quality of life measures in the clinical setting. *BMJ*. [Internet]. 2001 May 26;322(7297):1297–300. Available from: http://arxiv.org/abs/1712.01238

7. Efficace F, Rosti G, Aaronson N et al. Patient- versus physician-reporting of symptoms and health status in chronic myeloid leukemia. *Haematologica*. 2014;99(4):788–93.

8. Shapiro CL. Cancer Survivorship. Longo DL, editor. *N Engl J Med*. [Internet]. 2018 Dec 20;379(25):2438–50. Available from: http://www.nejm.org/doi/10.1056/NEJMra1712502

9. Lacouture ME, Anadkat MJ, Bensadoun RJ et al. Clinical practice guidelines for the prevention and treatment of EGFR inhibitor-associated dermatologic toxicities. *Support Care Cancer*. 2011;19(8):1079–95.

10. Cortes JE, Lipton JH, Miller CB et al. Evaluating the Impact of a Switch to Nilotinib on Imatinib-Related Chronic Low-Grade Adverse Events in Patients with CML-CP: The ENRICH Study. *Clin Lymphoma, Myeloma Leuk* [Internet]. 2016;16(5):286–96. Available from: http://dx.doi.org/10.1016/j.clml.2016.02.002

11. Khoury HJ, Williams LA, Atallah E, Hehlmann R. Chronic myeloid leukemia: What every practitioner needs to know in 2017. *Am Soc Clin Oncol Educ B* [Internet].

2017;37:468–79. Available from: http://meetinglibrary.asco.org/content/175712-199

12. Kroschinsky F, Stölzel F, von Bonin S et al. New drugs, new toxicities: Severe side effects of modern targeted and immunotherapy of cancer and their management. *Crit Care.* 2017;21(1):1–11.

13. (GEICAM) GE de I en C de M. Guía de Práctica Clínica para el diagnóstico y tratamiento de cáncer de mama metastásico [Internet]. 2015. 142 p. Available from: http://www.guiasalud.es/GPC/GPC_538_AF GUIA GEICAM_resumida.pdf

14. Brufsky AM. Long-term management of patients with hormone receptor-positive metastatic breast cancer: Concepts for sequential and combination endocrine-based therapies. *Cancer Treat Rev.* [Internet]. 2017 Sep;59:22–32. Available from: http://dx.doi.org/10.1016/j.ctrv.2017.06.004

15. De Miguel-Luken MJ, Mansinho A, Boni V, Calvo E. Immunotherapy-based combinations: Current status and perspectives. *Curr Opin Oncol.* 2017;29(5):382–94.

16. Tralongo P, Pescarenico MG, Surbone A, Bordonaro S, Berretta M, DI Mari A. Physical needs of long-term cancer patients. *Anticancer Res.* 2017;37(9):4733–46.

17. De Marchi F, Medeot M, Fanin R, Tiribelli M. How could patient reported outcomes improve patient management in chronic myeloid leukemia? *Expert Rev Hematol* [Internet]. 2017;10(1):9–14. Available from: http://dx.doi.org/10.1080/17474086.2017.1262758

18. Parás-Bravo P, Paz-Zulueta M, Santibañez M et al. Living with a peripherally inserted central catheter: The perspective of cancer outpatients—A qualitative study. *Support Care Cancer.* [Internet]. 2018 Feb 13;26(2):441–9. Available from: http://link.springer.com/10.1007/s00520-017-3815-4

19. Flynn KE, Atallah E. Quality of life and long-term therapy in patients with chronic myeloid leukemia. *Curr Hematol Malig Rep.* [Internet]. 2016 Apr 15;11(2):80–5. Available from: http://link.springer.com/10.1007/s11899-016-0306-5

20. Castañeda de la Lanza C, O'Shea C. GJ, Narváez Tamayo MA, Lozano Herrera J, Castañeda Peña G, Castañeda de la Lanza JJ. Calidad de vida y control de síntomas en el paciente oncológico. *Gac Mex Oncol* [Internet]. 2015;14(3):150–6. Available from: http://linkinghub.elsevier.com/retrieve/pii/S1665920115000449

14

Interactions with Medical-Aesthetic Treatments

Silvia Gabriela Ortiz Zamorano and Victoria Zamorano Triviño

Introduction

The oncology patient is a complex patient from the medical point of view. Precision medicine—with its directed or personalized therapies consisting in the design of the most selective possible drugs against molecular targets directly involved in the tumoral processes—opens a wide range of treatment options. Additionally, on occasion, various pathologies occur together, in which case the oncological patient could receive various additional treatments and medication. All these options increase the possibility of interactions between treatments and aesthetic-medical procedures [1].

It is therefore important to know the interactions that may exist in order to act with a margin of safety when performing aesthetic medicine in an oncological patient. For this, it is important to know the stages of the disease, the treatments that the patient follows, which treatments may specifically be contraindicated, and how they can affect the evolution of the disease. The range of treatments in the cancer patient is so wide that for this chapter we selected those that are most commonly followed by patients who, in our experience, also request medical-aesthetic treatments.

Interaction between Radiotherapy Treatments and Treatments in Aesthetic Medicine

The first side effects of radiotherapy are usually manifested in tissues with high proliferative activity. The cells of the basal layer of the skin epidermis divide rapidly and, therefore, are very prone to cell death after radiotherapy. Secondary to the death of the basal cells, an inflammatory reaction develops that results in an erythematous reaction. Dry desquamation is caused by the rapid production of cells in the basal layers, and wet desquamation appears after high doses of radiation because cell production in the basal layers cannot compensate for the loss of cells in the basal layers, and exudate is released [2]. In addition, hair follicle loss can occur as another early side effect. We can differentiate two stages of toxicity, an early or acute stage that can occur for up to 6 months of exposure and a late stage after 6 months of exposure to radiation (Table 14.1).

To take care of the treated area skin if external radiotherapy is received, there are a series of recommendations that the medical team should know, aimed at basic recommendations about soaps, lotions, deodorants, medications, perfumes, cosmetics, powders, or any other product in the treated area. Some of these products can irritate sensitive skin [3]. From a practical point of view, we can temporarily differentiate acute radiodermatitis from chronic

TABLE 14.1

Clinical Manifestations of Acute and Chronic Radiodermatitis

Acute Toxicity	Chronic Toxicity
Manifests in the 6 months after exposure to radiation.	Present after 6 months of final exposure to radiation; it can follow up to 4 years after treatment.
Phases	
First phase: Erythema scarcely visible in the 24 hours after exposure	**Characteristics** Atrophy
Second phase: Erythema visible after a period of latency of 6–12 days from exposure	Fibrosis Telangiectasias Modification of pigmentation Alopecia
Characteristics	
Erythema	
Edema	
Hyperpigmentation	
Erosion	
Desquamation (dry or damp)	
Alopecia	
Xerosis	

radiodermatitis according to the time at which the lesions caused by radiation due to cancer treatments appear [4] (Figure 14.1).

Several studies have shown the benefit of using a kit with treatment creams during radiotherapy. Product users had significantly fewer early skin reactions (within 10 days after the start of radiotherapy) compared to patients who did not use them [5,6].

Some clinical studies have demonstrated the improvement of erythema induced by ultraviolet radiation with topical application of melatonin, depending on the moment of its application [7]. Treatment with conventional creams enriched with melatonin seems to prevent the onset of radiodermatitis and would be a treatment to be considered in patients who are going to undergo radiotherapy [8].

Low-level light therapy (LLLT), also known as photobiomodulation (PBM) or "soft laser" (red or infrared light, power less than 150 mW), is best known in dermatology to treat ulcers. However, the biological mechanisms behind the therapeutic effect are currently not well known. Recent molecular and cellular research suggests that LLLT has biostimulant properties that allow tissues to regenerate and heal faster [9].

Chronic radiodermatitis after radiotherapy for breast carcinoma is a common sequel to treatment and can be distressing for the patient. The skin is atrophic and shows prominent telangiectasia due to dilation of a reduced or poorly supported skin vasculature. Pulsed dye laser is an established treatment for cutaneous telangiectatic disorders, including facial telangiectasia and spider veins, and is safe and effective. Pulsed dye laser treatment

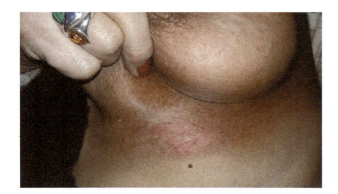

FIGURE 14.1 Radiodermatitis in breast area.

has been shown to be beneficial in eliminating radiation-induced telangiectasia. The first prospective study reported by Lanigan et al. was conducted in eight individuals; this showed that lesions could be bleached using very short pulse durations (0.45 ms) using a 585 nm pulsed dye laser. [10]

Other researchers have determined that longer pulse durations may be more effective in more dilated vessels, typical of radio-dermatitis, according to the rules of selective photothermolysis. However, although efficacy has been satisfactory for both pulse times, shorter pulse durations seem more effective [11].

Dermatological and cosmetic recommendations for patients during the acute phase of radiotherapy can prevent or mitigate its adverse effects, with a positive interaction between cosmetic recommendations and radiotherapy treatment.

In the event of radiodermatitis, aesthetic and dermatological medical treatments to alleviate their consequences should be administered after 6 months of radiation exposure, ensuring their safety and efficacy.

Botulinum Toxin Type A Interaction with Cancer Treatment and Its Implications

Botulinum toxin administration is the most popular nonsurgical cosmetic procedure worldwide, according to data from the International Society of Aesthetic Plastic Surgery (ISAPS). The aesthetic result obtained with botulinum toxin is generally highly satisfactory with a good safety profile. However, in the cancer patient, it is particularly important to know the interactions, complications, side effects, and adverse reactions of the application of botulinum toxin both locally and systemically.

Botulinum toxin achieves a neuromuscular block by translocating its light chain, released into the intracellular medium that acts by highly specific zinc-dependent endopeptidases with proteolytic activity, which divide one or more of the SNARE proteins of each neurotoxin, inhibiting the coupling and fusion between vesicles and receptors, and thereby blocking the release of exocytotic neurotransmitters [12]. In any situation where neuromuscular transmission is compromised, therefore, the injection of botulinum toxin could theoretically increase the underlying clinical picture [13].

Paraneoplastic Neurological Syndrome and Botulinum Toxin

Oncological patients sometimes present with neurological syndromes as part of their cancer symptoms. The pathogenesis is

unknown. Among the different theories proposed to explain its appearance, the autoimmune hypothesis stands out, whereby the different neurological syndromes would be secondary to the production of autoantibodies against nervous system cells with antigens common to tumor cells [14].

A paraneoplastic syndrome can occur in any type of tumor; however, it is more common in lung cancer and could affect 1% of patients with neuroendocrine tumors [15].

Diagnosis is often difficult. In patients previously diagnosed with cancer, in the presence of neurological symptoms, it is necessary to first rule out the presence of metastases, due to their higher incidence. Physical examination, the study of cerebrospinal fluid, and imaging techniques (computed tomography, magnetic resonance imaging) are all essential for its diagnosis. Considering that botulinum toxin for aesthetic use is contraindicated in patients with neurological disorders, chronic diseases that affect the muscles, and preexisting autonomic dysfunction, it does not seem advisable to use botulinum toxin for aesthetic use in cancer patients with symptoms of paraneoplastic neurological syndrome.

Neurotoxicity of the Aminoglycosides and Botulinum Toxin

Of the antibiotics, aminoglycosides in particular are known to inhibit neuromuscular transmission as a result of muscle weakness. The effect depends on the dose. Aminoglycosides can affect the release of acetylcholine (e.g., tobramycin) or block the binding of acetylcholine to receptors (e.g., netilmicin) [16].

Muscle paralysis as a result of a presynaptic inhibition of acetylcholine, as well as the postsynaptic blockade of acetylcholine, may be increased by the action of healing agents, magnesium, and botulism, and in patients with myasthenia gravis.

Despite the great safety profile of botulinum toxin, there have been some cases of botulism after botulinum toxin injection in the treatment of blepharospasticity and other cases of spasticity [17].

The use of botulinum toxin aesthetically in patients receiving aminoglycoside treatment should be deferred until the end of the treatment.

Conversely, the extensive use of large doses of botulinum toxin in other areas of medicine that are not aesthetic has verified the safety of its use in cancer patients. Several publications assess its effectiveness in pain control [18,19].

Various observations indicate that botulinum toxin injected subcutaneously can inhibit directly the primary sensory fibers, which leads to a reduction of the peripheral sensitization, with botulinum toxin transported retrogradely to the central nervous system. In one reported case, botulinum toxin injection had a significant analgesic effect on neuropathic pain induced by a brain tumor with no apparent side effects [20].

With the information we have available today, we can conclude that the use of botulinum toxin is safe in the cancer patient with active disease, without significant interactions with their medication; however, this is always in the context that the cancer patient is a heterogeneous patient, and that treatment may be contraindicated in a patient taking many medications or with neurological diseases such as paraneoplastic neurological syndrome (see Table 14.2).

TABLE 14.2

Botulinum Toxin Type A Interactions with Other Treatments: Aesthetic Use in Oncology Patients

Is botulinum neurotoxins (BoNTs) treatment safe for patients with coronary heart (CD) using anticoagulants?	The risk of hematoma with BoNT due to concomitant use of coumarin is low.
Is it safe to use BoNT in oncological patients with concomitant neurological comorbidities?	Patients with concomitant deterioration in neuromuscular transmission may experience clinical deterioration after treatment, although in selected cases treatment with BoNT may be beneficial. In case of aesthetic BoNT, it should be contraindicated.
Is treatment with BoNT safe for patients with cancer and paraneoplastic syndrome?	The deterioration of neurological function in oncological patients and the aesthetic benefit of BoNT do not outweigh the risk.
Is treatment with BoNT safe in patients with active disease?	Although there are *in vitro* studies with BoNT in tumors and some *in vivo* studies of the use of therapeutic BoNT in oncological patients with active disease without presenting adverse effects, we must balance treatment against the context of a patient with heterogeneous disease, in polymedicated patients, or in the presence of neoplastic syndrome.

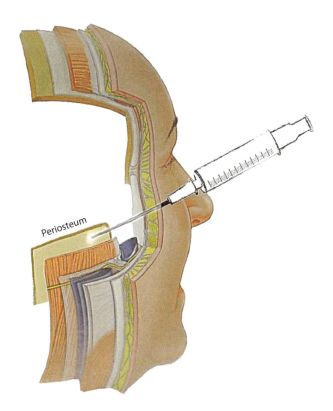

FIGURE 14.2 The injection of filling material in contact with the bone surface is relatively contraindicated in patients being treated with bisphosphonates.

Bisphosphonates and Interaction with Medical-Aesthetic Treatments

Bisphosphonates are a group of medicines that have a common antiosteoclast and antiresorptive biological effect, allowing an irreversible inhibition of the osteoclast cells (apoptosis); they have an affinity of places where there is active osseous refill, and in the centers of growth, which is why they have been used as markers in bone scans as a radionuclide carrier specific for bone [21]. In 1960, the first bisphosphonate was introduced in the market for therapeutic purposes: Etidronate, a potent antimineralizer, was used for the treatment of hypertrophic calcifications and to limit excess bone production in Paget disease; it is currently known to decrease serum calcium levels and to prevent the release of morphogenetic protein and growth factor [22].

Bone involvement is a common complication of various solid and hematologic tumors. In multiple myeloma, almost all patients develop bone metastases. In the case of solid tumors, the incidence is variable, developing mainly in breast and prostate (65%–75%), thyroid gland (60%), lung (40%), bladder (30–40%), and kidney cancers [23].

The use of bisphosphonates has been widely disseminated in the management of cancer-related conditions, such as hypercalcemia, in the management of lytic lesions (multiple myeloma), and in stabilizing bone pathologies such as osteopenia and osteoporosis, thus preventing pathological fractures [24].

Bisphosphonates, and especially zoledronic acid, are used in the prevention of bone metastases and their possible complications in breast, prostate, lung, renal, thyroid, bladder, colorectal, and multiple myeloma cancer. In addition, in the case of prostate cancer, lung cancer, and multiple myeloma, they improve overall survival [25]. Zoledronic acid is the most potent bisphosphonate, followed by neridronate, risedronate, ibandronate, alendronate, and finally, pamidronate; it is one of the most used in patients with breast cancer during their treatment [26].

Although there are no publications about the safety of aesthetic-medical treatments in patients receiving bisphosphonates, it seems prudent not to carry out any type of treatment that puts an implant of hyaluronic acid, calcium hydroxyapatite, or other compounds used in aesthetic medicine in contact with the bone surface in these patients (Figure 14.2). In recent years, treatments with fillers have been extended to volumize facial areas directly over the periosteum. As these often involve techniques in which contact of the needle with the periosteum can produce small bone lesions, the use of these techniques is not recommended in cancer patients who are receiving bisphosphonate. It would be prudent in these cases to use other infiltration techniques that do not involve direct contact with a bone surface that may have reduced turnover, with decreased blood supply and increased risk of bacterial aggression; the reduction of blood supply, decreased bone turnover, and bacterial aggression of oral flora are routinely cited as the main reasons for the occurrence of osteonecrosis in these patients.

Patients with a Catheter and/or Anticoagulant and Medical-Aesthetic Treatments

The central venous catheter (CVC) is a permanent catheter of prolonged use; to ensure good maintenance it is necessary to bond it with heparin and take into account a number of aspects. Thromboembolic complications represent the second most important issue that accompanies catheter insertion. Cancer patients are at great risk for thromboembolism, mainly due to the nature of their disease [27].

If the CVC is at rest, it should be periodically heparinized every 6–8 weeks with a volume of 10 mL of a heparin solution at a concentration of 100 IU/mL (1 mL of 1% sodium heparin + 9 mL physiological saline solution (SSF) 0.9%) or based on the protocol of the center.

The CVC will be left sealed with heparin whenever it is not used or if it is anticipated that nothing will be administered in 1–5 minutes, to prevent clot formation at the distal end of the catheter.

Patients under anticoagulant treatment with subcutaneous heparin of low molecular weight can undergo interventional procedures but cannot leave the consultation until it is certain that there is no bleeding; although there is no absolute contraindication, it is recommended to assess the benefit of the intervention.

In general, the existence of a catheter is not a contraindication of aesthetic, facial, or body medical treatments that avoid the implant area.

Interaction of Manual Treatments, Massages, and Lymphatic Drainage with Oncological Treatments

Patients undergoing cancer treatment can get great relief when they receive massage or lymphatic drainage massage. Some patients manage to reduce anxiety with massage treatments [28] and even to decrease skeletal muscle pain [29], which brings benefits to the quality of life. However, few doctors recommend massage, and many advise against it.

The Spanish Association Against Cancer (AECC) affirms the following in reference to massage:

> There are positive results in the management of pain and anxiety, as well as in the treatment of lymphedema (manual lymphatic drainage). Massage should be used with caution in patients with bone metastases due to the risk of fractures, and in those with thrombocytopenia or taking anticoagulant medication as they may lead to bruising. Massages should be avoided directly on tumors, on prostheses (due to possible displacement), on thrombi, and on tissues damaged by surgery and/or radiotherapy.

We should bear in mind that certain conditions could be worsened by the performance of treatments that involve the direct

TABLE 14.3

Limitations and Interactions of Cancer Treatments and Massage Modalities

- Skin lesions caused by radiotherapy, chemotherapy, and/or surgery (mastectomy, breast reconstruction, etc.)
- Malignant lymphedemas
- Discomfort caused by chemotherapy (nausea, weakness, etc.)
- Appearance of hematoma or seroma after surgery
- Presence of reservoirs under the skin for chemotherapy or phlebitis
- Carotid sinus syndrome
- Hyperthyroidism
- Erysipelas or lymphangitis
- Postsurgical inflammation
- Metastasis in bones (increased fracture risk)

mobilization of body areas by manual pressure or with apparatus. The presence of a reservoir under the skin is a contraindication to performing massages in that area (see Table 14.3), as is the presence of bone metastases, due to the risk of fractures [30].

In certain oncological treatment, there are other things that can interfere with the aesthetic-medical treatments and the performance of massages, such as radiation implants, which would cause a problem for the safety of the therapist who performs the aesthetic treatment.

Chemotherapy can be both an indication and a contraindication depending on, among other factors, the reaction that the patient has, since the use of massages can be comforting or inconvenient, depending on the general condition of the patient.

REFERENCES

1. Grumann M, Schlag PM. Assessment of quality of life in cancer patients: Complexity, criticism, challenges. *Onkologie.* 2001;24:10–5.
2. Balagula E, Rosen ST, Lacouture ME. The apparition of the oncodermatología of support: Andl studio of the adverse events dermatológicos to the therapies against the cancer. *J Am Acad Dermatol.* 2011;65:624–35.
3. American Cancer Society. Coping with radiation treatment. From https://www.cancer.org/treatment/treatments-and-side-effects/treatment types/radiation/coping.html (Date busqueda 28/07.
4. Seité S, Bensadoun R-J, Mazer J-M. Prevention and treatment of acute and chronic radiodermatitis. *Breast Cancer (Dove Med Press).* 2007;551–7.
5. Berger A, Regueiro C, Hijal T et al. Interest of supportive and barrier protective skin care products in the daily prevention and treatment of cutaneous toxicity during radiotherapy for breast cancer. *Breast Cancer (Auckl).* 2018;2:12.
6. Potenza MS et al. *Hypericum perforatum* and neem oil for the management of acute skin toxicity in head and neck cancer patients undergoing radiation or chemo-radiation: To single-arm prospective observational study. *Radiat Oncol.* 2014;9:297.
7. Bangha E, Elsner P, Kistler GS. Suppression of UV-induced erythema by topical treatment with melatonin (N-acetyl-5-methoxytryptamine). To dose response study. *Arch Dermatol Animal* 1996; 288:522–6.
8. Fernández-Tresguerres Rye AC. Radiodermitis prevention, Service of Dermatology, University Hospital Sanitas The Moralej. ANNALS RANM.13–19.
9. Hashmi JT, Huang YY, Sharma SK et al. Effect of pulsing in low-level light therapy. *Lasers Surg. Med* 2010;42:450–66.
10. Lanigan SW, Joannides T. Pulsed dye laser treatment of telangiectasia after radiotherapy for carcinoma of the breast. *Br J Dermatol.* 2003;148(1):77–9.
11. Nymann P, Hedelund L, Hædersdal M. Intense pulsed light Vs. long-pulsed dye laser treatment of telangiectasia after radiotherapy for breast cancer: To randomized split-lesion trial of two different treatments. *Br J Dermatol.* 2009;160(6): 1237–41.
12. Sollner T, White heart SW, Brunner M, Erdjument- Bromage H, Geromanos S, Tempst P. SNAP receptors implicated in vesicle targeting and fusion. *Nature.* 1993;362: 318–24.
13. Huang W, Foster JA, Rogachefsky ACE. Pharmacology of botulinum toxin. *J Am Acad Dermatol.* 2000;43(2):249–59.
14. Chunyang Li, Xiaolei Wang, Lihua Sun et al. Anti-SOX1 antibody-positive paraneoplastic neurological syndrome presenting

with Lambert-Eaton myasthenic syndrome and small cell lung cancer: To it marry report. *Thorac Cancer.* 2019;11(2):465–9.

15. Tannoury J, Mestier L, Hentic Or et al. Contribution of immune-mediated paraneoplastic syndromes to neurological manifestations of neuroendocrine tumours: Retrospective Study. *Neuroendocrinology* 2020;23(6):1–10.

16. Elsais A, Popperud TH, Melien Y, Kerty E. *Journal Nor Legeforen* 2013;133: 296–9.

17. Coban A, Matur Z, Hanagasi H, Parman Y. Iatrogenic Botulism after Botulinum Toxin type to injections. *Clin Neuropharmacol.* 2010:33(3):158–60.

18. De Groef An, Devoogdt N, Van Kampen M et al. The effectiveness of Botulinum Toxin A for treatment of upper limb impairments and dysfunctions in breast cancer survivors: A randomised controlled trial. *Eur J Cancer Care.* 2020;29(1):1–10.

19. Wang L, Lei QS, Liu YY, Song GJ, Song CL. A case report of the beneficial effects of botulinum toxin type A on Raynaud phenomenon in a patient with lung cancer. *Medicine (Baltimore).* 2016;95(40):e5092.

20. Oliver M, MacDonald J, Rajwani M. The use of botulinum neurotoxin type A (Botox) for headaches: a case review. *J Can Chiropr Assoc.* 2006;50(4):263–70.

21. Rogers MJ, Crockett JC, Coxon FP, Mönkkönen J. Biochemical and Molecular mechanisms of action of bisphosphonates. *Bone.* 2011;49(1):34–41.

22. Giger EV, Castagner B, Leroux JC. Biomedical applications of bisphosphonates. *J Control Release.* 2013;167(2):175–88.

23. Tolia M, Zygogianni A, Kouvaris JR et al. The key role of bisphosphonates in the supportive care of cancer patients. *Anticancer.* 34(1):23–37.

24. Aapro M, Saad F, Coast L. Optimizing clinical benefits of bisphosphonates in cancer patients. *Oncologist.* 2010;15(11): 1147–58.

25. Wirth M, Tammela T, Cicalese V et al. Prevention of bone metastases in patients with high-risl nonmetastasic prostate cancer treated with zoledronic acid: Efficacy and safety results of the Zometa European Study (ZEUS). *Eur Urol.* 2015;67(3):482–91.

26. Ottewell PD, Wang N, Brown HK et al. Zoledronic acid has differential anti-tumour activity in the pre-and post-menopausal bone microenvironment in Alive. *Clin Cancer Animal* 2014;20(11):2922–32.

27. Granic M, Zdravkovic D, Krstajic S et al. Totally implantable central venous catheters of the port-a-cath type: Complications due to its use in the tratamients of cancer patients. *J BUON.* 2014;19(3):842–6.

28. Genik LM, McMurtry CM, Marshall S, Rapoport A, Stinson J. Massage therapy for symptom reduction and improved quality of life in children with cancer in palliative care: A pilot study. *Complement Ther Med.* 2020;48.

29. Pinheiro da Silva F, Moreira GM, Zomkowski K, Amaral de Noronha M, Flores Sperandio F. Manual therapy as treatment for chronic musculoskeletal pain in female breast cancer survivors: A sSystematic review and meta-analysis. *J Manipulative Physiol Ther.* 2019;42(7):503–13.

30. Keilani M, Kainberger F, Pataraia A et al. Typical aspects in the rehabilitation of cancer patients suffering from metastatic bone disease or multiple myeloma. *Wien Klin Wochenschr.* 2019;131(21–22):567–75.

15

Medical-Aesthetic Treatments in the Survivor Patient

Manuela Sánchez-Cañete

Introduction

A cancer survivor is a person who is free from disease or in remission from disease or undergoing treatment over a long period [1]. Therefore, this pathology should be seen as part of a *continuum*, and there should be established a particular medical care that tackles the late side effects derived from oncology therapies, the physical effects of the cancer (scars, lymphedema), and the psychosocial impact involving acceptance of a chronic disease with a fear of relapse [2]. Professional participants are required, from multidisciplinary backgrounds, to help these patients to recover their body image in order to let them improve their quality of life, minimizing the oncological effects and integrating back into their routine activities.

For many of the treatments specified in this section, there are no bibliographical references to consult for their use in an oncological patient. It therefore seems prudent to follow the recommendations and opinions from relevant experts in the subjects, who because of their experience with these therapies are aware that they produce a suitable tissue response and the correction of those problems without any excessive increase of risks or side effects. Even so, the oncologist should always be consulted for approval, if in doubt.

Skin

The skin and adnexa are often the most damaged tissues because they have the most active cell replacement.

Direct Cutaneous Toxicity

Dehydration and Xerosis

These side effects remain for some time after oncological treatment has finished or do not disappear at all. Treatments for this might include the following:

- Hyaluronic acid for hydration.
- *Mesotherapy (vitamins/homeopathy)*: It must be confirmed that no component in these could interfere with the pharmacokinetics of the oncological medicines, in the event that the patient—even if in disease remission—had to continue to take them.
- *Carboxytherapy*: This treatment restores microcirculation and helps collagen formation [3]; it is used safely in the treatment of digestive pathologies [4].
- *Superficial/medium peelings*: These should start with the least irritating.
- *Platelet-rich plasma (PRP)*: There is no evidence that the use of growth factors could constitute a danger for neoplastic growth or tumor progression or metastatic spread in patients with previously diagnosed malignant oncologic process [5]; certainly, it has been used in mammary reconstruction after conservative surgery for mammary cancer [6].

In spite of that, it is not appropriate to use this in patients who receive antitumor treatment or are likely to still have disease.

- *Topical hydration treatment*: The use of face masks has a moisturizing, antiaging, and antioxidant effect; body treatments can help patients reactivate the circulation and blood flow, which will contribute, apart from hydration, to the feeling of comfort and well-being.

Hyperpigmentation

Hyperpigmentation usually disappears spontaneously after finishing the treatment, and it only requires ultraviolet (UV) protection. In cases where it continues for 6 months, other kinds of treatment can be used, although there are no studies in the oncological patient:

- *Intense pulsed light (IPL)*: This is not invasive but is effective for those kinds of lesions [7].
- *Depigmentation peelings:* These should commence with the least irritating types, based on kojic acid or arbutin.
- *Laser (mode Q-switched, fractional CO_2)*: In the initial phases (6–12 months), we would use lasers that maintain the epidermis intact (the nonablative systems in Q-switched mode); from 12 months onward, we would use ablative lasers, based on prior diagnosis of the state of the skin.

Facial Volume Changes

The patient's face may lose mass as a consequence of either the oncological process or the physiological aging process. In the superior third of the face (temporal zone and dark circles), there may be volume loss; in the inferior two-thirds (malar area), there may be reduction of the fatty compartments or an increase of volume produced by the corticoid treatment [8].

The materials most used in these cases are the absorbable soft tissue implants, which generate a mechanical filler effect that provides an improvement of the facial volume. Those are as follows:

- *Hyaluronic acid*: This is the most used and is the only one that provides a clinical study linking the concept in the use of the aging patient with use in an oncological patient [9] and with reconstruction after oncological surgery for the head and neck [10].
- *Methylcellulose*: Some studies with the oncological patient show the possible role of this treatment in the prevention of the adverse effects after radiotherapy [11].
- *Polylactic acid*: There are no specific studies on the oncological patient.
- *Hydroxyapatite calcium*: There are no specific studies on the oncological patient, but it is important to be aware that this material is visible with x-ray. Patients who require a radiologic study should be informed of this in order to dismiss false-positive tests, raising the suspicion of cancer.
- *Polycaprolactone*: There are no specific studies on the oncological patient.

Bisphosphonate treatment will benefit the appearance of osteonecrosis, but it would be prudent not to undertake any type of treatment that puts such filler materials or compounds in contact with bone.

Autologous fat implantation: Removing adipose tissue from the abdomen or thighs (lipofilling) is also a good alternative to using a soft tissue filler. It is used in mammary reconstruction after mastectomy in cancer and treatment for tissue damage caused by radiotherapy [12,13].

Expression Lines

As the first choice for dynamic wrinkles in the superior third of the face, we would use botulinum toxin [9].

Facial Skin Flaccidity

- *Radiofrequency*: This produces heat in the deep dermal layer and the subcutaneous tissue, restructuring the collagen and creating new fibers.
- *Nonablative fractional laser mode Q-switched* [14]: This penetrates to the deep dermal layer and stimulates the production of collagen, with improvement in the quality and skin tension.

- *No fractional ablation laser*: CO_2 laser or erbium:YAG 2940 nm. This is not recommended until a year after the end of all treatments, because they affect the capacity for tissue repair, thus increasing possible side effects.
- *Absorbable threads (polydioxanone [PDO] or Polycaprolactone [PLC])*: Patients should wait approximately 6 months after finishing treatments (1 year for those that generate a bigger tissue response such as a higher degree of inflammation that will require greater effort in recovering).

Acne

In the event that acne remains after finishing the treatments or appears with the use of hormonal treatment, the choice of treatment will depend on the previous condition of the skin.

Treatment should commence with a cosmetic approach using sebum regulators, retinoids, and adequate skin hygiene, continuing with treatments of the following:

- Superficial chemical peels (starting with the least irritating, such as azelaic acid and salicylic acid)
- Phototherapy with light-emitting diodes (LEDs) with an anti-inflammatory effect (used for patients to prevent dermatitis induced by radiation in breast cancer) [15]
- Intense pulsed light (has a bactericide effect, besides reducing red spots and improving skin texture and tone) [7]

Vascular Alterations

These can occur as a consequence of chronic radiodermatitis in an area up to 6 months after treatment has finished or in any other area with no relation with the oncology process. The treatment, in both situations, will be the same:

- *Intense pulsed light*: The chromophore corresponds to the oxyhemoglobin [7]
- *Pulsed dye laser*: Safe and effective in telangiectasias after radiodermatitis [16]
- *Laser KTP Nd:YAG 532 nm*: Highly selective in superficial vascular injuries [17]
- *Laser Nd:YAG 1064 nm*

Scars

These can present as a result of surgery or as a side effect of some therapies.

Hypertrophic and/or keloids:

- *Intraregional corticotherapy*: A first-line treatment with complete remission of 50% [18]
- *Cryotherapy*: Less selective, with a risk of residual hypopigmentation [18]
- *Light sources*: CO_2 [10], Nd:YAG, and IPL

Atrophic or hypotrophic:

- Sublative fractionated radiofrequency (restructures dermal collagen)
- Hyaluronic acid implants [10]
- Carboxytherapy (increases collagen density) [3]
- Intense pulsed light
- Micropigmentation (allows camouflage of scars)

Radiotherapy Tattoo Removal

Nd:YAG laser in mode Q-switched has a high level of safety and effective results [19].

Hair

Scalp Alopecia

The evolution and duration of alopecia will depend on the agent used in treatment. *Radiotherapy* will cause permanent alopecia from 35 Gy, and temporary below that, whereas *chemotherapy* causes temporary alopecia in most cases, and hair will appear again from 3 to 6 months after the last session.

- Topical drugs: Minoxidil, especially indicated in long-term hormonal treatments
- Mesotherapy for hair loss
- Carboxytherapy
- Micropigmentation
- Hair transplantation

Eyebrow Alopecia

- Micropigmentation
- Eyebrow implant

Hair Increase

- *Photodepilation*: Provided that the skin does not have any prior injury

Mucosa

Vaginal Atrophy

Infiltration in the vulvovaginal area:

- Hyaluronic acid [20]
- Carboxytherapy [21]
- PRP
- Lipofilling

Microablative fractional CO_2 laser. It stimulates the connective tissue cellularity, promotes the synthesis of collagen and elastin, favors angiogenesis of the lamina propria and increased epithelial thickness [22].

Circulatory System

Telangiectasias and Varicose Veins from Lower Limbs

These problems require the same treatment as in the healthy patient; with chemical sclerosis in those patients on treatment with tamoxifen, their thromboembolic risk should be evaluated [12], although it has not been proved to be an absolute contraindication due to the lack of clinical studies.

Lymphedema

This is a common side effect to oncological treatments.

Complex physical therapy: Manual lymphatic drainage, bandage, pressotherapy, skin care, and exercises (the initial treatment of choice in all degrees of lymphedema) [23].

Cellulitis and Localized Adiposity

The presence of lymphedema in lower limbs, even in the initial stages, must always be ruled out:

- Mesotherapy
- Carboxytherapy
- Ultrasonic cavitation
- HIFU (a secure method to use in the treatment of solid tumors) [24]
- Hydrolipoclasia
- Lipolysis laser (selective photothermolysis to break up adipocytes, preferably without affecting the surrounding structures) [25]
- Cryolipolysis (controlled and located cooling of the adipocytes that cause their destruction in the area of treatment) [26]

All these nonsurgical techniques for the treatment of localized fat cause a reduction of the thickness of the treated fat tissue [27].

Overweight

The advice is to follow a healthy diet, as is recommended in healthy people: eat a balanced diet, try to maintain a steady weight, and exercise (according to the particular characteristics of each patient) [28].

Controlling weight is very important for cancer survivors because it affects their quality of life, and obesity is associated with a risk of secondary cancers and recurrences [29].

REFERENCES

1. Ferro T, and Borràs JM. Una bola de nieve está creciendo en los servicios sanitarios: Los pacientes supervivientes de cáncer. *Gac Sanit* 2012;25(3):240–5.

2. Vivar CG. Impacto psicosocial del cáncer de mama en la etapa de larga supervivencia: Propuesta de un plan de cuidados integral para supervivientes. *Aten Primaria*. 2012;44(5):288–92.

3. Arellano Salazar M. Aplicación subcutánea de dióxido de carbono para atenuación de cicatrices. *Rev ECIPerú*. 2013;9(2):42–5.

4. Hombrados E, Virto C, Ma E, Sánchez C, and Collado V. Beneficios de la infusión de CO 2 en pacientes sometidos a una colonoscopia. *Enferm Endosc Dig [Internet]*. 2015;2(1):20–5. Available from: http://aeeed.com/documentos/publicos/revista/abril2015/Enferm Endosc Dig. 2015;2(1)20–25.pdf

5. Martínez González JM, Cano Sánchez J, Gonzalo Lafuente JC, Campo Trapero J, Esparza Gómez GC, and Seoane Lestón JM. Existen riesgos al utilizar los concentrados de Plasma Rico en Plaquetas (PRP) de uso ambulatorio? *Med Oral*. 2002;7:375–90.

6. Navine J, Botey M, Pascual I, Balibrea M, and Grı JR. Reconstrucción de la mama con gel de plaquetas en la cirugía conservadora del cáncer. *Cirugía Española*. 2012;90(9):58.

7. Murillo RM. Luz pulsada intensa: Aplicaciones en dermatología. *Rev Hosp Jua Mex*. 2011;78(4):240–3.

8. Schiff D, Lee EQ, Nayak L, Norden AD, Reardon DA, and Wen PY. *Neuro Oncol*. 2015;17:488–504.

9. Shamban AVA. Safety and efficacy of facial rejuvenation with small gel particle hyaluronic acid with lidocaine and abobotulinumtoxinA in post-chemotherapy patients. *J Clin Aesthet Dermatol*. 2014;7(1):31–6.

10. Hernández BA, Santana LVG, Galimberti DR, and Galimberti GN. Reparación con láser y ácido hialurónico de cicatriz facial secundaria por cirugía oncológica. *Dermatologia Cosmet Medica Y Quir*. 2016;14(4):284–8.

11. Tan A, Argenta P, Ramirez R, Bliss R, and Geller M. The use of sodium hyaluronate-carboxymethylcellulose (HA-CMC) barrier in gynecologic malignancies: A retrospective review of outcomes. *Ann Surg Oncol*. 2009;16(2):499–505.

12. Clinicos E, La EN, and Farmacologica P. Enfoques en la prevenci Ûn Moduladores Selectivos de Receptores. *Clin Trials*. 2004;64:66–72.

13. Mu V. Revista de Senología y Patología Mamaria de la cirugía de la mama. *Nuestra Experiencia*. 2014;27(3):119–22.

14. Beasley K, Iii JMD, Brown P, Lenz B, and Hivnor CM. Ablative fractional versus nonablative fractional lasers—where are we and how do we compare differing products? *Curr Derm Rep*. 2013;2:135–43

15. DeLand MM, Weiss RA, McDaniel DH, and Geronemus RG. Treatment of radiation-induced dermatitis with light-emitting diode (LED) photomodulation. *Lasers Surg Med*. 2007;39(2):164–8.

16. Ruiz-Genao DP, Córdoba S, García-F-Villalta MJ, Dorado JM, and Fernández-Herrera J. Telangiectasias posradioterapia. Tratamiento con láser de colorante pulsado. Estudios histológicos secuenciales. *Actas Dermosifiliogr [Internet]*. 2006;97(5):345–7. Available from: http://dx.doi.org/10.1016/S0001-7310(06)73416-0

17. Tagle ET. Láser Ktp en el Tratamiento de Lesiones Vasculares Superficiales. *Revista Médica Clínica Las Condes*. 2002;13:3–7.

18. Zaballos P, Morales A, Navarro A, Salsench E, Garrido A, and Montañés J. Los queloides y las cicatrices hipertróficas. *Med Integr*. 2001;38(9):385–9.

19. Castro T, Velez M, and Trelles MA. Tatuajes y su eliminación por láser Tattoos and their removal by laser. *Cir Plástica Ibero-Latinoamericana*. 2013;39(2):195–205.

20. Berreni N, Marès P, Tan N, and Couchourel D. Correction of female genital deficiencies through a new specific product range of hyaluronic acid gels. *Isdin*. 2014;85(1):2014.

21. Scilletta DA. Carboxiterapia de nueva generación: un enfoque prometedor para el rejuvenecimiento vulvovaginal no quirúrgico Dra Alessandra Scilletta.:7–8. Available from: file:///J:/Articulos Trabajo Máster/Atrofia vaginal/Carboxiterapia-rejuvenecimiento-vulvovaginal.pdf

22. Adabi K, Golshahi F, Niroomansh S, Razzaghi Z, and Ghaemi M. Effect of the fractional CO_2 laser on the quality of life, general health, and genitourinary symptoms in postmenopausal women with vaginal atrophy: A prospective cohort. *Journal of lasers in medical sciences*, 2020;11(1):65–9. doi:10.15171/jlms.2020.11.

23. López Jiménez RM, and Carolina Muriel López SLJ. Tratamiento fisioterápico del linfedema en las pacientes tratadas de Cáncer de mama. *Enfermería Docente [Internet]*. 2015;1(103):55–9. Available from: http://www.revistaenfermeriadocente.es/index.php/ENDO/article/view/80/pdf_44

24. Orsi F, Zhang L, Arnone P et al. High-intensity focused ultrasound ablation: Effective and safe therapy for solid tumors in difficult locations. *Am J Roentgenol*. 2010;195(3):245–52.

25. Leal-Silva H, Carmona-Hernández E, López-Sánchez N, and Grijalva-Vázquez M. Reducción de grasa subcutánea, técnicas invasivas y no invasivas. *Dermatologia Rev Mex*. 2016;60(2):129–41.

26. Anmat. Informe Ultrarrápido De Evaluación De Tecnología Sanitaria Criolipólisis: Su Aplicación En La Medicina Estética Programa Evaluación De Tecnología Sanitaria-Anmat. 2017;22. Available from: http://www.anmat.gov.ar/ets/Criolipolisis.pdf

27. Nipoti I, and Ja F-T. Artículo Original Tratamiento de adiposidades localizadas mediante técnicas no quirúrgicas Techniques for the treatment of localized fat without surgery. *Nutrición clínica y dietética hospitalaria*. 2012;32(2):37–43. Available from: http://www.nutricion.org/publicaciones/revista_2012_32_2/TRATAMIENTO-ADIPOSIDADES.pdf

28. San H, Dios J De, Ali R, and Reyes E. TEMA-2017: Prescripción del ejercicio en el paciente con cáncer ISSN. *Revista Clínica de la Escuela de Medicina UCR – HSJD*, 2017;7(II):11–8.

29. Solano Santos LV, Martínez Moreno AG, Salazar Estrada JG, and López Espinoza A. Conducta alimentaria y estado nutricional: Antes, durante y después del cáncer. *Actual en Nutr [Internet]*. 2017;18:20–5. Available from: https://www.researchgate.net/profile/Antonio_Lopez-Espinoza/publication/318761654_Conducta_alimentaria_y_estado_nutricional_Antes_durante_y_despues_del_cancer/links/597c9076aca272d568f8d32b/Conducta-alimentaria-y-estado-nutricional-Antes-durante-y-despues

16

Medical-Aesthetic Treatments in Oncology Patients

Karina Díaz Bustamante and Paloma Tejero

Introduction

Given the increase in the number of cancer patients worldwide, it is important to increase medical efforts to offer a wide range of treatments, both curative and aesthetic-medical treatments that cover the psychosocial needs of patients. We therefore need a multidisciplinary response to meet the needs and demands of cancer patients. Early detection plus advances in cancer treatments have increased the survival rate. In the United States, there are about 4 million women living with a history of breast cancer, and this figure is expected to increase [1,2]. In addition to improving diagnostic and therapeutic procedures, we must consider factors such as the patient's age, nutritional status, living conditions, and family and social factors. It is increasingly important to know the perception of individuals about their health and their image, to ensure a good quality of life, and to maintain a good mental state. A better relationship between health professionals, patient, family, and medical institution would guarantee greater adherence to treatment [2,3]. The experiences of patients about the disease and the treatments received lead to great challenges in their lives that imply a process of acceptance and adaptation. It is important to evaluate and support patients with a specific approach to improve their image, as a means to improve their quality of life [4,5].

The *self-perception of aging* is an important parameter of health and longevity. The study by Schroyen and colleagues [6] showed that patients with a negative perception of self-aging showed a lower functional health than those who had a positive parameter and demonstrated the association with longevity of this parameter (the self-perception of aging with value). Those with a positive association lived 7.5 years longer than those with a negative value [6]. It should be remembered that during physiological aging, there is an increase in DNA damage, shortening of telomeres, reduction in the reserve of stem cells, and so on, and that these are the same routes affected by antineoplastic treatments [7].

During oncological disease, the sudden change in body image creates confusion and negative changes in the way patients perceive themselves [5]. Cancer patients are more likely to be *depressed and report a lower quality of life*; if this is associated with a negative perception of aging, we are faced with a double stigmatization. This is a marker of vulnerability in oncology that affects negatively the evolution of the physical and mental health of the patient, and it is important to treat it in a personalized way [6]; after the changes experienced by the fight against the disease and the side effects of the treatments received, cancer survivors

frequently present with somatic effects, neurological, emotional, sleep dysfunction, fatigue, and worry about the possibility of a shorter life and fear of relapse [7], all of which can cause great psychological impact and negative feelings.

The perception of a patient's body image will be altered with their new life condition, which in the majority requires a readjustment after treatment [3,8]. In patients who suffered lymphedema in the upper and lower extremities as an adverse effect of chemotherapeutic treatments, and in those undergoing surgical procedures that leave scars or amputations, the impact is greater and more lasting, decreasing their quality of life and their social and functional well-being [9].

Different studies [3,8,9] show how people with high self-esteem feel safe and appreciated for their positive feelings toward themselves and believe in their capacity to be able to face and adapt better to the challenges imposed in different situations.

Having a *positive attitude and a supportive social environment* significantly influences the return to work of survivors [10].

Medical-aesthetic treatments should be aimed at preventing disease and its recurrences through the promotion of healthy habits, early diagnosis, and prevention of recurrences (adequate weight, correct nutrition, sun protection, etc.) to prevent and mitigate the adverse effects of the treatments; where they become more important is in the maintenance of the patient's perception of their body image, making them improve their self-esteem and their conditions to face the fight with the disease and the survival process.

We also know that physical activity in a lifestyle has been associated with a significant improvement in self-esteem in cancer survivors, for all patients and especially with breast cancer. The study "Influence of an Adaptive Physical Activity Program on Self-Esteem and Quality of Life of Breast Cancer Patients after Mastectomy" also assessed the benefits of performing a weekly session of 1 hour of muscle strengthening, balance, and flexibility; self-esteem and physical self-perception improved significantly, and additional positive effects on quality of life, overall health status, and physical functioning were observed, leading to the conclusion that exercise is a useful tool to counteract the detrimental effects of surgery and antineoplastic treatments [10].

Approximately 3.5 million people are diagnosed with cancer annually in Europe, and 50% of these figures are part of the active population. With the advances made by medicine—early detection as well as available treatments—we have increased the rates of survival as well as the ability to return to work or even continue while receiving treatment; however, this ability may be altered by factors related to the disease and treatment such as fatigue, pain, or physical appearance [11].

The demand of patients for a multidisciplinary team for the treatment of their disease and follow-up is increasing, involving in addition to the treatment of the disease the approach and repair of the sequelae, the recovery of self-image, and improvement to the quality of life. Patient groups are achieving great challenges through different organizations—for example, in Spain, micropigmentation of the postmastectomy areola is already included in the public health system—but there is still a lot of work to do, and that will only be possible with interrelation between the different health and non-health preprofessionals, research, family, and patients [12,13].

Medical-Aesthetic Treatments

In the different chapters of this book, several treatments that aesthetic physicians can perform for cancer patients at different stages of the disease are described, and the role of aesthetic medicine as a preventive medicine is discussed.

> The origin of cancer is usually silent, barely noticeable to the cell and much less to the whole organism. Years, or even decades before a tumor forms, the appearance of mutations in the DNA of some cells of the body initiates a cascade of molecular events that, if not counteracted, culminates with the transformation of healthy cells into growing cells which proliferate without control. [14]
>
> In some cases, cancer is hereditary and occurs due to the presence of mutations transmitted from parents to children. In most cases, however, cancer occurs due to the action of external agents that induce mutations, such as radiation, or errors when copying DNA during cell division. Whatever the origin of the mutation, if the cell does not identify and repair the error, it becomes part of the genome of the cell permanently and will be transmitted to the daughter cells when the cell divides. [14]

These quotations give us an idea of the importance of adopting healthy lifestyles in trying to avoid environmental factors and life behaviors, which through epigenetic mechanisms contribute to initiate mutations that cause cancer.

The results of the Pan-cancer project are that "The new findings are key to the development of personalized medicine, once the genome sequencing of a cancer is common in the clinical setting," as indicated by Ivo Gut, director of the Centro Nacional de Análisis Genómico of the Centre for Genomic Regulation (CNAG-CRG). "In the not too distant future we can diagnose the type of tumor accurately, predict with more certainty the progression of a cancer and what treatment should be chosen" [15].

This gives cause for optimism, and since the number of survivors will increase, aesthetic medicine and medical-aesthetic treatments must adapt increasingly and be a reality within the global approach to prevention programs, early diagnosis, cancer treatment, relapse prevention, image recovery, and in summary, in the search for a better quality of life.

To summarize, aesthetic medicine consists of the following:

1. *Prevention of the illness*: Healthy habits, photoprotection, skin care, diet, and exercise
2. *Prediagnosis*: Clinical history, research, skin

3. *Prevention and treatment of side effects of treatment*: Cutaneous side effects, the power of image therapeutic treatment
4. *Healing process after oncology treatment*: Physical appearance, mental stability, avoiding stigmas and sequelae

The creation of oncological aesthetic medicine units must become a reality in order to be able to treat the patient in an integral way. Physicians should be trained, create consensus protocols, and adapt their treatments for better outcomes. In Spain, the Spanish group of experts in aesthetic medicine has been created for this purpose, and the first university studies are already consolidated as their own degrees from the University of Alcalá de Henares—the master's degree in quality of life and medical-aesthetic care of the oncological patient.

REFERENCES

1. Awick EA, Phillips SM, Lloyd GR, McAuley E. Physical activity, self-efficacy and self-esteem in breast cancer survivors: A panel model: Physical activity and self-esteem in breast cancer survivors. *Psychooncology*. octubre de 2017;26(10):1625–31.
2. Maciel PC, Veiga-Filho J, de Carvalho MP Fonseca FEM, Ferreira LM, Veiga DF. Quality of life and self-esteem in patients submitted to surgical treatment of skin carcinomas: Long-term results. *An Bras Dermatol*. julio de 2014;89(4):594–8.
3. Leite MAC, Nogueira DA, Terra de FS. Evaluation of self-esteem in cancer patients undergoing chemotherapy treatment. *Rev Lat Am Enfermagem*. diciembre de 2015;23(6):1082–9.
4. Tonsing KN, Ow R. Quality of life, Self-Esteem, and future expectations of adolescentand young adult cancer survivors. *Health Soc Work*. 1 de febrero de 2018;43(1):15–21.
5. Ferreira da EC, Barbosa MH, Sonobe HM, Barichello E. Self-esteem and health-related quality of life in ostomized patients. *Rev Bras Enferm*. abril de 2017;70(2):271–8.
6. Schroyen S, Missotten P, Jerusalem G, Van den Akker M, Buntinx F, Adam S. Association between self-perception of aging, view of cancer and health of older patients in oncology: A one-year longitudinal study. *BMC Cancer*. diciembre de 2017;17(1):614.
7. Arndt J, Das E, Schagen SB, Reid-Arndt SA, Cameron LD, Ahles TA. Broadening the cancer and cognition landscape: The role of self-regulatory challenges: Self-regulation, cancer, and cognition. *Psychooncology*. enero de 2014;23(1):1–8.
8. Mayer S, Teufel M, Schaeffeler N et al. The need for psycho-oncological support for melanoma patients: Central role of patients' self-evaluation. *Medicine (Baltim)*. septiembre de 2017;96(37):e7987.
9. Cromwell KD, Chiang YJ, Armer J et al. Is surviving enough? Coping and impact on activities of daily living among melanoma patients with lymphoedema. *Eur J Cancer Care (Engl)*. septiembre de 2015;24(5):724–33.
10. Landry S, Chasles G, Pointreau Y, Bourgeois H, Boyas S. Influence of an adapted physical activity program on self-esteem and quality of life of breast cancer patients after mastectomy. *Oncology*. 2018;95(3):188–91.
11. Duijts SFA, van Egmond MP, Gits M, van der Beek AJ, Bleiker EM. Cancer survivors' perspectives and experiences regarding

behavioral determinants of return to work and continuation of work. *Disabil Rehabil.* 9 de octubre de 2017;39(21):2164–72.

12. Johansen S, Cvancarova M, Ruland C. The sffect of cancer patients' and their family caregivers' physical and emotional symptoms on caregiver burden. *Cancer Nurs.* 2018;41(2):91–9.

13. Lawn S, Fallon-Ferguson J, Koczwara B. Shared care involving cancer specialists and primary care providers—What do cancer survivors want? *Health Expect.* octubre de 2017;20(5):1081–7.

14. Tolosa A. Los genomas del cáncer Genotipia https://genotipia.com/genetica_medica_news/los-genomas-del-cancer/ 6–02–2020.

15. Campbell PJ, Getz G, Korbel JO et al. Pan-cancer analysis of whole genomes. *Nature.* 2020;578, 82–93. https://doi.org/10.1038/s41586-020-1969-6

17

Facial Medical-Aesthetic Treatments in Oncology Patients

Victoria Zamorano Triviño and Silvia Gabriela Ortiz Zamorano

Introduction

The face is presented as the letter of introduction of any individual, and any modifications suffered will change that individual's self-image. The changes that the face and its frame (the hair) can undergo in patients suffering oncological treatments can cause rapid and acute alterations in the image of women and men suffering from cancer. Although some of these changes are transient, and not clinically serious, they are important to the patient. The word *cancer* should not be associated with death, since currently more than 60% of all serious malignant tumors (excluding nonmelanoma skin cures) are cured [1].

Cancer therapies have resulted in remarkable results due to improved survival. While chemotherapy treatments, radiation, surgery protocols, and new immune therapies are primarily responsible for these notable improvements, an unexpected constellation of toxicities has emerged where dermatological adverse events have gained considerable attention due to their high frequency, visibility, and impact on physical and psychosocial health, depending on the intensity of the dose and the clinical outcome. Consequently, greater attention to cutaneous health in oncology has resulted in dermatological oncology support, promoting toxicity programs and research, with the aim of mitigating these adverse events and allowing the development of continuous optimization of cancer treatments [2].

Focusing on the total facial approach of women with an oncological history involves knowing our patient's medical history; working closely with her oncologist and knowing what type of treatments she has or continues to undergo will give us security in our work.

Needless to say, in cancer patients, we must know perfectly the concerns that they present to us—fears regarding the safety of the treatment and how this could affect not only their health but also their image in the face of others and a society that still regards as frivolous aesthetic treatments in patients who have endured serious diseases.

The face is the most visible body area of our anatomy, which is why patients generally have concerns about the results of facial aesthetic-medical treatment. In the case of the cancer patient, this concern may be more evident, driven by a series of physical changes that the patient does not usually want to perceive and certainly does not want to add to with other obvious changes; they request mostly natural, nonstrident facial treatments, with only a few momentary sequelae such as bruises or marks to show that treatment has been performed.

Knowing the particularities presented by the cancer patient gives us security in our work. Knowing the complexity of this patient and what we should and should not do about the treatments we have, working in a framework of safety and satisfaction is a necessity and a commitment to the cancer patient.

Facial Involvement by Long-Term Cancer Therapies

Everyone knows the complexity of cancer and the cancer patient. Antineoplastic therapies, although decreasing in toxicity, remain aggressive in the context of a patient who may also suffer from other concomitant pathologies.

On the other hand, some patients continue to receive antineoplastic treatments for long periods of time. Some of these treatments may be aimed at treating long-standing cancer pathologies such as some proliferating myeloid neoplasms. Other treatments are aimed at increasing the years of survival of the patient, such as adjuvant therapies for stage IV cancer, and others are part of the curative or preventive treatment of some tumors such as breast cancer, with long hormonal treatments that can last 5 or more years (Table 17.1).

Cancer treatment may involve surgery, chemotherapy, radiotherapy, hormone therapy, immunotherapy, and in some cases, the combination of several. Although the trauma of more radical surgery may be lessened, alternative treatments can be extremely harmful to physical and psychological health. Some of the facial side effects in relation to the treatment are skin alterations, alterations of facial volumes, facial scars, and alterations of the aging process, accelerated by adjuvant treatments.

Chemotherapy can affect the function of the ovaries and cause sterility. Therefore, women who are associated with chemotherapy with premature menopause may have negative results on the skin [3]. The skin and its adjoining structures represent an important component of such events; menopause has a known influence on the skin, making it dehydrated and presenting a dry and rough appearance. It loses freshness and luminosity, and its tone is no longer uniform; it decreases its thickness, loses elasticity, and becomes

TABLE 17.1

Causes of Complexity with the Cancer Patient

- Multiple pathologies
- Combination of several treatments
- Requests by the patient

Source: Presented in the master's thesis on Quality of Life and Medical-Aesthetic Care of the Cancer Patient by Dr. Mª Victoria Zamorano Triviño.

brittle and prone to injury. The number and depth of wrinkles intensifies [4]. When the elastin and collagen fibers break down, the skin loses firmness and slips. Flaccidity can be seen, especially in the lower part of the face and neck, as well as in the inner part of the arms and legs. Hyperpigmentation is a frequent event.

All these events can be exacerbated in a patient who, in addition to suffering from early menopause, may require hormonal antiestrogenic treatments that worsen these symptoms [5].

When treating these patients from the aesthetic-medical point of view, it is important to know what stage of the disease they are in and what treatments they are receiving that may cause interactions with the aesthetic-medical treatments.

Facial Approach of the Oncological Patient

Ideally, you should start aesthetic-medical treatments and general care before receiving cancer treatments, care and follow-up during them, and once the treatment is finished, consider what to do (Table 17.2).

First Phase: Facial Medical Aesthetic treatments before the introduction of antineoplastic therapies

For the patient confronting a diagnosis of cancer, in an unexpected situation involving a change in life and self-image, one of the most important concerns is hair loss and dryness or skin involvement [6]. We must therefore carry out prevention and support accordingly (Table 17.3), offering treatments that prepare the skin of the face before the main consequences of cancer treatments, such as dehydration, alterations of the thickness of the dermis, and pigmentary alterations. At this stage, aggressive treatments should be avoided, but aesthetic and beauty support should be given.

In this phase, comfortable treatments that provide well-being and information about the consequences of cancer treatments and how to minimize their effect should prevail.

As a way of prevention, hydration can be performed before starting treatment; the use of hyaluronic acid (topical or injected) can have a preventive effect. The decision about the route of administration depends on the physical and emotional condition of the patient.

It is important to give support about home facial treatments and home creams that provide hydration. Creams containing glycolic

acids, retinol, and similar components should not be indicated. Neither should abrasive cleaners be used, since, if an immediate onset of chemotherapic-type treatments is anticipated, we could be inflicting dermal aggression that does not have sufficient recovery time before cancer treatment.

Second Phase: Facial Medical-Aesthetic Treatments during Treatment

In the second phase, any aesthetic-medical treatment should be carried out in absolute coordination with the responsible oncologist, since during this phase the presence of complications before aesthetic treatments or aggressive treatments is multiplied.

It is necessary to know the contraindications of the aesthetic-medical treatments during the oncological treatment in its first stage, since the complexity of the cancer patient merits specialized attention (Table 17.4).

The most common dermatological toxicities include acneiform rashes, paronychia, alopecia, and xerosis. Many of these side effects can be controlled, which can increase compliance and help reduce the physical and emotional burden patients face [7]. In most cases, the rash is a maculopapular rash that affects the face, arms, or trunk of the body, and less frequently, the lower extremities, scalp, and intertriginous areas. The lesions appear about 2 months after the start of treatment, while the edema begins about 15 days before the skin lesions. Edema predominates in the area of the face, especially in the periocular region, and may be associated with epiphora [8].

A group of expert oncologists, radiotherapists, and dermatologists published a consensus document that determined the guidelines for the treatment of cutaneous lesions secondary to concomitant chemoradiotherapy with epidermal growth factor receptor (EGFR) inhibitors [9]. If radiodermatitis and acneiform lesions concur in the clinic, the management will be based on the most serious injuries. If radiodermatitis predominates, it is essential to instruct the patient in hygiene. The irradiated area should be washed and dried daily, even if it is ulcerated. The application of antiseptics, hydrocolloid gels, anti-inflammatory emulsions based on hyaluronic acid or trolamine, and zinc oxide pastes is recommended. Topical antibiotics should not be used prophylactically but reserved for cases where there is a superinfection.

Acneiform lesions related to local lesions but without any association to other symptoms may not require treatment. Daily washing with antiseptic soap is recommended, and local corticosteroid treatment may be included. When the lesions are more severe, antihistamines and antibiotic treatment can be added and assessed. In some cases, the use of isotretinoin in low doses (10–20 mg) daily could be assessed in patients who do not respond to the previous measures, bearing in mind that this medicinal

TABLE 17.2

Phases of Intervention in Aesthetic-Medical Care

- First Phase: Special techniques to alleviate the possible adverse effects of the medical treatment to be initiated
- Second Phase: What to do during treatment
- Third Phase: What to do once cancer treatment is finished

TABLE 17.3

First Phase Approaches

- Prepare the skin
- Avoid aggressive treatments
- Aesthetic and beauty support

TABLE 17.4

Second Phase Approaches

- Reassure the patient that most side effects of cancer treatments disappear shortly after the end of treatment.
- Provide conservative and supportive treatment during treatment.
- Know the contraindications of aesthetic-medical treatments during this phase.
- Aesthetic treatments performed by estheticians must be supervised by the medical team.

product may worsen xerosis. If necessary, the patient will have to be transferred to a specialized unit [10].

Photosensitivity and hyperpigmentation are the most common side effects presented by cancer patients and concerning to patients during their treatments. Increased sensitivity to ultraviolet radiation may occur after exposure to multiple chemotherapies. This photosensitivity can manifest itself as a tendency to erythema, burns, hyperpigmentation, and rash after sun exposure. The recommendation for the use of photoprotectors is mandatory in these patients, in addition to avoiding exposure to the sun, as far as possible [8].

The xerosis and skin atrophy that we observe in these patients may be related to the antiproliferative and cytostatic action of the drugs in the epidermis, particularly in the basal layer, the basal lamina, and the microfibrils of the papillary dermis.

Other factors that affect hydration of the skin in the cancer patient are malnutrition, immunosuppression, and anemia or hypoproteinemia processes that some individuals may experience [11].

Proper treatment of these side effects at the time of first presentation prevents more aggressive treatments in the future to restore skin health. Major side effects—severe acne and severe xerosis—should be treated during treatment. However, pure aesthetic-medical treatments, which do not treat side effects but are part of the beautifying or antiaging treatments, should be evaluated at this stage of the disease on an individual basis. Since, depending on the pathology and the stage, they can be received routinely or not, always remain in close contact with the oncologist and know the oncology treatment.

Third Phase: Cancer Treatment Is Finished

Once the cancer treatment is finished, it is the ideal time to start the aesthetic-medical treatments that repair the skin and facial attachments of the cancer patient. At this time, patients come more frequently to our office looking for supportive treatments that help them look good, recover their appearance before the disease, and help them to quickly reinsert themselves into social and work life.

It is time to make a good aesthetic-medical diagnosis and evaluate the changes that the patient may present and that are associated with cancer treatments (Table 17.5). Assessing the state of the skin and scalp and changes in facial volumes gives us an idea of those points to prioritize treatment.

TABLE 17.5

Third Phase Approaches

---
1. Evaluate changes associated with oncological treatments
   A. Skin and scalp
   - Cutaneous xerosis
   - Hyperpigmentation
   - Rashes (acne)
   - Hair alterations (alopecia; facial hypertrichosis)
   B. Volume changes
   - Upper third of the face
     - May suffer volume loss in temporal region linked to weight loss
   - Lower two-thirds of the face
     - Increase in volume due to weight gain or linked to steroid use
     - Decrease in malar fatty compartments due to weight loss
2. Evaluate changes linked to the physiological aging process
   A. Photoaging
   B. Volume changes in fat and bone compartments

We should not forget that, in addition to the changes associated with cancer treatment, this patient, like any other, will have changes linked to their own physiological aging that should also be considered at the time of diagnosis.

In the ideal scenario, the cancer patient should be attended by a multidisciplinary group in which the aesthetic doctor should have room. In that case the information would flow between the components of the team, and the treatment would be carried out within a comprehensive treatment format.

In the cancer patient, we should always know the medical history, what treatments have been followed, and the current state of disease. If the oncological treatment has only finished a short time before or the patient continues with some type of treatment, we must contact the responsible oncologist or request a medical history summary, since in many cases, the patient does not know exactly the detailed staging of the disease, which may lead to mistakes.

For the proper care of the cancer patient, we must

- Know closely the medical history of our patient
- Work closely with the cancer team
- Determine current disease status
- Determine what types of treatments have been followed
- Determine what treatments are currently being followed

Hyperpigmentation and How to Address It

Skin care products that contain highly active, but stable, ascorbic acid forms such as magnesium ascorbyl phosphate (MAP) can be used in pigmented areas if the skin is healthy and healed. It must also be ensured that the patient uses sunscreen every day for added protection [12].

When the dermis has recovered, we can start depigmenting treatments.

- Patients should not expose their skin to the sun even after the end of the treatment, for at least the first 3 months.
- Patients should avoid peeling procedures; while it may occasionally be necessary to use superficial peels, do not perform medium or deep peeling.
- The use of appliances (Q switch, pulsed dye, intense pulsed light) is indicated as long as the skin is healthy and the treatment localized.

Invasive Facial Treatments in Oncology Patients

There are several points that we must consider when using injectables in the cancer patient:

1. Consult with the oncologist whenever there is doubt about the state of the disease.
2. Perform the recommended blood testing in a patient with less than 1 year of completion of treatment (Table 17.6).
3. Do not start treatment until immune competence has been recovered.
4. Choose a treatment that can be administered safely and is safer to restore and can still achieve adequate aesthetic results.

TABLE 17.6

Absolute Contraindications to Injectable Treatments

- Cancer treatments with immune system suppression
- Neutropenia
- Platelets in the range 50,000–80,000/mm³

TABLE 17.7

Questions to Have in Mind before Starting Injectable Aesthetic-Medical Treatment on Oncological Patient

- What is the total blood count, including neutrophils and platelets?
- If aesthetic invasive interventions are to be performed, are there adequate coagulation actors?
- Does the patient have a central venous catheter?
- What is the timing of treatments (for cancer), to plan a safe aesthetic-medical treatment?

It should be noted that there are contraindications to the use of injectables in the cancer patient (Tables 17.6 and 17.7). It is evident that in the case of a patient with immune depression due to an oncological treatment, the use of injectables for aesthetic use should be weighed against the consequences of possible complications.

The use of injectables in the cancer patient should prioritize patient safety with the use of medical devices or medications that involve a low risk of complication and the assessment of the appropriate timing of treatment.

Several published studies show that the results of facial rejuvenation with botulinum toxin significantly improve self-esteem and components of quality of life in noncancer patients. In addition, facial rejuvenation can contribute to the improvement of physical health, mood, household activities, general satisfaction with life and the body, self-perception of intellect, self-esteem, appearance, attractiveness, the sense of doing well, self-esteem related to appearance, and self-esteem related to society [13]. The efficacy and safety of facial rejuvenation with hyaluronic acid and botulinum toxin in postchemotherapy patients have been observed; both products have been well tolerated by the patients, achieving an improvement in the severity of wrinkles after treatment [14].

Patients in aesthetic medicine may receive a combination of abotulinumtoxin A and small particles of hyaluronic acid gel with lidocaine. There is currently a growing trend in the combined use of these products. It is suggested that the combination treatment with botulinum toxin and dermal fillers may produce a natural and refined improvement. With dermal fillers, the volume, which can be lost due to the natural aging process and/or weight loss as a result of the process of the cancer disease or from undergoing chemotherapy, is restored with the use of injectable hyaluronic acid.

A prudent time lag equal to or greater than 6 months after the end of the treatment with chemotherapy allows us to treat these patients safely, achieving a high degree of satisfaction with no adverse effects.

Regarding the botulinum toxin in the treatment of wrinkle lines of the upper third of the face in the cancer patient, it should be noted that the cancer patient generally requests naturalness in the treatment, an effective treatment, and the evaluation of contraindications to offer a safe treatment [15] (Figure 17.1). Botulinum toxin has been safely used in the treatment of oncological surgery scars and in the treatment of tumor-induced neuropathic pain with no parallel side effects [16].

Among the contraindications of botulinum toxin for aesthetic use are hypersensitivity to botulinum toxin, infections at the injection site, preexisting autonomic dysfunction, and myasthenia gravis and Eaton-Lambert syndrome.

In the cancer patient, we must be aware of the possibility of other pathologies with neuromuscular involvement (paraneoplastic syndromes). However, although the majority of cancer patients have a mild degree of neuromuscular dysfunction, only in a small percentage of patients is there a diagnosis of a neurological paraneoplastic syndrome that would contraindicate the aesthetic use of botulinum toxin.

Regarding the suspension threads and fillers, there is a wide variety of sanitary products that should comply with the sterility and biocompatibility safety standards. When using them, we must use low reactive materials. As there is a risk of complications, suspension threads whose complications are easily resolved should be used.

(a)

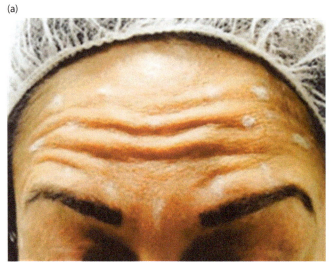

(b)

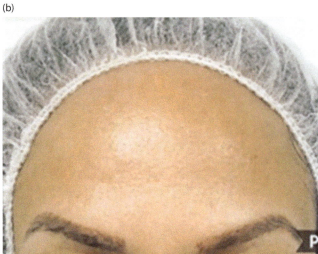

FIGURE 17.1   (a) Before and (b) after treatment with botulinum toxin. (Courtesy of Dr Zamorano Triviño.)

In the case of fillers, materials should be used that are biocompatible, induce minimal reaction to a foreign body, remain stable in the implanted place, maintain volume and do not make protrusions in the skin, do not migrate at a distance, and are not phagocyted [17].

Different dermal fillers have very different properties, associated risks, and injection requirements. All dermal fillers have the potential to cause complications, most related to volume and technique, but some associated with the material itself. The majority of adverse reactions are mild and transient, such as bruises and trauma-related edema. Serious adverse events are rare, and most are avoidable with proper planning and technique.

Conclusions

Cancer treatments can produce side effects that affect the skin, hair, and general physical appearance, and although the symptoms are not clinically important, they are important for the well-being of the patient. Facial aesthetics is a focal point in the individual, as it is a body area exposed to the vision of others as well as the patient. That is why cancer patients demand the attention and resolution of facial problems that may arise from cancer treatments, or that are increased by them in conjunction with the aging process of the individual.

Additionally, advances in oncology have meant a change in the healing and survival of many patients, and cancer patients now demand greater attention to their physical and psychological well-being. Advances in aesthetic medicine also mean there is a greater range of safer and more effective treatments.

Choosing the right time to perform such treatment is vital to the good performance of facial medical treatments in the cancer patient. In the services of aesthetic medicine, we must be prepared to attend patients in a safe and viable way, offering the patient comprehensive medical care and teamwork. Every day, this attention to aesthetic medicine starts earlier to be timely. Knowing the patient's medical conditions, being aware of the contraindications to certain treatments, and offering the most appropriate treatment in a timely manner constitute the pillars of aesthetic treatment for the cancer patient.

REFERENCES

1. Miller KD, Nogueira L, Mariotto AB. Cancer Survivorship Research Collection. *Cancer J Clin.* 2019;365–85.
2. Balagula Y, Rosent ST. The emergence of supportive oncodermatology: The study of dermatologic adverse events to cancer therapies. *J Am Acad Dermatol.* 2011;65:624–35.
3. Harcourt D, Frith H. Women's experiences of an altered appearance during chemotherapy: An indication of cancer status. *J Health Psychol.* 2008 Jul;13(5):597–606.
4. Duarte GV, Trigo A, Paim de Oliveira Mde F, Cutis. Skin disorders during menopause. *MDedge(Internet).* 2016;97(2):E16–23.
5. Noushin H, Haley N. Chemotherapeutic agents and the skin: An update. *J Am Acad Dermatol.* 2008;58:545–70.
6. Allevato M. Efectos adverso cutanea from antineoplastic therapy. *Act Terap Dermatol* 2008;31:78.
7. Oliveri S, Faccio F, Pizzoli S, Monzani D, Redaelli C, Indino M, Pravettoni G. A pilot study on aesthetic treatments performed by qualified aesthetic practitioners: Efficacy on health-related quality of life in breast cancer patients. *Qual Life Res.* 2019;28(6):1543–53.
8. Esmaeli B, Diba R, Ahmadi MA, Saadati HG, Faustina MM, Shepler TR, Talpaz M, Fraunfelder R, Rios MB, Kantarjian H. Periorbital edema and epiphora as ocular side effects of imatinib mesylate (Gleevec). Eye (London, England), 18(7):760–2.
9. Califano R, Tariq N et al. Expert consensus on the Management of adverse events from EGFR tyrosine kinase inhibitors in the UK. *Am J Clin Oncol.* 2015. 39(4):75(12): 1335–1348.
10. Blasco A, Caballero C. Toxicidad de los tratamientos oncológicos. *SEOM* 2019.
11. Valentine J, Reddy V, Duran J, Ciccolini K. Incidence and risk of xerosis with targeted anticancer therapies. *J Am Acad Dermatol.* 2015;72(4):656–67.
12. Telang PS. Vitamin C in dermatology. *Indian Dermatol Online J.* 2013;4(2):143–6.
13. Dayan SH, Arkins JP, Patel AB, Gal TJ. A double-blind, randomized, placebo-controlled health-outcomes survey of the effect of botulinum toxin type A injections on quality of life and self-esteem. *Dermatol Surg.* 2010;36:2088–97.
14. Shammban A. Safety and efficacy of facial rejuvenation with small gel particle hyaluronic acid with lidocaine and abobotulinumtoxin A in post-chemotherapy patients in a phase IV investigator-initiated Study. *Clinical L Aesthetic Dermatology.* 2014;7(1):31–6.
15. Kassir M, Gupta M, Galadari H, Kroumpouzos G, Katsambas A, Lotti T, Vojvodic A, Grabbe S, Juchems E, Goldust M. Complicaciones de la toxina botulínica y sus rellenos: Revisión narrativa. *J Cosmet Dermatol.* 2020;19:570–3.
16. Nam E, Kim S et al. Ann Rehabil. Botulinum toxin type A injection for neuropathic pain in a patient with a brain tumor: A case report. *Med.* 2017;41(6):1088–92.
17. Funt D, Pavicic T. Rellenos dérmicos en estética: Una visión general de los eventos adversos y los enfoques de tratamiento. *Clin Cosmet Investig Dermatol.* 2013;6: 295–316.

18

Filler Materials: Indications, Contraindications, and Special Considerations in Oncology Patients

Paloma Tejero

Introduction

The use of fillers in oncological patients is widely accepted as an adjuvant to prevent the risk of therapies such as radiotherapy [1] or chemotherapy [2]; they have also been used in the reconstructive approach, especially in the breast, where there are great controversies [3], and in the repair of scars [4].

However, there are hardly any studies on treatment in these patients, and there is some concern about the use of fillers to improve their aesthetic problems and signs of aging. An increasing number of cancer survivors want to recover their self-image and demand these treatments, which requires a physician to review products, treatments, and techniques to apply them to these patients. We currently know that fillers can produce inflammatory reactions and immune reactions even in healthy patients [5], which causes concern for an oncology patient who can also be undergoing treatments that interfere with the response.

It is also important to remember that there are cancer patients who were treated with filler materials before their diagnosis, so it is necessary to know what interaction their presence can have, especially in the case of permanent materials, with the diagnostic methods [6], and whether the presence of the disease and its treatments will influence the response of the tissues to the implanted material.

Hyaluronic acid (HA) is a major component in the extracellular matrix, and there is increasing evidence that the high concentration of HA in the extracellular matrix in tumors is related to poor prognosis in patients with advanced cancer, because HA creates a "specific microenvironment" [7] that is favorable for tumor angiogenesis, invasion, and metastasis.

This raises several questions that oblige doctors to investigate and work as a team to be able to respond to the demand of patients who request treatments with fillers.

Objectives

A. Know the different types of dermal filler materials that are in the market and their indications and contraindications.

B. Assess the possible interactions with cancer treatments.

C. Discern which is the best option depending on the stage of the disease and indication.

D. Prevent complications and adverse effects and resolve them if they occur.

Filling Materials

Implanting is the action of introducing a foreign element into the organism. An immediate or innate immune response can develop against the implant, which normally limits itself if there are no adjuvant factors, although it can progress in an overlapping manner to manifest itself late, thus developing a specific immune response (granulomas) [8]. All filler materials are foreign elements, but the response will depend on the physical-chemical properties of the product, the technique in which it has been used, and the response of the recipient [9].

The feature that best defines the possible response is the permanence of the implant in the tissues, which is why we classify them as resorbable or nonpermanent fillers and nonresorbable fillers, although there is increasing evidence that some fillers considered as resorbable are found in the tissues long after expected, depending on their characteristics.

A thorough medical examination includes carrying out an exhaustive medical history of the current situation of the patient, his or her immunological competence, and the state of the area that we are going to treat. Even so, we must not forget that it is always the oncologist who must give his or her approval in case of doubt.

As general considerations before performing any aesthetic-medical procedure, we must confirm certain clinical and analytical data:

- Good general condition of the patient, which guarantees the correct response to the different treatments.
- Hemoglobin of 10 g/dL, which ensures the repair process occurs without complications; with less than this amount, the oxygenation of the tissues will be deficient.
- Neutrophil count: 50,000–80,000/mm^3
- Normal platelet count greater than 100,000/mm^3

We must remember that many of our patients, before being diagnosed, have undergone aesthetic-medical treatments that in some way may also be affected by different cancer treatments or may interfere with the results of some diagnostic tests. For example, patients with long-term implants such as polyalkylimides (Bio-Alcamid) or polyacrylamides (Aquamid) can present cases of infection and even biofilm formation due to alterations in the immune system, despite having the implant for years in the tissue [10–12].

On the other hand, calcium hydroxyapatite carriers should warn the professional when performing certain tests, because the image will be hyperintense on computed tomography (CT), will appear as hypermetabolic in ^{18}F-fludeoxyglucose–positron emission tomography (FDG-PET), and will have an intermediate signal intensity in magnetic resonance imaging (MRI), which will be a possible cause of a false-positive interpretation.

The main fillers commonly used are discussed in the next sections.

Hyaluronic Acid

HA is the most used product in our practice.

This is synthesized in the cell membrane of many of our cells, such as fibroblasts, endothelial cells, synovial cells, muscle fibers, oocytes, and by the synthases Has1, Has2, and Has3, and then extruded out of the cell. It is metabolized by endocytosis mediated by receptors and by specific enzymes, hyaluronidases, which degrade it. Its catabolism is very fast, lasting on average in our tissues between 12 hours and a few days. Inflammatory processes increase its catabolism. The concentration of HA in the tissues usually remains constant, and the residency time is only slightly dependent on its molecular weight.

The cellular interaction of HA is mediated by the CD44 receptor. This receptor has a wide tissue distribution and is responsible for modulating cellular metabolism, particularly in synoviocytes and hematopoietic cells. This association between the HA and the CD44 receptor can explain the apparent ability of HA to modulate the inflammatory response, pain, normalization of GAG (glycosaminoglycans) and production of PG (prostaglandins), cellular metabolism, and stimulation of cellular cleanliness of oxygen free radicals [14,15]. Not all products with HA are the same, but all are formed by chains of polymers of glucuronic acid and *N*-acetylglucosamine disaccharides. This molecule is repeated several times, differentiating itself because it is the only nonsulfated polymer, which gives it rigidity and linearity.

HA plays an important role in the physiology of normal tissue but also intervenes in inflammatory processes, resistance to certain medications, processes of angiogenesis and tumorigenesis, homeostasis and cellular mobility, and changes in the viscosity of the extracellular matrix. These activities will depend on the size of HA and cell receptors.

It has been estimated that the half-life of HA in the skin is approximately 24 hours, in the eye 24–36 hours, in the cartilage 1–3 weeks, and in the vitreous humor 70 days. One of the properties of HA is its ability to degrade into safe products, CO_2, and water.

There is a delicate balance between production by synthetase and degradation by hyaluronidases and oxidative processes, which condition the composition in HA of the extracellular space; the balance of HA varies according to specific cells and tissues and in normal and pathological conditions.

In addition, before complete degradation, you can see the following:

- *High-molecular-weight HA fragments in heavy chains*: Mw (Mw >500 kDa) are "space-filling" molecules involved in normal biological processes, with anti-angiogenic and "immunosuppressive" properties.

Generally, they are associated with inhibition of cell differentiation by suppressing cell-cell interactions or by binding to cell surface receptors.

- *Shorter fragments of HA (Mw = 20–200 kDa)*: These have pro-inflammatory activity, immunostimulants, and angiogenic properties.

For aesthetic medicine, we use HA synthesized by genetic engineering techniques in bacteria. The main difference is the length of the HA chain, which is lower in the derivative of nonanimal origin (10,000–15,000 monomer units per chain in animal origin versus 4000–6000 per chain in nonanimal origin). The process involves fermentation bacteria, which reduces the antigenic risk and its ability to produce hypersensitivity reactions. It is vital to have proper manufacturing for a safe raw material that meets the standards of the European Pharmacopoeia, which is then handled and distributed safely [16]. For the different types, a cross-linking process (see later) adds substances such as butanediol diglycidyl ether (BDDE) that have demonstrated their safety at the doses used. From the first patented products from QMed in 1987 to the present day, different manufacturing processes have led to about 200 HA products being currently registered with AGEMED (the Spanish Medicines and Medical Devices Agency).

Synthetic HA has a variable duration of months to years; their molecular weight is very varied. Our body can absorb HA in a variable time after subcutaneous injection, by enzymatic digestion, or through disintegration with facial mimicry movements. The time it takes to be eliminated directly influences the duration of treatment and has individual variability, in addition to being influenced by lifestyle (smoking habit, alcohol intake, sun exposure) [17]. Most of the HAs currently used last between 2 and 18 months, depending on the complexity and molecular weight of the implanted molecule, although it has been reported to be present more than 10 years after being implanted (and we have verified its presence). With the use of ultrasound, we can modify the concept of duration of HA, and distinguish instead between permanence of HA in the tissue and the duration of treatment effectiveness, which is usually much shorter.

The physicochemical properties of HA—its solubility and the availability of reactive functional groups—facilitate performing chemical modifications to obtain biocompatible materials for use in tissue regeneration. Bioscaffolds and dermal injectables are manufactured in different forms including hydrogels, tubes, meshes, among others [18]. One of these modifications is the so-called cross-linking, which consists of the union of several HA molecules, generating bonds difficult to separate by hyaluronidases, thus increasing the time of permanence in the tissue. Each commercial company uses a cross-linking method, but all coincide in the use of cross-linking agents such as BDDE or divinyl sulfone (DVD). Although they are toxic products, the dose used is very low and guarantees their safety [19]. In addition, the competition to achieve the ideal filler has caused other substances such as mannitol, dextranomers, lidocaine, and so on, to be added in order to attribute better properties to the implant.

The HA have a natural antidote—hyaluronidase, an enzyme that opportunely absorbs only the injected HA, restoring the pretreatment situation in a short time interval in most cases, without affecting the HA present in the body. The hyaluronidase injection is approved by the U.S. Food and Drug Administration as a temporary drug dispersion agent for joining the HA between the C1 of an *N*-acetylglucosamine molecule, and the glucuronic C4; however, its action as an agent that degrades HA is today an "off-label" indication, despite evidence of its effectiveness, in the reversal of HA fillers. It is important to remember, as Rao [20] points out, that due to the different biochemical compositions of the different HA products, each product can respond differently to hyaluronidase.

Methylcellulose

This is widely used as a vehicle in many fillers (polycaprolactone, hydroxyapatite). At present, a material based on the crosslinking of methylcellulose has been marketed under the name Erelle. Its main advantage is that we have an enzyme, cellulase, capable of degrading it, and that it can be used in the event of an adverse reaction, although that indication is also off-label and difficult to achieve.

This is a material for which we also have some studies linked to the cancer patient, exploring its possible role in the prevention of adverse effects after radiotherapy [21–23]. Some authors consider it a safe alternative to HA [24], although it does not have the same number of studies, experience, and versatility. However, in the cancer patient, it could have as an additional advantage that it does not join the CD44 receptor or is present in the tumor microenvironment.

Calcium Hydroxyapatite

The reason for interest in the use of these substances is simple: calcium hydroxyapatite (CHA) is the major component of the mineral part of bone and dental tissue, so it is expected that materials prepared from this substance will be more biocompatible when implanted in bone. It is a product synthetically formed as one of the bioceramics, which involves the ionic binding of calcium and phosphate. It becomes an integral part of living tissue and is the most commonly used calcium phosphate biomaterial.

Calcium phosphate ceramics have been used as implant materials in bone tissue for approximately 30 years. The first application of these as bone substitutes is attributed to Albee (1920) with the use of calcium phosphate compounds in bone defects to promote osteogenesis and the formation of new bone. CHA implants are calcium phosphate compounds, which, like others of the same composition, are used essentially to increase bone parts; subsequently, its use has been extended into specialties such as stomatology, surgery, and orthopedics. In Spain, the first filler product to be marketed was Radiesse, composed of microspheres (of 25–45 nm) suspended in glycerin and sodium hydroxycellulose gel. Currently, there are other products marketed, as well as a presentation that includes CHA and HA; however, we do not have experience to evaluate them.

CHA acts by generating a foreign body–type reaction, where the carrier compound is absorbed between 6 and 8 weeks, with the phagocytized and encapsulated CHA preventing its migration. This waterfall stimulates neocollagenogenesis, guaranteeing longevity between 2 and 5 years. It has FDA approval for correction of oral and maxillofacial defects, vocal cord insufficiency, and tissue radiographic marking, as well as for treatment in HIV-induced lipodystrophy. The size of the particles, the porosity of the material, its composition, and the tissue in which it is inserted influence the speed of resorption.

Its use as a treatment for HIV-associated lipoatrophy is relatively recent, so there are still no data on its long-term safety, especially in the amounts used for lipoatrophy corrections. Overcorrection must be avoided due to the capacity for formation of palpable nodules of bone consistency. The rate of formation of labial nodules is relatively high, so it should not be used in this region. Its use is more indicated in correction of deep wrinkles. It is also widely used in bioplasty and rhinomodelation techniques.

Numerous studies have shown that soft tissue CHA implants, such as in facial tissue, remain soft and in place for long periods of time. Unlike implants based on silicone, polytetrafluoroethylene, and similar materials, CHA particles undergo degradation through the same metabolic pathways as the bone fragments that remain after a common fracture over a period of time: they undergo degradation by dissolution in the aqueous environment and dissolve from the outside to the inside, and the remaining submicron unit is reduced to calcium and phosphate ions at the site of the original particle. These ions are subjected to normal homeostatic processes.

It should be remembered that CHA is visible on x-rays, and patients should be informed if they require a radiological study; it also produces changes in MRI and CT scans and may lead to false positives.

We have not found reports or experience on the use of other resorbable materials such as polylactic acid, agarose, polycaprolactone, or other materials in the oncologic patient.

Permanent Materials

There are currently several permanent, authorized and marketed products, despite the severe adverse effects that may occur. The main ones are methacrylates, silicones, and alkylamides. In 1991, the FDA declared the use of injectable silicone illegal; however, silicone oil is still widely used in some countries. It is important to be aware of them, even if they are not used, because many patients come to our consultations having been implanted with these products and, on many occasions, bearing the consequences of the adverse effects they have produced.

There is also a whole group of unauthorized substances injected without proper medical guidance that are part of the syndrome we know as "iatrogenic allogenosis." In relation to the oncological patient, the main problem is the possible interaction with diagnostic methods [26], although there is also suspicion that the chronic inflammation the patient maintains may promote the triggering of cell mutations. Some articles on the use of polyacrylamide in breast reconstruction guarantee its safety, and although there is reaction to a foreign body and chronic inflammation, no atypia or changes to stromal malignancy have been found [27].

Silicone can interfere with diagnosis and is similar to some granulomas, with metastases that require biopsy. The appearance of a type of anaplastic large cell lymphoma in relation to silicone breast implants is known [28].

Comprehensive study is mandatory in patients with ruptured silicone prostheses [29]. Although the use of liquid silicone for breast augmentation is now prohibited, it is still used illegally. Although very rare, carcinomas on granulomas have been described [30].

Indications for Use of Fillers in Cancer Patients

The main aesthetic indication is the correction of the signs of aging and the changes in volume that may occur as a result of the disease, such as loss of volume in the upper facial third, in the temporal zone, or in the area of the dark circles due to weight loss. In the lower two-thirds, we will see increases in volume generated by corticosteroid treatment [31], alterations of the fatty compartments, and decrease in the malar fatty compartment due to weight loss. We use dermal filler implants as the main therapy for facial volume in aesthetic medicine, with materials that generate a mechanical filling effect providing an improvement of facial volume. In order to perform these treatments, we should be sure of the patient's immunological competence, thoroughly review the patient's history, contact the oncologist if the patient has not finished the treatment, and assess the possible interaction of possible medications.

The most recommended material would be autologous fat (lipofilling, for which see Chapter 1), but resorbable materials such as HA can also be used. We have only found one author (Shamban) [33] who endorses the use of HA as filler material for aesthetic purposes, but in my personal experience, when well indicated, it is a safe treatment that improves the quality of life of patients.

We should observe the usual precautions and care that we would have with any patient, taking a thorough clinical history, confirming that enough time has passed for the skin to have recovered from the sequels of cancer treatments, and monitoring the immunocompetency state to prevent infectious complications. On the other hand and in the case of patients who are being treated with bisphosphonates, due to the reduction in blood supply, decreased bone turnover, and bacterial aggression of the oral flora that will favor the appearance of osteonecrosis in these patients, it seems prudent not to perform any type of treatment that puts fillers or other compounds in contact with bone.

Patients under anticoagulant treatment with subcutaneous heparin of low molecular weight can undergo interventional procedures, taking precautions during the procedure and making sure that they do not leave the consultation until we are certain that there is no active bleeding. There is no absolute contraindication, but it is recommended that the physician assess the risk-benefit balance of the intervention.

In general, the patient with a port-a-cath does not present an express contraindication for aesthetic-medical treatment, so long as the implant area is avoided [32].

Other important indications include the application of dermal fillers with HA to correct atrophic scars after cancer surgery [34,35].

HA has been used in the treatment of vaginal dryness and atrophy, through the topical application of intravaginal gels whose main function, due to its high hydrophilic power, is simply to hydrate. Since 2014, it has been used as a cross-linked HA gel for rejuvenation of the vulvovaginal area: It is used in the vestibule area, labia majora for correction of hypotrophy, and vaginal mucosa for rehydration and biostimulation of the middle to deep dermis. It restores the volume, rehydrates the skin and the mucosa, due to its hygroscopic effect, and stimulates the fibroblasts (favoring the synthesis of collagen) of the labia majora, the vestibule, and/or the vagina [36]. It can be considered a good treatment alternative for vulvovaginal atrophy (VVA) and atrophy of the labia majora pending further studies [25].

Contraindications

The main contraindication would be its use in the following:

- Oncological patients who do not meet the immunocompetence requirements that we have established so do not present the good general condition that guarantees their response to treatment.
- Patients under treatment with systemic chemotherapy in general, until they have finished the treatment (the approval of treatment by the oncologist is advised).
- Patients with drugs that alter the immune response, and in chemotherapies such as those performed with kinase inhibitors. Hibler et al. describe the case of a patient who presented facial edema and nodule formation with granulomatous reaction to a foreign body when starting treatment with tyrosine kinase inhibitors (neratinib) in the cheekbones area, where a year earlier, it had been treated with HA [13]; the authors conclude by saying that "doctors who evaluate patients with facial nodules/swelling and a history of cosmetic procedures should be aware that late reactions to fillers are possible."
- Patients under treatment with radiotherapy; it should not be used on skin with radiodermatitis.
- Anticoagulated patients, although in some heparinized patients it can be used with caution after assessing the risk-benefit ratio.

There is a relative contraindication to the use of bisphosphonates. Physicians must also take care in conjunction with hormonal therapies and corticosteroid treatments.

It is essential to maximize aseptic conditions due to the increased risk of infection in these patients.

Prevention and Treatment of Complications and Adverse Effects

The main preventive measure is carrying out a proper clinical history, which allows us to know the suitability of the patient.

Even so, as we have seen, granulomatous reactions to the foreign body may appear and nodule formation in patients carrying filler materials, which will require the usual treatment, including corticosteroids, surgical excision, and/or hyaluronidase injection, if the material is hyaluronic acid (HA).

It is essential to maximize aseptic conditions due to the increased risk of infection in these patients.

Conclusions

Resorbable fillers such as HA and methylcellulose can be used in an oncological patient, but their use must be determined by their state of health and time of illness, and an individual evaluation should always be done.

Studies are needed that allow us to evaluate the safety of products such as HA in these patients and the possible development of HA as a therapeutic agent in these patients.

REFERENCES

1. Guimas V, Quivrin M, Bertaut A, Martin E, Chambade D, Maingon P, Mazoyer F, Cormier L, and Créhange G. Focal or whole-gland salvage prostate brachytherapy with iodine seeds with or without a rectal spacer for postradiotherapy local failure: How best to spare the rectum? *Brachytherapy.* 2016;15(4):406–11.

2. Zhao G, Yan G, Cheng J, Zhou X, Fang T, Sun H, Hou Y, and Hu Y. Hyaluronic acid prevents immunosuppressive drug-induced ovarian damage via up-regulating PGRMC1 expression. *Sci Rep.* 2015;5:7647.

3. McCleave MJ. Is breast augmentation using hyaluronic acid safe? *Aesthetic Plast Surg.* 2010;34(1):65–8; discussion 69–70. Epub 2009 Dec 5.

4. Hasson A, and Romero WA. Treatment of facial atrophic scars with Esthélis, a hyaluronic acid filler with polydense cohesive matrix (CPM). *J Drugs Dermatol.* 2010;9(12):1507–9.

5. Wollina U, and Goldman A. Dermal fillers: Facts and controversies. *Clin Dermatol.* 2013;31(6):731–6.

6. Feeney JN, Fox JJ, Akhurst T et al. Radiological impact of the use of calcium hydroxylapatite dermal fillers. *Clin Radiol.* 2009;64(9):897–902. Epub 2009 Jul 5.

7. Chanmee T, Ontong P, and Itano N. Hyaluronan: A modulator of the tumor microenvironment. *Cáncer Lett.* 2016;375(1):20–30. Epub 2016 24 de febrero. 28 de mayo de.

8. Ercilla Gonzalez G. Informe de bioseguridad inmunológica de implantes: ácido hialurònico. *SEME.* 2010;24:7–13.

9. Tejero P. Efectos secundarios de los implantes tisulares Tesis doctoral UCM 2013.

10. Christensen L, Breiting V, Bjarnsholt T et al. Bacterial infection as a likely cause of adverse reactions to polyacrylamide hydrogel fillers in cosmetic surgery. *Clin Infect Dis.* 2013;56:1438–44.

11. Bjarnsholt T, Tolker-Nielsen T, Givskov M, Janssen M, and Chrsitensen L. Detection of bacteria by FISH in culture-negative soft tissue filler lesions. *Dermatol Surg.* 2009;35:1620–4.

12. Pallua N, and Wolter T. A 5-year assessment of safety and aesthetic results after facial soft-tissue augmentation with polyacrylamide hydrogel (Aquamid): A prospective multicenter study of 251 patients. *Plast Reconstr Surg.* 2010;125:1797–804.

13. Hibler BP, Yan BY, Marchetti MA, Momtahen S, Busam KJ, and Rossi AM. Facial swelling and foreign body granulomatous reaction to hyaluronic acid filler in the setting of tyrosine kinase inhibitor therapy. *J Eur Acad Dermatol Venereol.* 2018;32(6):e225–7. Epub 2018 Jan 3.

14. Day AJ, and de la Motte CA. Hyaluronan cross-linking: A protective mechanism in inflammation. *Trends Immunol.* 2005;26:637–43.

15. Tian X, Azpurua J, Hine C, Vaidya A, Myakishev-Rempel M, Ablaeva J, Mao Z, Nevo E, Gorbunova V, and Seluanov A. High-molecular-mass hyaluronan mediates the cancer resistance of the naked mole rat. *Nature.* 2013;499:346–9.

16. Aguilar Donis A. et al. Filler materials: A review. *DCMQ.* 2015;13(1).

17. Marinelli E, Montanari Vergallo G, Reale G, di Luca A, Catarinozzi I, Napoletano S, and Zaami S. The role of fillers in aesthetic medicine: Medico-legal aspects. *Eur Rev Med Pharmacol Sci.* 2016;20(22):4628–34.

18. Hemshekhar M et al. Emerging roles of hyaluronic acid bioscaffolds in tissue engineering and regenerative medicine/*International Journal of Biological Macromolecules* 86 (2016) 917–928. *Clin Cosmet Investig Dermatol.* 2017;10:239–47.

19. De Boulle K, Glogau R, Kono T, Nathan M, Tezel A, Roca-Martinez JX, Paliwal S, and Stroumpoulis D. A review of the metabolism of 1,4-butanediol diglycidyl ether-cross-linked hyaluronic acid dermal fillers. *Dermatol Surg.* 2013;39(12):1758–66. Epub 2013 Aug 13.

20. Rao V, Chi S, and Woodward J. Reversing facial fillers: Interactions between hyaluronidase and commercially available hyaluronicacid based fillers. *J Drugs Dermatol.* 2014;13(9):1053–6.

21. Patel R, Modi PK, Elsamra SE, and Kim IY. Long-term outcomes of using hyaluronic acid-carboxymethylcellulose adhesion barrier film on the neurovascular bundle. *J Endourol [Internet].* 2016;30(6):709–13. Available from: http://online.liebertpub.com/doi/10.1089/end.2016.0046

22. Tan A, Argenta P, Ramirez R, Bliss R, and Geller M. The use of Sodium Hyaluronate–Carboxymethylcellulose (HA-CMC) barrier in gynecologic malignancies: A retrospective review of outcomes. *Ann Surg Oncol [Internet].* 2009;16(2):499–505. Available from: http://www.springerlink.com/index/10.1245/s10434-008-0235-1

23. Yang EJ, Kang E, Jang JY et al. Effect of a mixed solution of sodium hyaluronate and carboxymethyl cellulose on upper limb dysfunction after total mastectomy: A double-blind, randomized clinical trial. *Breast Cancer Res Treat [Internet].* 2012;136(1):187–94. Available from: http://link.springer.com/10.1007/s10549-012-2272-5

24. D'Aloiso MC, Senzolo M, and Azzena B. Efficacy and safety of cross-linked carboxymethylcellulose filler for rejuvenation of the lower face: A 6-month prospective open-label study. *Dermatol Surg.* 2016;42(2):209–17.

25. Berreni N, Marès P, Tan N, and Couchourel D. Correction of female genital deficiencies through a new specific product range of hyaluronic acid gels. *IMCA Scientific Program.* 2014;85(1):2014.

26. Phan SyO, Rouchy RC, De Leiris N, Nika E, and Djaileb L. FDG PET/CT of a supraclavicular silicone granuloma at follow-up of a breast carcinoma. *Clin Nucl Med.* 2020;45(3):e169–e170. doi: 10.1097/RLU.0000000000002894. [Epub ahead of print].

27. Leung KM, Yeoh GP, and Chan KW. Breast pathology in complications associated with polyacrylamide hydrogel (PAAG) mammoplasty. *Hong Kong Med J.* 2007;13(2):137–40.

28. Yim N, Parsa F, and Faringer P. The first confirmed case of breast implant-associated anaplastic large cell lymphoma in Hawaii Hawaii. *J Health Soc Welf.* 2019;78(11):338–40.

29. Sutton EJ, Dashevsky BZ, Watson EJ et al. Incidence of benign and malignant peri-implant fluid collections and masses on magnetic resonance imaging in women with silicone implants. *Cancer Med.* 2019;00:1–7. https://doi.org/10.1002/cam4.2189

30. Nakahori R, Takahashi R, Akashi M, Tsutsui K, Harada S, Matsubayashi RN, Nakagawa S, Momosaki S, and Akagi Y. Breast carcinoma originating from a silicone granuloma: A case report. *World J Surg Oncol.* 2015;13:72.

31. Schiff D, Lee EQ, Nayak L, Norden AD, Reardon DA, and Wen PY. Medical management of brain tumors and the sequelae of treatment. *Neuro Oncol.* 2015;17(4):488–504.

32. Delltell Canales J, and Sanchez-Cañete Valenzuela M. Propuesta de protocolo de actuación del médico-estetico en el pacietne Oncológico. *TFM master de Calidad de vida y cuidados Medico-esteticos del paciente Oncologico.* UAH 2016.

33. Shamban AVA. Safety and efficacy of facial rejuvenation with small gel particle hyaluronic acid with lidocaine and Abobotulinumtoxin A in post-chemotherapy patients. *J Clin Aesthet Dermatol.* 2014;7(1):31–6.

34. Kasper DA, Cohen JL, Saxena A, and Morganroth GS. Fillers for postsurgical depressed scars after skin cancer reconstruction. *J Drugs Dermatol [Internet].* 2008;7(5):486–7. Available from: http://www.ncbi.nlm.nih.gov/pubmed/1850514

35. Cooper J, and Lee B. Treatment of facial scarring: Lasers, filler, and nonoperative techniques. *Facial Plast Surg [Internet].* 2009;25(5):311–5. Available from: http://www.thieme-connect.de/DOI/DOI?10.1055/s-0029-1243079

36. Gwrs. *Technical Brochure.* 2013;15. https://doi.org/10.1002/bapi.201390039

19

Aesthetic-Medical Treatments during the Disease: What Is the Plan?

Juana Deltell

According to the U.S. National Cancer Institute, the number of new cancer cases is estimated to increase to 23.6 million by 2030 [1], but we should not be pessimistic; thanks to great scientific progress, patient survival is growing at an annual rate of 1%, in many cases even reaching the stage of being considered "merely" a chronic disease [2]. This has changed the needs of oncological patients; cancer is no longer synonymous with death but, after the impact that the diagnosis has on them, patients must make a significant adaptive effort to confront and accept a series of physical, personal, and somewhat permanent changes that will condition their entire reality and that of the people around them [3]. Body image and aesthetic care are becoming increasingly important—even being demanded from the hospital [4]—and will represent a means of accepting or bearing the burden of the treatments and their side effects, providing patients with hope and optimism for the future and thereby improving their quality of life [5–7].

This means that aesthetic medicine must be included in the care of oncological patients from a scientific perspective, contributing to the recovery of health, the latter being defined by the World Health Organization as, "A state of complete physical, mental, and social well-being and not merely the absence of disease or infirmity" [8].

There is currently a trend toward the customization of the different treatments available, which variously combine drugs that are so new that some of their potential adverse effects are only just starting to be known; this makes the development of a general protocol for action complex, with the aesthetic doctor having to deal with each case individually based on expert consensus and his or her own personal experience, since in many cases there is no scientific evidence available [9]. In order to align that customized treatment with the patient's well-being and quality of life, an effective communication between the aesthetic doctor, the patient, and the oncologist during the whole process will be particularly important [10] because, in this disease, the oncologist becomes the "director of the orchestra" for a large number of professionals who will help meet all the patient's needs from a true multidisciplinary approach [9].

As shown in Figure 19.1, the oncological process is a continuum where all stages are related with one another, and through which we can accompany, guide, and advise patients about their best therapeutic options to take care of their aesthetic needs (see further Dulaney et al. [11]). Prevention is a constant at all times; we can also guide patients with recommendations to prevent the occurrence of new cancers and/or comorbidities, which are closely analyzed in chapters of this book.

Our action plan will always begin by properly preparing a medical history, in which will be included the most complete information gathered about the patient's current health status, as well as all aesthetic-medical procedures that were previously conducted. It is essential to request medical reports of their oncological process; however, we must be able to understand the different terms and know the several treatments, as well as speak a common language, which is fundamental to maintaining the previously mentioned communication between the aesthetic doctor, the patient, and the oncologist. In this respect, there are dictionaries of oncological terms for nononcologists that can make our interpretation of them easier [12].

If it is confirmed that a patient has undergone an aesthetic-medical procedure, such as permanent filler implant (regardless of the time of the implant) or resorbable implant (close to the start of the oncological treatment), the patient must be warned about the importance of telling his or her oncologist, since these procedures may interfere with the results of some diagnostic tests and even facilitate the occurrence of adverse effects that may complicate their progress. Those patients with long-lasting implants, such as polyalkylimides (Bio-Alcamid) or polyacrylamides (Aquamid), may present with infections and even formation of biofilm due to alterations of the immune system [16], despite it having been in the tissue for years without any issues; or those with liquid silicone implants, even if they got them over 25 years ago, may present with reactions to a foreign body after using immunotherapy [17]. Edematous and granulomatous reactions to a foreign body after treatment with tyrosine kinase inhibitors have recently been described in patients who underwent infiltration with hyaluronic acid months before receiving their cancer treatment [18]. We should also not forget that some oncological treatments and their different combinations are very recent, and we are just starting to see some of their middle- and long-term effects and interactions. Additionally, those with recent calcium hydroxyapatite implants must inform their health professional about them before certain tests, because these implants may appear hyperattenuated on computed tomography (CT) scans, hypermetabolic on ^{18}F-fludeoxyglucose–positron emission tomography (FDG-PET) scans, and with an intermediate signal intensity on magnetic resonance imaging (MRI), being a potential cause of a false-positive image [19].

After the history taking, it is essential to perform a proper exploration, since it is known that, during the oncological process, there are organs and body structures that will be more affected by the disease itself and/or by the several treatments; some of these belong to the field of action of the aesthetic doctor,

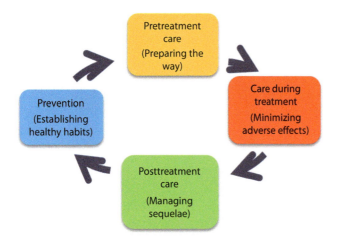

FIGURE 19.1 The continuum of aesthetic-medical treatment of cancer.

such as hair, skin, or nails, which play a significant cosmetic and functional role, with a psychological impact on patients to the extent that certain treatments are rejected due to the aesthetic impact they may have (e.g., about 8% of patients with breast cancer reject a treatment because they are afraid of losing their hair) [13].

We must expressly confirm the absence of toxicities generated by the different treatments, if the patient were undergoing any at that time; if these were at the skin level, Dreno et al. have proposed an action protocol that we could follow, which highlights the need to daily apply cosmetic moisturizers, as well as regularly use sun protection on photoexposed areas to keep the skin in its best state, always remembering to refer the patient to a dermatologist if toxicities reach a grade higher than 2 [14].

In the face, we will particularly assess those alterations that can be expected based on the patient's medical situation and treatments received, such as accelerated signs of aging [15] (most frequent), loss of volume in all thirds of the face, the presence of skin flaccidity, wrinkles, hyper- or hypopigmentations, or based on its sequelae, such as scarring, signs of radiodermatitis, and so on.

In the body, due to the metabolic stress that the organism is subject to, there will be about 40%–80% of cases associated with malnutrition [21], accompanied with an increase in morbidity/mortality, so it will be necessary to evaluate the body composition to provide relevant nutritional recommendations. During the exploration, we will confirm the lack of structures or the presence of devices such as stomas, prosthetics, catheters, and so on, since these clearly condition the selection of some of our body treatments.

Before we begin any aesthetic-medical procedure as part of that initial assessment, we will make sure that the patient's general status is good enough as to ensure a proper response to potential infections, as well as appropriate coagulation. If necessary, we will request supplementary tests (analytics, ultrasounds, etc.), although we will consult with the oncologist at the slightest doubt.

At the time of signing the informed consent, we must expressly warn our patients that we do not have a lot of scientific evidence to support the use of many of our usual treatments in them—and even less with the new oncological therapies—so the occurrence of adverse effects described earlier is feasible, forcing us to thoroughly weigh the risk-benefit balance of our procedures.

It is important to know what to do, but also to know and inform the patient about what not to do during the process of acute treatment, or while their skin status is not optimal; for example, the use of waxing; facial or body exfoliation; use of hair dyes, solvents, or decolorant; use of products with direct hormone activity on the affected organ; or use of fake eyelashes and fingernails, among other general recommendations [13,20].

Therefore, aesthetic doctors must know the oncological treatments and their potential adverse effects, how to act in each case, when to refer the patient to a specialist, and all that while listening and meeting their patients' needs, which will significantly condition their quality of life (Figure 19.2).

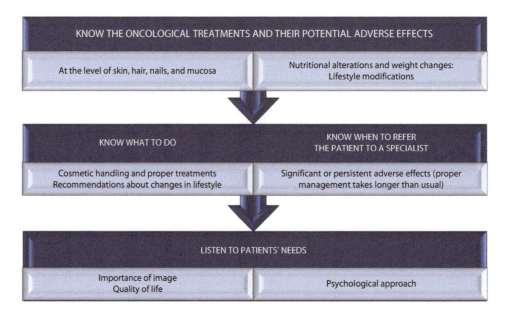

FIGURE 19.2 How must the aesthetic doctor proceed?

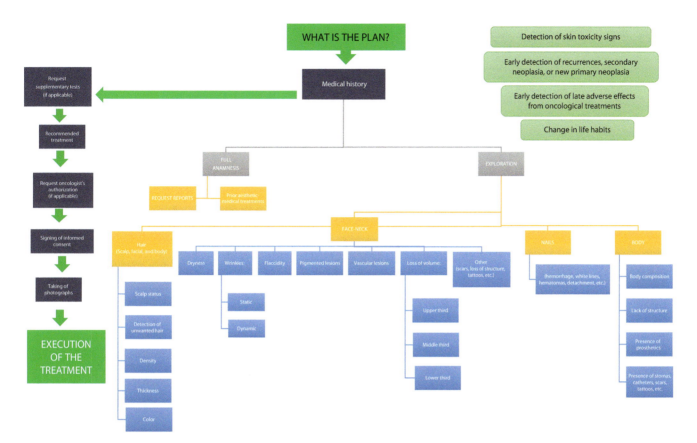

FIGURE 19.3 What is the plan?

In conclusion, we insist on the need to exhaustively assess each patient. A complete medical history is our fundamental tool to understand the reality of our patients, allowing us to guide them on the best solution for their aesthetic disorder. This solution is a part of the multidisciplinary approach of integral care that oncological patients require, and "oncological aesthetic medicine" is introduced as a response to the demands of patients themselves in order to reestablish and improve their quality of life with the highest scientific rigor [21]. See further Figure 19.3.

REFERENCES

1. Instituto Nacional del Cáncer de los Institutos nacionales de Salud de Estados Unidos (NIH). Estadísticas del cáncer. Naturaleza del cáncer. [cited 2019 Jan 27]. Available from: https://www.cancer.gov/espanol/cancer/naturaleza/estadisticas

2. Phillips JL, Currow DC. Cancer as a chronic disease. *Collegian.* 2010;17(2):47–50. Available from: http://dx.doi.org/10.1016/j.colegn.2010.04.007

3. Solana C. Aspectos psicológicos en el paciente superviviente. *Oncol.* 2005;28(3):157–63.

4. Amiel P, Dauchy S, Bodin J et al. Evaluating beauty care provided by the hospital to women suffering from breast cancer: Qualitative aspects. *Support Care Cancer.* 2009;17(7):839–45.

5. Hidalgo DA, Baranski J, Sinno S. Aesthetic surgery in patients with lung cancer. *Plast Reconstr Surg - Glob Open.* 2016 Oct;4(10):e1086. Available from: http://insights.ovid.com/crossref?an=01720096-201610000-00004

6. Di Mattei VE, Carnelli L, Taranto P et al. Health in the mirror: An unconventional approach to unmet psychological needs in oncology. *Front Psychol.* 2017 September;8:Available from: http://journal.frontiersin.org/article/10.3389/fpsyg.2017.01633/full

7. Tischer B, Huber R, Kraemer M, Lacouture ME. Dermatologic events from EGFR inhibitors: The issue of the missing patient voice. *Support Care Cancer.* 2017;25(2):651–60. Available from: http://dx.doi.org/10.1007/s00520-016-3419-4

8. OMS. Preguntas más frecuentes. WHO. 2017 [cited 2017 Dec 10]; Available from: http://www.who.int/suggestions/faq/es/#.Wiz5Q9H-iIc.mendeley

9. Shapiro CL. Cancer Survivorship. *N Engl J Med.* 2018 Dec 20;379(25):2438–50. Longo DL, editor. Available from: http://www.nejm.org/doi/10.1056/NEJMra1712502

10. de Cáceres Zurita M, Ruiz Mata F, Germà Lluch J, Busques C. Manual para el paciente oncológico y su familia. 2007;201 p. Available from: http://fecma.vinagrero.es/documentos/pacientes.pdf

11. Dulaney C, Wallace AS, Everett AS, Dover L, McDonald A, Kropp L. Defining health across the cancer continuum. *Cureus.* 2017 Feb 15;9:Available from: http://www.cureus.com/articles/6377-defining-health-across-the-cancer-continuum

12. Lacosta P, Ramos M, Ugarte L. *Diccionario de términos oncológicos para los no oncólogos.* Edición Punto D, ed. Madrid; 2018, 178.

13. Sibaud V, Delord J-P, Robert C. *Dermatología de los tratamientos contra el cáncer.* Guía práctica. Editions P. 31080 Toulouse Cedex 6;2015;231 p.

14. Dreno B, Bensadoun RJ, Humbert P et al. Algorithm for dermocosmetic use in the management of cutaneous side-effects
associated with targeted therapy in oncology. *J Eur Acad
Dermatol Venereol* 2013;27(9):1071–80.

15. Cupit-Link MC, Kirkland JL, Ness KK et al. Biology of premature ageing in survivors of cancer. *ESMO Open.* 2017 Nov
18;2(5):e000250. Available from: http://esmoopen.bmj.com/
lookup/doi/10.1136/esmoopen-2017-000250

16. Rostom M, Brendling L, Stewart K. Bio-Alcamid complications: A 10 year review. *J Plast Reconstr Aesthetic Surg.*
2019;72(5):848–62. doi:10.1016/j.bjps.2018.12.047.

17. Bisschop C, Bruijn MS, Stenekes MW, Diercks GFH, Hospers
GAP. Foreign body reaction triggered by cytotoxic T lympho-
cyte-associated protein 4 blockade 25 years after dermal filler
injection. *Br J Dermatol.* 2016;175(6):1351–3. doi:10.1111/
bjd.14674

18. Hibler BP, Yan BY, Marchetti MA, Momtahen S, Busam KJ,
Rossi AM. Facial swelling and foreign body granulomatous
reaction to hyaluronic acid filler in the setting of tyrosine
kinase inhibitor therapy. *J Eur Acad Dermatol Venereol* 2018
Jun;32(6):e225–7. doi: 10.1111/jdv.14749. Epub 2018 Jan 3.
PMID: 29224214; PMCID: PMC6685169.

19. Feeney JN, Fox JJ, Akhurst T. Radiological impact of the use
of calcium hydroxylapatite dermal fillers. *Clin Radiol.* 2009
Sep;64(9):897–902. doi: 10.1016/j.crad.2009.05.004. Epub
2009 Jul 5. PMID: 19664480.

20. Jaén P, Truchuélo MT, Sanmartin O, Soto J. Dermatosis
frecuentes en oncología y su cuidado específico. In: AEDV
(Asociación Española de Dermatología y Venereología)
AECC (Asociación Española Contra el Cáncer). El cáncer
y la piel. Guía de cuidados dermatológicos del paciente
oncológico [Internet]. 2012. p. 11–21. Available from: http://
gedet.aedv.es/wp-content/uploads/2015/09/El_cancer_y_la_
piel.pdf

21. Deltell J, Lacosta P, Mota S, Tejero P. Medicina Estética
Oncológica: Retos y futuro. *Rev EME (Expertos en Med
Estética).* 2017;19:60–4. Available from: http://www.gemeon.
org/retos-y-futuro/

20

The Role of the Aesthetic Doctor in Follow-Up of the Oncology Patient

Sheila K. Mota Antigua

Oncological disease affects all spheres of life for the patient—the physical, emotional, social, and occupational—causing changes that could be temporary or permanent, resulting in the oncological patient having to adapt to his or her new life and then start a recovery phase.

Aesthetic medicine can influence this group in terms of aesthetics, image, quality of life in general, and prevention, depending on the stage of the disease, as follows:

1. If the patient has already gone through the active phase of treatment, we can intervene for *the recovery of the image and treat those setbacks* that have been generated as a result of the treatments.

2. Before starting the antineoplastic therapies and during treatment, the aesthetic doctor can intervene by carrying out actions that will *improve the image and quality of life* of the patient.

3. Another action for the aesthetic doctor who works with cancer patients is to *help in the prevention and early detection of recurrences and other primary tumors* as well as to positively influence the *prevention and elimination of risk factors.*

Image Recovery and Treatment of Aesthetic Problems

Cancer therapies such as radiotherapy, chemotherapy, hormone therapy, immunotherapy, targeted therapies, and surgical interventions can leave temporary or permanent sequelae in cancer patients, and it is here that aesthetic medicine plays its main role in trying to restore the patient's image prior to the disease through minimally invasive aesthetic-medical procedures.

Aesthetic-medical intervention can be performed in three moments:

- Before starting antineoplastic therapies, minimizing the occurrence of adverse effects, such as by performing micropigmentation of eyebrows to cope with their falling out or recommend the use of the cooling helmet during the chemotherapy to minimize the hair loss.

- During antineoplastic treatments, taking care of the skin and skin adnexa: we refrain from performing aggressive procedures or ones that may interfere with the antineoplastic therapies the patients receive, but we do undertake a dermocosmetic protocol to preventing and treating, if necessary, dermatological adverse effects caused by those therapies.

- After finishing the therapies, treating the adverse effects that may have presented: aesthetic-medical interventions will be performed, such as treatments for hyperpigmentation, improvement of skin quality, skin repair, volume replacement, among others.

Improvement of Quality of Life

Quality of life comprises the set of conditions that contribute to the well-being of individuals and the realization of their potential in social life, including both subjective and objective factors. Among the subjective factors is the perception by each individual of his or her well-being on a physical, psychological, and social level. The objective factors would be material well-being, health, and a harmonious relationship with the physical environment and the community [1].

For the World Health Organization, quality of life would imply a person's perception of his or her life situation in relation to context (culture and value system), goals, aspirations, and concerns [2].

Based on these definitions, we can emphasize the role of aesthetic medicine in improving quality of life in cancer patients through the implementation of nonpharmacological measures, lifestyle habits, and minimally invasive interventions aimed at recovering harmony lost because of the disease, which will provide the patient with well-being on a physical, psychological, and social level.

Prevention and Early Detection of Recurrences and New Primary Tumors

The aesthetic doctor who works with cancer patients should use part of his or her efforts to prevent recurrences and even eliminate risk factors that can trigger the appearance of a new tumor. This involves implementing measures such as a balanced diet, moderate exercise, sunscreen use, smoking cessation, decreased alcohol intake, dermatoscopic examination of skin lesions, and early detection of physiological or morphological alterations through recall, physical exploration, and complementary tests. The aesthetic doctor in most cases cares for healthy patients who want to improve facial, body, or hair aesthetics, but in many cases do not have frequent contact with their family physician, so it is somewhat common for the aesthetic doctor to be the first to detect certain anomalies and be responsible for referring the patient to other specialists for other assessments that are considered appropriate.

Prevention and Elimination of Risk Factors

The prevention and elimination of risk factors are aimed at both the cancer patient and the healthy patient. The aesthetic doctor's interventions will be made with the intention of preventing, eliminating, or reducing the risk factors related to life habits.

The prevention of obesity and overweight, combined with the implementation of healthy eating habits, will be two fundamental pillars of this intervention, since obesity is related to numerous chronic pathologies, such as hypertension, hypercholesterolemia, diabetes mellitus, among others, and with more than ten types of cancers.

Stopping smoking is another pillar of this intervention, since in addition to being a cause of premature aging, it is also associated with the appearance of cancer of the lung, larynx, and others.

The use of sunscreen and primary measures of sun protection, as well as the review of nevus and benign lesions, are habits that should be instilled in patients with the intention of preventing the appearance of premalignant lesions, such as actinic keratosis and malignant skin cancer (melanoma, squamous cell carcinoma, basal cell carcinoma, etc.). Frequent chemical peelings have also been associated according to various studies with the prevention of skin cancer [3–5]. The use of nutraceuticals and antioxidants by mouth, such as melatonin, has been shown to help prevent and treat some cancers [6–8].

The implementation of physical exercise as a prevention of pathologies and improvement of the musculoskeletal system is another of the measures developed by aesthetic doctors.

REFERENCES

1. Calidad de vida. 2017. Available at: https://www.significados.com/calidad-de-vida/ (Accessed Feb 2020).
2. Calidad de vida. Available at: https://www.ecured.cu/Calidad_de_vida. (Accessed Feb 2020).
3. Hakim IA, Harris RB, Ritenbaugh C. Citrus peel use is associated with reduced risk of squamous cell carcinoma of the skin. *Nutr Cancer.* 2000;37(2):161–8.
4. Abdel-Daim M, Funasaka Y, Kamo T et al. Preventive effect of chemical peeling on ultraviolet induced skin tumor formation. *J Dermatol Sci.* October 2010;60(1):21–28.
5. Nair SA, Rajani Kurup SR, Nair AS, Baby S. Citrus peels prevent cancer. *Phytomedicine.* 2018 Nov 15;50:231–237. Epub 2017 Aug 17.
6. Li Y, Li S, Zhou Y et al. Melatonin for the prevention and treatment of cáncer *Oncotarget* 2017 Jun 13;8(24):39896–39921.
7. Hanikoglu A, Kucuksayan E, Akduman RC, Ozben T. A review on melatonin's effects in cancer: Potential mechanisms. *Anticancer Agents Med Chem.* 2018;18(7):985–992.
8. Zhang L, He Y, Wu X et al. Melatonin and (−)-epigallocatechin-3-gallate: Partners in fighting cancer. *Cells* 2019 Jul;8(7):745. Published online 2019 Jul 19.

21

Medico-Aesthetic Collaboration

Margarita Esteban

Relation between the Aesthetician and the Aesthetic Doctor

An aesthetic doctor is a medical-aesthetic professional who uses minimally invasive, nonsurgical procedures to rejuvenate, maintain, or correct unsightly facial and body features. Their work is aimed at the promotion and maintenance of health, as well as the diagnosis of diseases.

The aesthetician is a nonmedical aesthetic professional who uses body procedures such as lymphatic drainage, facial treatments such as cleaning and moisturizing, and facial and body appliances to maintain the integrity of the aesthetic patient's image. The aesthetician must have the necessary knowledge for postmedical treatment care, but they must also have informed professional ethical principles to avoid intruding into the sphere of the medical-aesthetic doctor.

The relationship in daily practice between the aesthetic doctor and the aesthetician is essential, both in the use of knowledge and in the optimization of resources. In addition, continuous improvement in job performance is very important to ensure the best possible assistance, and service, and collaboration with all the professionals for the welfare of the population.

Differences between the Aesthetician and the Aesthetic Doctor

Both aesthetician and aesthetic doctor are professionals who work under very different administrations; aesthetic medicine belongs to the sphere of health, while aesthetics is included in that of the consumer. This administrative separation, at the population level, is more difficult to interpret, because both act on the human body.

Action limits are clearly differentiated both at the level of professionals who carry them out and at the level of the patients and users. The function of aesthetic medicine is the diagnosis and subsequent treatment, while the aesthetician is responsible for the care and maintenance of the body. Additionally, the aesthetician does not take part in diagnosis.

The border that limits and separates the aesthetic doctor and aesthetician consists of the training and the profession. The limits are clearer with better training on both sides, but it is necessary to emphasize the procedures performed by the aesthetician must

not cross the skin barrier. This means the aesthetician should not perform any type of invasive procedure (breaching the integrity of the skin barrier).

The most important difference in training is that the aesthetician is not prepared in the academic and technical way as is a graduate in medicine. A graduate in medicine has deep knowledge in anatomy, physiology, physiopathology, pharmacology, dermatology, and the principles of surgery, among others. The aesthetician will be aware of this knowledge and is generally instructed in anatomy, physiology, and dermatology, since the field of action includes the skin and adnexa, subcutaneous cellular tissue, and muscles. Obviously, scientific knowledge is needed to be able to know how patients should be treated, what active principles should be applied, and how to apply them depending on the need of the patient in the booth.

The aesthetician should therefore be dedicated only to care, beautification, and body maintenance; the diagnosis, treatment, and procedures that cross the skin barrier should be left at the hands of the aesthetic doctor; they have complementary actions, both at the beginning and at the end of the treatment.

Regulations

It is necessary to adequately regulate the designations of the aesthetician and the aesthetic doctor at a legal level, because any lack of legislation gives space to many unqualified people to carry out fraudulent practices that generally belong to other areas of aesthetic practice.

In some cases, the poor training they have leads to practices that in most cases have no beneficial result in the patient. Poorly trained professionals discredit the profession and reflect badly by association on professionals who are properly trained and accredited by educational and health authorities.

It should be noted that people carrying out these practices have easy access to laboratory products and aesthetic appliances. This situation leads to more people who want to work without any kind of training, which results in malpractice in the nonmedical aesthetic sector.

Therefore, in these matters, it is necessary to regulate not only the professional aesthetic doctor but also the entire sector of the aesthetic and cosmetic industry, laboratory products, and all the equipment that is required for a beauty center to function.

Definition of Aesthetic (Royal Spanish Language Academy)

1. Belonging to or related to aestheticism
2. Adept to aestheticism
3. Person who is professionally dedicated to aesthetics (a set of techniques for the beautification of the body)

Aesthetician is a word that comes from the French *esthéticien* which was later coined as a Gallicism "aesthetician."

Currently, the aesthetician is a professional who is responsible for the beautification of the human body, with special emphasis on the face.

A professional beautician is academically qualified to perform skin, hair, and nail analysis. Additionally, when performing the analysis, the aesthetician has the ability to establish the most appropriate treatments to the patient's need, since he or she has the necessary knowledge to do so. The field of action is very wide, from the manipulation of appliances or micropigmentation, to the realization of manual techniques such as massage, facials, lymphatic drainage, manicure, and clinical pedicure.

It is necessary to delimit the functions and limits of the beautician: "The beautician is the base of the pyramid of the aesthetic offer: he or she is the closest person to the aesthetic user, the one who advises, the one who introduces the first treatments, and the one who projects the future treatments to maintain the beauty. On his or her behalf, the work of the cosmetic doctor is aimed at the promotion and maintenance of health, as well as the diagnosis of diseases" [1].

A beautician is a professional trained in the area of the aesthetic and beauty, who carries out methods and techniques in a comprehensive manner to care for and beautify the body and facial image. The aesthetician's work is directed to the application of procedures and cosmetic treatments such as after-care aesthetic-medical treatments, lymphatic drainage, massages, body modeling, masks, and makeup and advice on cosmetic products. The aesthetician should also reiterate the explanation of the healthy habits that patients must take on posttreatments and promote services that offer an improvement of the corporal aspect.

Treatments Aestheticians Should Perform

- Provide hygiene, care, and maintenance of the skin of the face and body, as well as beautification.
- Carry out patient need analysis and skin analysis.
- Cleanse the skin and apply facial and body treatments.
- Apply aesthetic techniques of hygiene and facial and corporal hydration.
- Wax hair removal.
- Laser depilation and photoepilation.
- Perform aesthetic treatments of hands and feet, including manicure and pedicure.
- Install and maintain sculpted and gel nails.
- Prepare cabins for work.
- Carry out treatments and massages in the office.

- Advise and sell products and services for the patient's personal image.
- Prepare treatment plans for patients.
- Perform specialized procedures such as acne treatment, electrotherapy, skin rejuvenation therapies, camouflage treatments, among others.
- Be trained to recognize problems and refer those patients to doctors who can resolve the conditions.

If the aesthetic procedure approaches a medical act, it should be reserved for physicians with training in aesthetic medicine. However, the fact that the beautician cannot carry out such procedures does not mean that he or she cannot collaborate with the doctor to provide a better-quality service to the patient. On the contrary, nowadays many aestheticians practice inside aesthetic-medical clinics where they form part of a team of professionals together with the aesthetic physician or other aesthetic professionals, offering much more complete and integrated treatments, since the treatments that the aesthetician realizes complement those that the aesthetic doctor undertakes in the clinic.

The aesthetician also has a responsibility for health: whatever his or her professional activity is, he or she must take care of preventive and educational aspects and the promotion of healthy lifestyle habits. If necessary, the aesthetician will refer to the relevant health personnel (nutritionist, dermatologist, etc.).

Relation to Other Areas

The field of aesthetics and cosmetics is very broad and continues to grow significantly. There are technological and scientific advances within the aesthetic industry, and at the same time as this industry grows, the beautician must be up to date with it and be at the forefront of all the novelties the sector brings with it. Therefore, the aesthetician must be aware of the best-quality and cutting-edge products on the market. He or she must be knowledgeable about most of the key features of the products that are offered to them to provide quality services within their station.

This relates not only to having links with manufacturers or distributors of the wide range of products that exist in their market, it also involves having links with other professionals who are dedicated to medical and nonmedical aesthetics.

Relationship with Health Professionals

Aesthetic medicine and the aesthetician's work are intimately intertwined, as the beautification provided by the aesthetician's services is a fundamental part of the well-being achieved by aesthetic medicine. However, the aesthetician should remain in close relation not only with aesthetic medicine, but all the branches of medicine that ensure the care, embellishment, and conservation of the body.

Plastic surgery and dermatology are two branches of medicine that also have close ties to nonmedical aesthetics. The treatments carried out by these medical professionals are subsequently the object of the beautician's work. There is no doubt the aesthetician plays a definite role in the postoperative period for patients who make the decision to undergo cosmetic surgery.

"In addition, they are the professionals indicated for advising the patients who have taken the decision not to undergo procedures of invasive character but who wish to improve their physical aspect" [2].

Workplaces

Aestheticians carry out their activity in a variety of settings within the services sector and more specifically in the activity of aesthetic treatments, developing the processes of rendering aesthetic services:

- Aesthetic institutes
- Aesthetic departments of companies dedicated to the treatment of the integral personal image
- Aesthetic medicine clinics
- Rehabilitation centers
- Spas
- Teams of technicians, dependent on laboratories and commercial firms that develop their activity in the field of integral aesthetics, such as testers, instructors of application techniques, and sales personnel
- Hospitals
- Clinics
- Health institutes
- Geriatric centers
- Physical activity centers

Within these establishments, the beautician should carry out the following functions:

- Customer service
- Preparation and interpretation of technical documentation
- Advice to clients
- Surveillance and promotion of health and safety conditions at work
- Coordination of the professional team
- Use of technical equipment and products necessary for the provision of services and for the maintenance of the facilities and resources in optimal condition
- Processes/treatments of integral aesthetics
- Diagnosis of nonpathological alterations with aesthetic repercussion and application of the corresponding treatments
- Commercial planning
- Collaboration with doctors
- Quality control in the service delivery process and in the results obtained

Aesthetic Station

By the "aesthetic station," we refer to the place where the different aesthetic treatments are carried out.

Only simple procedures such as facials, massages, reduction treatments, and application of nonmedical appliances should be performed in the aesthetic station. A station does not have space for hydrotherapy treatments or aggressive treatments.

Aesthetic Clinic Medicine

Aesthetic clinics are health-care units in which a doctor is responsible for carrying out nonsurgical treatments with the aim of improving the body or facial aesthetic.

This establishment has stations in which diverse aesthetic treatments can be carried out—it can have offices, reception, and special areas.

Within the aesthetic clinic, there can be diverse teams of professionals, among them aesthetic doctors, dermatologists, aestheticians, and nutritionists. In addition, minimally invasive procedures are performed on patients, such as the application of botulinum toxin, fillers, threads, mesotherapy, medical devices, among others.

Functions of an Aesthetician in a Cosmetic Medicine Practice

All health professionals in the field of aesthetics should know that an aesthetician is there to help the physician, but under no circumstances should an aesthetician perform a minimally invasive intervention. However, the aesthetician should know the different techniques used in the field of aesthetic medicine and possess an adequate vocabulary and technical knowledge for interaction with the doctor.

When administering medications, the aesthetician must take into account the care to be given to the patient after the treatment the doctor has provided, so that if the doctor recommends the patient undergo any other therapy after this intervention, the aesthetician knows how to do it properly and carefully. Aestheticians should carry out the assistance function of their profession for care and maintenance of the skin; additionally, they must have knowledge of the work of cosmetic support in the skin with pathologies and injuries. The aesthetician must be aware of prevention techniques for the different dermatological problems, as well as know the pre- and postcosmetic support needed in aesthetic medicine procedures; they should also have the necessary skill and experience to work with patients after plastic surgery.

It is also important for the aesthetician to acquire the necessary skills to perform the procedures and techniques with dexterity and safety and to develop relevant attitudes to effectively manage interpersonal relationships with service users and, if necessary, in the work team.

Conclusions

No procedure or treatment for which the aesthetician is trained should cross the skin barrier under any circumstances. An aesthetician is therefore not able to carry out procedures that belong to the medical professional, not only because he or she does not have the knowledge to do so but also because at the time of a medical emergency, the aesthetician is not trained to solve it. Every aesthetician must therefore be aware of the objectives, fields of application, limits, and ethical principles of his or her profession, especially when they do not work in a center of aesthetic medicine.

However, the aesthetician can assist the doctor in minimally invasive procedures, so it follows that he or she should know the different treatments provided by the aesthetic doctor. Part of the aesthetician's assistance in a minimally invasive procedures in the aesthetic medicine clinic consists of providing treatments that help to enhance and maintain the results obtained in a procedure at the medical level.

Unqualified intruders are very common in this profession; they arise as a consequence of nonregulation of the profession within a country, so it can be common to see aestheticians performing procedures belonging to medical practitioners both in aesthetic medicine clinics and in nonmedical aesthetic clinics.

REFERENCES

1. Tufet DJ, (04 of 10 of 2016). Aesthetic world. Obtained from http://estheticworld.es/medicos-esteticos-y-esteticistas-unidos-por-la-belleza/
2. Minieducación. (29 de enero de 2006). Minieducación.gov. Obtenido de http://www.mineducacion.gov.co/cvn/1665/fo-article-93432.pdf

BIBLIOGRAPHY

Lopez PV. (2013). DPCMEC. Barcelona, España: METGES DE ESTETICA. Obtenido.

Pimentel AD. (2010). Médicina y Cirugía Estética en el Consultorio. Sao Paulo, Brasil: AMOLCA.

Royal Spanish Academy. (s.f.). Pan-Hispanic Dictionary of the Royal Academy.

Trelles DM. (10 de 09 de 2017). Centro Europeo de Cirugia Estetica.

al PV. (2014). Aesthetic and cosmetic medicine: optimization of results with mesotherapy.

22

Dietetics and Nutrition in Oncology Patients: Evaluation of Nutritional Status, Weight Control, and Nutrigenomics

Iris Luna-Boquera

Cancer-Related Malnutrition

Malnutrition is one of the most frequent causes of mortality and a major health problem worldwide, in both developed and economically disadvantaged countries. In order to distinguish malnutrition related to disease from that associated with social causes, famine, or environmental catastrophes, the term *disease-related malnutrition* (DRM) has been established in the last few years [1].

DRM especially affects specific groups such as oncological patients, in whom disability and functional limitations are frequent. It is important to point out that the concept of the oncological patient is quite general and encompasses patients throughout their trajectory from initial diagnostic stages to curative or palliative treatment, and also includes cancer recurrences and cancer survivors. In the oncological patient, DRM is the result of the complex interaction between disease, food, and nutrition. When the nutritional state is deficient, recovery is compromised, hospital stays are prolonged, the rate of premature readmissions is increased, there is greater susceptibility to infection, and autonomy and quality of life are significantly altered. All these factors increase morbidity and mortality and negatively affect health costs [2,3]. When chemotherapy and radiotherapy treatments are administered, a previously deficient nutritional state leads to worse tolerance and higher toxicity, with the need to reduce or fractionate the dosage and in some cases interrupt it. DRM leads to a worse survival prognosis that could be modified with specific nutritional interventions [4–6].

It has been argued that hospital morbidity and mortality and associated costs are primarily determined by the patient's underlying medical condition rather than by the presence or absence of malnutrition. However, recent studies about the economic impact of nutritional interventions show that the costs associated with hospitalization of malnourished patients are three times higher than for those with normal nutrition and that the risk of death at 3 years after discharge from hospital is up to four times higher in the group of malnourished patients [7]. A multicenter study (PREDyCES: Prevalence of Hospital Malnutrition and Associated Costs in Spain) evaluated the prevalence of malnutrition at Spanish hospitals [8]: the main factors associated with the presence of malnutrition were advanced age (>70 years), female gender, oncological disease, diabetes mellitus, dysphagia, and

polymedication—all common features in the population we usually treat.

Care practice in cancer must include nutritional intervention to identify patients with malnutrition or at high risk of nutritional complications caused by their own illness or by the treatments applied (surgery, chemotherapy, radiotherapy, and new approaches such as immunotherapy or hormone therapy). Nutritional screening tools help to identify patients at nutritional risk or who are malnourished and should receive an organized plan for nutritional care. Nutritional actions will be aimed at improving dietary intake, reducing the metabolic impact of disease, maintaining skeletal muscle mass and physical condition, minimizing the risk of reductions or interruptions of antineoplastic treatments, and improving quality of life [9].

Malnutrition related to cancer presents differential characteristics that require specific management. This chapter develops the evaluation of nutritional status in cancer patients, body weight control, and an overview of the complex relationship between genes and nutrients.

Evaluation of Nutritional Status

Nutrient deficiencies (proteins, energy, micronutrients) usually have many factors in cancer patients: they may be due to inadequate intake (loss of appetite, cachexia), increased digestive losses (diarrhea, malabsorptive syndromes), or increased requirements (linked to disease or treatments). In recent years, the relevance of the systemic inflammatory response in cancer has been described as responsible for changes in organs and tissues that contribute to malnutrition [10].

A nutritional assessment is recommended at the time of cancer diagnosis [11]. Although some kinds of neoplasms are rarely related to malnutrition, the clinical basal characteristics (advanced age, presence of comorbidities, polypharmacy) are determining factors in the nutritional state. For this reason, an initial evaluation is recommended in every patient, regardless of the type of tumor the patient has. The requirement for periodic reevaluation will vary depending on the medical situation.

The first step in nutritional assessment is to apply a screening test to identify patients at risk of malnutrition or the malnourished who require more comprehensive evaluation. Malnutrition is ideal for population screening because it is a high-prevalence entity with the potential for early treatment. The screening tests are validated in different clinical settings, reliable, reproducible, practical, and connected with specific protocols. According to the European Society of Parenteral and Enteral Nutrition (ESPEN) [1,4], every test must include three elements on nutritional status: current anthropometry (body weight or body mass index [BMI]), recent nonvoluntary weight loss, and evaluation of recent dietary intake. The latest consensus also introduces etiological criteria for undernutrition [12].

There are more than 70 nutritional screening methods for adult patients. The Nutrition Risk Screening (NRS-2002), the patient generated–subjective global assessment (PG-SGA), and the Malnutrition Screening Tool (MST) have been validated in cancer, each one with different strengths and weaknesses [13,14]. NRS-2002 [15] has two categories of simple questions validated for hospitalized patients. It is easy to apply, although it requires trained nurse teams. PG-SGA [16,17] is a structured process that integrates parameters of clinical history, current disease, and physical examination. It has a high predictive power and allows subsequent patient monitoring. However, it requires trained personnel and takes a long time (15 minutes). MST [18] is a brief and simple tool validated for outpatients receiving radiotherapy and chemotherapy. It includes weight loss and decreased energy intake. More specific tools for oncological patients are continually being developed: for example, NUTRISCORE [19] includes the location of the neoplasm and establishes a different nutritional risk depending on the oncological treatments administered. The selection of the screening method to be applied depends on the characteristics of each center, taking into account all these previous considerations.

Classic nutritional classifications were focused on the determination of biochemical parameters (mainly proteins like albumin) and on static anthropometric measurements (weight, BMI, skin folds) [20]. Marasmo-type caloric malnutrition was established when the loss of adipose tissue predominated in the absence of edema and without a significant decrease in albumin. This type was usually diagnosed in chronic cachexia diseases, prevalent in developed countries. Kwashiorkor-type protein malnutrition was established when the clinical setting was dominated by hypoproteinemia with important associated edema, alteration in cellular immunity with lymphopenia, delay in wound healing, and appearance of pressure ulcers, but with relatively preserved adipose panicle and little affectation on body weight. This clinical scenario is the most common in underdeveloped countries with cereal-based diets and protein source shortages. This dual approach did not adequately assess the initial stages of undernutrition or the combined calorie-protein malnutrition: the classic nutritional evaluation used static anthropometric parameters that do not adequately reflect body composition (alteration in sarcopenia, ascites, edemas, etc.) and therefore underdiagnose malnutrition in obese people. A new approach was therefore needed.

In 2019, the consensus of the Global Leadership Initiative on Malnutrition (GLIM) [12], convened by several of the major clinical nutrition societies worldwide, was published. This document is an important step forward because it establishes new diagnostic criteria for undernutrition and also assesses its severity. GLIM establishes the diagnosis of malnutrition if the patient meets at least one phenotypic criterion in addition to one etiological criterion. The phenotypic criteria are percentage of unintentional weight loss (with temporal criteria), BMI (adjusted for age and race), and loss of muscle mass (determined by validated body composition techniques, anthropometric measurements, physical examination, or grip strength). The determination of malnutrition severity is based exclusively on phenotypic criteria. The etiological criteria are decreased dietary intake or reduced absorption and inflammatory burden due to underlying disease (acute disease or inflammation related to chronic disease). Etiological criteria are used to guide nutritional interventions appropriately.

Once the diagnosis of undernutrition is established, a more comprehensive assessment should be carried out. It is recommended to combine medical, nutritional, and pharmacological history data with physical examination, anthropometric parameters, laboratory tests, and body composition methods. The main components of a complete nutrition evaluation are summarized in a practical way as follows:

- Assess the presence of systemic diseases that interfere with the feeding process (intestinal ischemia, heart failure, chronic renal or hepatic insufficiency), relevant surgical antecedents (particularly of the digestive tract), mental state of the patient (depression, cognitive deterioration), alcoholism, and drug addiction.

- Evaluate dietary intake (food intake history, 24-hour diet recall or food frequency questionnaire). If nutritional supplements are used, confirm that they have been taken properly. Ask about consumption of natural food supplements with or without official sanitary control. Inquire about the existence of food intolerances or allergies. Find out if there are any dietary restrictions of cultural origin.

- Ask about symptoms that may interfere with food intake (xerostomia, changes in smell and taste, swallowing disorders or dysphagia, nausea, vomiting, gastroesophageal reflux) or indicate malabsorption (depositional rhythm, stool characteristics), establishing a temporary relationship with the administration of oncological treatment, if any.

- Review the patient's medication and adapt it in case it produces digestive effects, interferes with the absorption of nutrients, or does not provide benefits at the present time. Liquid formulations offer absorption advantages in patients with quick digestive transit. In diabetes mellitus, it is essential to adapt the treatment regimen to avoid hypoglycemia and prevent hyperglycemia induced by corticosteroids.

- Conduct a nutrition-focused physical examination (icteric or dry skin, oral cavity abnormalities, dentition, mucositis, abdominal exploration, presence of edema or pressure ulcers, state of surgical wounds and stomas, etc.).

- Review and evaluate anthropometric measurements (height, body weight, BMI, muscular circumferences, body folds, bone mineral densitometry, and bioelectric impedance phase angle, if available). Muscle mass measurements provide information on the current functional status of the patient. It is of great value to have anthropometric information prior to the onset of the disease, as well as to establish a temporal profile.

- Calculate fluid requirements. Normal hydration is compatible with a wide range of fluid intake. Numerous factors can modify water needs (metabolism, climate, physical activity, diet, and extraordinary losses). The quantities required in cancer patients are normally 35–40 mL/kg weight/day [21,22]. Recommendations will be made regarding water and liquid intake and digestive (vomiting, diarrhea) and extradigestive losses (sweating, urine, drainages).

- Calculate energy requirements. Oncological patients present important modifications in their energy requirements. Needs are influenced by the clinical situation, the treatment applied, and the stage of evolution. The use of standard formulas such as Harris-Benedict's for the calculation of energy needs may be inaccurate given the metabolic differences in different cancer types. These formulas tend to underestimate requirements if a stress correction factor is not applied. For this reason, the most appropriate method for calculating the energy expenditure is indirect calorimetry. In the absence of this tool, calorie intake of 25–30 kcal/kg/day seems to be appropriate for most patients to help maintain or restore lean body mass [1,4]. In severely depleted patients, feeding is initiated slowly to avoid refeeding syndrome.

- Calculate protein requirements. The recommended protein intake is between 1.2 and 1.5 g/kg/day, depending on the characteristics of the clinical situation (0.8 in pre-dialysis, 1.2 in hemodialysis, 1.5 in sepsis or post-surgical stress). In patients over 65 years of age, a minimum of 1.2 g/kg/day is recommended [4,23].

- Review and evaluate biochemical measures. A complete laboratory assessment should be performed to detect early medical complications associated with malnutrition. It should include hemogram (lymphopenia is a marker of protein deficiency), renal and hepatic function, ionogram, glucose (in diabetes mellitus we request glycosylated hemoglobin), liposoluble vitamins (A, D, E, and prothrombin time to assess vitamin K status), hydrosoluble vitamins (folic acid, cobalamin, and others according to clinical suspicion), and visceral proteins (albumin, prealbumin, transferrin). In contrast to previous appraisals of undernutrition, biochemical parameters are losing relevance in favor of etiological criteria. Plasma albumin itself acts not only as a marker of the visceral protein reserve, but also as a negative acute phase reactant. The extent of systemic inflammation can be estimated by measuring serum C-reactive protein and albumin. Grading the inflammatory response according to the modified Glasgow Prognostic Score (mGPS) is highly predictive of morbidity and mortality in cancer patients [24,25]. Updated nutritional strategies now suggest considering nutrition with inflammation-suppressing ingredients such as omega-3 fatty acids.

- Determine the optimal route for nutrition support (i.e., oral, enteral, or parenteral). Be aware that the options can be complementary and can be modified throughout the disease evolution.

- Assess the degree of functional dependency and quality of life through validated scales at the time of diagnosis and on a regular basis in the follow-up. Data must be collected on physical and occupational activity, customs, and situations of loneliness.

- Explore patient and caregiver beliefs, academic skills, and economic resources, and offer tailored options as reasonable as possible.

- Develop an implementation and monitoring plan taking into account the treatment intention (curative, palliative) and the patient's life expectancy. In order to minimize duplicity in laboratory determinations and overdiagnoses, it is useful to reach a consensus within the medical team on the periodicity of revisions and to coordinate follow-up visits.

In summary, nutritional screening should be applied to all patients at the diagnosis of cancer. In those situations where nutritional risk or malnutrition is detected, a deep multimodal evaluation should be carried out. Current recommendations emphasize inflammation in the etiology of malnutrition over proteic parameters and body composition over classic weight parameters.

Weight Control in Cancer and Body Composition

Malnutrition involves changes in body composition (BC) (weight loss, loss of lean mass and fat mass) that will impair the function of different tissues and organs and negatively affect the clinical evolution of subjects.

Weight loss percentage is a sign of advancing malnutrition and thus needs to be detected and recognized early in cancer patients [26]. However, an approach based exclusively on body weight is insufficient. We have a better understanding of the metabolic alterations that occur prior to any measurable change in body weight. There is a reduction of the protein component with preferential use of muscle mass, especially branched amino acids, for gluconeogenesis leading to atrophy of muscle fibers. Different studies of BC in cancer indicate that the decrease in skeletal and cardiac muscle mass, associated or not with loss of fat mass, predicts a decrease in the ability to mobilize, predisposition to the development of pressure ulcers, postoperative complications, chemotherapy toxicity, and mortality [27,28]. An accepted value for severe depletion of muscle mass is a muscularity below the fifth percentile (age and gender adjusted).

Although some anthropometric measures, such as folds or circumferences, can estimate subcutaneous fat or muscle mass, there are more accurate techniques for determining BC [29].

Dual-energy x-ray absorptiometry (DEXA) is the reference technique in clinical practice. DEXA is primarily used for measurements of bone mineral content (hormonal blockages performed in some tumors and chronic use of corticosteroids directly affect bone mass). Total body DEXA scans can also accurately measure fat mass and lean mass (or free fat mass), both at the total body as well as at segmentary levels. DEXA does expose the patient and operator to ionizing radiation, but the dose is very small to both. The main limitations of DEXA are the cost and technical expertise [30,31].

It is also possible to use diagnostic imaging techniques already made to the patient, such as computed tomography and magnetic resonance imaging, to measure BC. Retrospective reviews of lumbar skeletal muscle index in patients with cancer can detect loss of muscle mass as well as fatty muscle infiltration (myosteatosis) [32,33].

Bioelectrical impedance (BIA) is an indirect method for measuring BC, based on the human body's ability to transmit electrical power. It obtains data on the body compartments and provides electrical values: impedance, resistance, reactance, and the phase angle (PA). The vectorial representation of PA has demonstrated its usefulness in identifying short-term body changes and serving as a specific marker of nutritional status. Absolute PA values are directly related to cell membrane health status and are an indicator of morbidity and mortality prognosis [34]. As weaknesses of this technique, we point out that PA is modified by the state of hydration (both dehydration and the presence of ascites and edema). In addition, it varies according to gender, age, BMI, and race, and we lack reference values for cancer population. The high interpatient variability requires careful interpretation of results, but it is a promising technique [35].

In some malignancies, there has been established a direct relationship between excess of adipose tissue and reduced cancer survival. Nevertheless, other research challenges this statement by demonstrating that overweight and early obese states are associated with improved survival [36]. The complex relationship between obesity, adipose tissue, and cancer is developed elsewhere.

Nutrigenomics

The Human Genome Project has changed the research of medical sciences including nutrition. The relationship between diet and genes has been studied for years, but until there was a better development and understanding of the mechanisms that activate selected genes, this link could not be completely defined. Nutritional genomics (or nutrigenomics) consist of genomic studies that relate nutritional factors in the regulation of genes that influence cellular processes genome-wide [37,38].

The comprehensive identification of human genetic variation will help us to explain the molecular basis of phenotypic differences among individuals that are mediated by nutrients. These genetic variations and their impact on metabolism address a new age of personalized nutrition [39]. The science of epigenetics focuses on the study of the nonmutational changes of a gene. Epigenetic changes occur throughout the life span and can be inherited in the next generation. They are modifiable by diet and lifestyle and are a target for cancer prevention. The Spanish working group PREDIMED (prevention with Mediterranean diet) has carried out multiple studies that indicate that the Mediterranean diet has a potential protective factor against cancer, with promising results that must be confirmed by long-term follow-up studies [40,41].

The processes through which nutrients are able to regulate gene expression, by modifying chromatin structure, and induce epigenetic changes (DNA methylation, posttranslational changes such as acetylation and glycation), are being defined [42]. Cancer cells exhibit greater metabolic plasticity and are able to alter their tissue microenvironment to elude physiological regulation and immune control [43]. Some cell lines are also able to avoid the pharmacological effect of chemotherapy by modifying nutrient use. If the nutrients that limit the survival of cancer cells are identified, we will have new therapeutic goals that can recover sensitivity to chemotherapy or even induce selective apoptosis of cancer cells [44,45].

Some current lines of research are focused on the interaction between diet, genes, and gut microbiome. Evidence suggests that toxic metabolites produced by dysbiosis—the activation of the immune system by pathogenic microorganisms and the proinflammatory state produced by the altered microbiome—participate in cellular oncogenesis [46,47].

Another main line of research links chronic exposure to inflammatory elements in the food and cancer [48,49], especially colorectal [50,51] and head and neck cancers [52,53]. Studies indicate that a Mediterranean-pattern diet may be preventive for these types of cancer.

Unfortunately, many of these studies need more follow-up time to confirm the findings and do not yet have translation into clinical practice [54]. It will still be some time before the studies of gene-nutrient interaction can be translated into generalized guidelines.

REFERENCES

1. Arends J, Bachmann P, Baracos V et al. ESPEN guidelines on nutrition in cancer patients. *Clin Nutr.* 2017;36(1):11–48.
2. Agarwal E, Ferguson M, Banks M, Bauer M, Capra J, Isenring S. Malnutrition and poor food intake are associated with prolonged hospital stay, frequent readmissions, and greater in-hospital mortality: Results from the Nutrition Care Day Survey 2010. *Clin Nutr.* 2013;32(5):737–45.
3. Van der Schueren M, Elia M, Gramlich L et al. Clinical and economic outcomes of nutrition interventions across the continuum of care. *Ann N Y Acad Sci.* 2014;1321:20–40.
4. Arends J, Baracos V, Bertz H et al. ESPEN expert group recommendations for action against cancer-related malnutrition. *Clin Nutr.* 2017;36(5):1187–96.
5. Stratton RJ, Hebuterne X, Elia M. A systematic review and meta-analysis of the impact of oral nutritional supplements on hospital readmissions. *Ageing Res Rev.* 2013;12(4):884–97.
6. Somanchi M, Tao X, Mullin GE. The facilitated early enteral and dietary management effectiveness trial in hospitalized patients with malnutrition. *JPEN J Parenter Enteral.* 2011;35(2):209–21.
7. Lim SL, Ong KC, Chan YH, Loke WC, Ferguson M, Daniels L. Malnutrition and its impact on cost of hospitalization, length of stay, readmission and 3-year mortality. *Clin Nutr.* 2012;31(3):345–50.
8. Álvarez-Hernández J, Planas M, León-Sanz M et al. Prevalence and costs of malnutrition in hospitalized patients; the PREDyCES Study. *Nutr Hosp.* 2012;27:1049–59.
9. Garcia de Lorenzo A, Alvarez Hernandez J, Planas M, Burgos R, Araujo K. The multidisciplinary consensus work-team on the approach to hospital malnutrition in Spain. Multidisciplinary consensus on the approach to hospital malnutrition in Spain. *Nutr Hosp.* 2012;26(4):701–10.
10. Jensen GL, Mirtallo J, Compher C et al. Adult starvation and disease-related malnutrition: A proposal for etiology based

diagnosis in the clinical practice setting from the International Consensus Guideline Committee. *JPEN J Parenter Enter Nutr.* 2010;34(2):156–9.

11. Marin Caro MM, Gómez-Candela C, Castillo Rabaneda R et al. Nutritional risk evaluation and establishment of nutritional support in oncology patients according to the protocol of the Spanish Nutrition and Cancer Group. *Nutr Hosp.* 2008;23(5):458–68.

12. Cederholm T, Jensen GL, Correia MITD et al. GLIM criteria for the diagnosis of malnutrition: A consensus report from the global clinical nutrition community. *Clin Nutr.* 2019;38(1):1–9.

13. Castillo-Martinez L, Castro-Eguiluz D, Copca-Mendoza ET et al. Nutritional Assessment Tools for the Identification of Malnutrition and Nutritional Risk Associated with Cancer Treatment. *Rev Invest Clin.* 2018;70(3):121–5.

14. Kondrup J, Allison SP, Elia M, Vellas B, Plauth M. ESPEN guidelines for nutrition screening 2002. *Clin Nutr.* 2003;22(4):415–21.

15. Kondrup J, Rasmussen HH, Hamberg O, Stanga Z. Nutritional Risk Screening (NRS 2002): A new method based on an analysis of controlled clinical trials. *Clin Nutr.* 2003;22:321–36.

16. Abbott J, Teleni L, McKavanagh D, Watson J, McCarthy AL, Isenring E. Patient-Generated Subjective Global Assessment Short Form (PG-SGA SF) is a valid screening tool in chemotherapy outpatients. *Support Care Cancer.* 2016;24(9):3883–7.

17. Rodrigues CS, Lacerda MS, Chaves GV. Patient generated subjective global assessment as a prognosis tool in women with gynecologic cáncer. *Nutrition.* 2015;31:1372–8.

18. Shaw C, Fleuret C, Pickard JM et al. Comparison of a novel, simple nutrition screening tool for adult oncology inpatients and the malnutrition screening tool (MST) against the patient-generated subjective global assessment (PG-SGA). *Support Care Cancer.* 2015;23:47–54.

19. Arribas L, Hurtós L, Sendrós MJ et al. NUTRISCORE: A new nutritional screning tool for oncological outpatients. *Nutrition.* 2017;33:297–303.

20. Álvarez J, Del Río J, Planas M et al. SENPE-SEDOM document on coding of hospital hyponutrition. *Nutr Hosp.* 2008;23(6):536–40.

21. Jéquier E, Constant F. Water as an essential nutrient: The physiological basis of hydration. *Eur J Clin Nutr.* 2010;64(2):115–23.

22. Ortiz Leyba C, Gómez-Tello V, Serón Arbeloa C. Requeriments of macronutrients and micronutrients. *Nutr Hosp.* 2005;20(2):13–7.

23. Volkert D, Beck AM, Cederholm T et al. ESPEN Guideline on clinical nutrition and hydratation in geriatrics. *Clin Nutr.* 2019 Feb;38(1):10–47.

24. McMillan DC. The systemic inflammation-based Glasgow Prognostic Score: A decade of experience in patients with cancer. *Cancer Treat Rev.* 2013;39(5):534–40.

25. Dolan RD, McSorley ST, Horgan PG, Laird B, McMillan DC. The role of the systemic inflammatory response in predicting outcomes in patients with advanced inoperable cancer: Systematic review and meta-analysis. *Crit Rev Oncol Hematol.* 2017;116:134–46.

26. Sotelo Gonzalez S, Sánchez Sobrino P, Carrasco Álvarez JA, González Villaroel P, Páramo Fernández C. Anthropometric parameters in evaluating malnutrition in oncological patients; utility of body mass index and percentage of weight loss. *Nutr Hosp.* 2013 May–Jun;28(3):965–8.

27. Baracos V, Kazemi-Bajestani SM. Clinical outcomes related to muscle mass in humans with cancer and catabolic illnesses. *Int J Biochem Cell Biol* 2013;45:2302–8.

28. Martin L, Birdsell L, Macdonald N et al. Cancer cachexia in the age of obesity: Skeletal muscle depletion is a powerful prognostic factor, independent of body mass index. *J Clin Oncol* 2013;31:1539–47.

29. García Almeida JM, García García C, Bellido Castañeda V, Bellido Guerrero D. Nuevo enfoque de la nutrición. Valoración del estado nutricional del paciente: Composición y función. *Nutr Hosp.* 2018;35(3):1–14.

30. Sheperd JA, Ng BK, Sommer MJ, Heymsfield SB. Body composition by DXA. *Bone.* 2017 Nov;104:101–5.

31. Marra M, Sammarco R, De Lorenzo A et al. Assessment of body composition in health and disease using bioelectrical impedance analysis (BIA) and dual energy x-ray absorptiometry (DXA): A critical overview. *Contrast Media Mol Imaging.* 2019 May;29:1–9.

32. Mourtzakis M, Prado CM, Lieffers JR, Reiman T, Mc Cargar LJ, Baracos VE. A practical and precise approach to quantification of body composition in cancer patients using computed tomography images acquired during routine care. *Appl Physiol Nutr Metab.* 2008 Oct;33(5):997–1006.

33. Yip C1, Dinkel C, Mahajan A, Siddique M, Cook GJ, Goh V. Imaging body composition in cancer patients: Visceral obesity, sarcopenia and sarcopenic obesity may impact on clinical outcome. *Insights Imaging.* 2015 Aug;6(4):489–97.

34. Hui D, Dev R, Pimental L et al. Association between multifrequency phase angle and survival in patients with advanced cancer. *J Pain Symptom Manage.* 2017 Mar;53(3):571–7.

35. Grundmann O, Yoon SL, Williams JJ. The value of bioelectrical impedance analysis and phase angle in the evaluation of malnutrition and quality of life in cancer patients: A comprehensive review. *Eur J Clin Nutr.* 2015 Dec;69(12):1290–7.

36. Lennon H, Sperrin M, Badrick E, Renehan AG. The Obesity Paradox in Cancer: A Review. *Curr Oncol Rep.* 2016 Sep;18(9):56–64.

37. Ross SA. Evidence for the relationship between diet and cancer. *Exp Oncol.* 2010 Sep;32(3):137–42.

38. Murgia C, Adamski MM. Translation of nutritional genomics into nutrition practice: The next step. *Nutrients.* 2017 Apr 6;9(4):366–70.

39. San-Cristobal R, Milagro FI, Martínez JA. Future challenges and present ethical considerations in the use of personalized nutrition based on genetic advice. *J Acad Nutr Diet.* 2013 Nov;113(11):1447–54.

40. Serra-Majem L, Román-Viñas B, Sanchez-Villegas A, Guasch-Ferré M, Corella D, La Vecchia C. Benefits of the Mediterranean diet: Epidemiological and molecular aspects. *Mol Aspects Med.* 2019 Jun;67:1–55.

41. Toledo E, Salas-Salvadó J, Donat-Vargas C et al. Mediterranean diet and invasive breast cancer risk among women at high cardiovascular risk in the PREDIMED Trial: A Randomized Clinical Trial. *JAMA Intern Med.* 2015 Nov;175(11):1752–60.

42. Ballestar E, Esteller M. The epigenetic breakdown of cancer cells: From DNA methylation to histone modifications. *Prog Mol Subcell Biol.* 2005;38:169–81.

43. Wang YP, Lei QY2. Metabolic recoding of epigenetics in cancer. *Cancer Commun (Lond).* 2018 May 21;38(1):25–33.

44. Wong CC, Qian Y, Yu J. Interplay between epigenetics and metabolism in oncogenesis: Mechanisms and therapeutic approaches. *Oncogene.* 2017 Jun 15;36(24):3359–74.

45. Hatziapostolou M, Iliopoulos D. Epigenetic aberrations during oncogenesis. *Cell Mol Life Sci.* 2011 May;68(10):1681–702.

46. Rajagopala SV, Vashee S, Oldfield LM et al. The human microbiome and cancer. *Cancer Prev Res (Phila).* 2017 Apr;10(4):226–34.

47. Gopalakrishnan V, Helmink BA, Spencer CN, Reuben A, Wargo JA. The influence of the gut microbiome on cancer, immunity, and cancer immunotherapy. *Cancer Cell.* 2018 Apr 9;33(4):570–80.

48. Garcia-Arellano A, Martínez-González MA, Ramallal R et al. Dietary inflammatory index and all-cause mortality in large cohorts: The SUN and PREDIMED studies. *Clin Nutr.* 2019 Jun;38(3):1221–31.

49. Fowler ME, Akinyemiju TF. Meta-analysis of the association between dietary inflammatory index (DII) and cancer outcomes. *Int J Cancer.* 2017 Dec 1;141(11):2215–27.

50. Ravasco P, Monteiro-Grillo I, Vidal PM, Camilo ME. Dietary counseling improves patient outcomes: A prospective, randomized, controlled trial in colorectal cancer patients undergoing radiotherapy. *J Clin Oncol.* 2005;23:1431–8.

51. Fasanelli F, Giraudo MT, Vineis P et al. DNA methylation, colon cancer and Mediterranean diet: Results from the EPIC-Italy cohort. *Epigenetics.* 2019 Oct;14(10):977–88.

52. Salvatore Benito A, Valero Zanuy MÁ, Alarza Cano M et al. Adherence to Mediterranean diet: A comparison of patients with head and neck cancer and healthy population. *Endocrinol Diabetes Nutr.* 2019 Aug–Sep;66(7):417–24.

53. Ravasco P, Monteiro-Grillo I, Marques Vidal P, Camilo ME. Impact of nutrition on outcome: A prospective randomized controlled trial in patients with head and neck cancer undergoing radiotherapy. *Head Neck* 2005;27:659–68.

54. Camp KM, Trujillo E. Position of the Academy of Nutrition and Dietetics: Nutritional genomics. *J Acad Nutr Diet.* 2014 Feb;114(2):299–312.

23

Nutrition: Diet Therapy and Nutritional Supplements

Margarita Esteban

Introduction

The oncological patient presents malnutrition associated with both the characteristics that define the malignant tumor and the treatment that needs to be applied. Cancer produces a direct decrease in intake, interfering mechanically with the normal transit of the digestive tract, or indirectly through the secretion of substances that act on peripheral receptors or on the hypothalamus. Likewise, the different types of treatments applied to cancer patients are an important cause of alteration in their nutritional status.

Functional and Mechanical Alterations

Tumors located in the digestive tract (pharynx, esophagus, stomach, and pancreas) cause direct obstruction or early satiety due to limited gastric capacity. A similar effect may be seen in tumors from other organs that produce extrinsic compression.

The location of the tumor at any point of the digestive system may induce mechanical and/or functional alterations that will affect the patient's diet:

- *Esophageal tumors*: Dysphagia
- *Head and neck tumors*: Alteration in chewing, salivation, or swallowing and associated pain
- *Gastric tumors*: Anorexia, early satiety, or obstruction of transit at the gastric level
- *Intestinal tumors*: Occlusive or subocclusive pictures, maldigestion, and malabsorption

Metabolic Alterations

There are a series of metabolic and endocrine changes that generate a catabolic state in which lipolysis and proteolysis are induced, resulting in loss of lean mass, fat, and insulin resistance.

- *Tumor factors (generated by the tumor itself)*: Proteolysis-inducing factor (PIF) or lipid mobilization factor.
- *Humoral factors (generated by the host in response to the presence of the tumor)*: Cytokines (tumor necrosis factor [TNF]-α, interleukin [IL]-1 and IL-6, and interferon [IFN]-γ), neuropeptides (neuropeptide Y,

serotonin, and melanocortins), and hormones (insulin and glucagon). In these cases, cancer induces anorexia by producing substances with remote effect on the central nervous system and without mechanical involvement of the digestive tract. For example, there are tumors that can produce substances that alter the perception of taste, generating an aversion toward meat (traditionally described in gastric cancer). Various mechanisms have been proposed to explain these situations. In this sense, various substances have been involved that exert a peripheral effect on neuroendocrine cells or directly on the hypothalamus, causing anorexia.

Alterations due to Treatment

Oncological treatments often lead to malnutrition. Surgery, chemotherapy, and radiotherapy treatments used in cancer patients can have side effects that have a negative impact on nutritional status.

Surgery

The surgery that patients undergo, even for palliative purposes, can involve losses that greatly limit their ability to feed themselves:
- *Head and neck*: Surgeries on head and neck tumors result in significant limitations in oral intake.
- *Digestive system*: In surgery on the esophagus, there is associated gastric stasis and fat malabsorption associated with the vagal section. Interventions on gastric tumors produce fat and protein malabsorption, as well as limitation in the absorption of vitamin B_{12} by reduction of intrinsic factor, dumping, and early sensation of satiety. These effects are similar to those occurring after pancreatic surgery, to which must be added diarrhea and diabetes mellitus. Surgical therapy on the small and large intestine produces fat and protein malabsorption, mineral and vitamin deficiencies, diarrhea, and excessive loss of fluids and electrolytes.
- *Genitourinary system*: Effects are similar to those from treatment of tumors of the digestive area. Infections, dehiscences, and fistulas as general complications of surgery also have multiple nutritional implications.

Chemotherapy

Chemotherapy causes nausea and vomiting, abdominal pain, mucositis, ileus, and malabsorption. Many of the cytostatic commonly used in the clinic, such as cisplatin, vinca alkaloids, 5-fluoruracil, and doxorubicin, can induce severe intestinal symptoms. The frequency and severity of these depend on the drug, the combination in which it is included, and the association with other types of therapy. Chemotherapy treatment has been shown to generate changes in body status in both breast and lung cancers.

Additionally, the administration of chemotherapy produces alteration in the perception of taste with a negative impact on appetite.

Radiotherapy

Radiotherapy can induce acute and chronic complications with very important nutritional implications. Side effects depend on the irradiated area, dose, fractionation, duration, and volume irradiated. Most are acute, begin around the second or third week of treatment, and disappear 2 or 3 weeks after the treatment is completed.

- In the irradiation of head and neck tumors, important mucositis, gingivitis, trismus, alterations of taste, and a characteristic xerostomia are produced, causing an important limitation to oral intake.
- Thoracic irradiation is associated with the development of radic esophagitis, fungal, or viral esophagitis; dysphagia; and gastroesophageal reflux.
- Abdominal and pelvic radiotherapy have as side effects proctitis, enteritis, and cystitis, depending on the location of the lesion to be irradiated.

Nausea, vomiting, and anorexia are common effects of irradiation to any location. Stenosis, bridle obstruction, chronic enteritis, and malabsorption can develop as chronic conditions.

Treatment with Immune Response Modulators

Immune response modulators such as IFN or IL-2 are associated with the development of anorexia, probably secondary to a central effect. However, this symptom is not by itself capable of inducing malnutrition and is part of a much larger symptom constellation. In this sense, it should be noted that on many occasions, these drugs are included in chemotherapy schemes for very advanced clinical situations in which it is practically impossible to determine the influence of each variable on the nutritional situation of the patient.

Nutritional Support

In cancer-associated malnutrition, there is low intake and metabolic alterations derived from the inflammatory response. Nutritional support can partially reverse this situation and has been associated with an improvement in the patient's body weight, functional status, and quality of life. Although it has not shown results in terms of survival, some studies suggest a better tolerance to treatment.

Nutritional support is indicated in malnourished patients or those at risk of malnutrition, and in those in whom the development of anorexia or gastrointestinal defects due to the toxicity of the treatment is foreseen. It can be classified, according to its complexity and invasiveness, into the following categories:

- *Nutritional recommendations or dietary advice*: When the patient is capable of ingesting more than 75% of his or her nutritional requirements with the oral diet and no risk, therapy is foreseen in the near future. The main objective of these nutritional recommendations is to control the symptoms caused by the tumor itself or the treatments, through changes in eating habits and oral supplements.
- *Artificial nutrition*:
  - Oral enteral nutrition or supplementation is recommended if the patient is only able to ingest between 50% and 75% of his or her requirements with the usual diet for more than 5 consecutive days, or has mild malnutrition; it is recommended to start supplementation with standard formulas, administered outside mealtimes.
  - Enteral nutrition by probe is recommended if the patient ingests less than 50% of his or her requirements for more than 5 days, or presents a moderate severe malnutrition; tube enteral malnutrition is specially indicated if dysphagia is present or severe mucositis is anticipated and can be administered by nasoenteric tube or ostomy.
  - Parenteral nutrition is recommended when enteral nutrition is contraindicated.

Food Supplements in Oncology

Food supplements in cancer patients can be useful as an instrument to provide the recommended daily amount of vitamins and minerals in patients with low intake.

After a diagnosis of cancer, it is known that dietary supplements are used by 20%–80% of individuals. Supplements are most commonly used by breast cancer survivors, followed by patients with prostate, colorectal, and lung cancers, which is not surprising, as these are the most common types of cancer diagnosed in adults. The reasons cited for that use include improving quality of life, reducing symptoms related to the treatment and/or disease process, and physician recommendation; family and friends might also be an influence. However, there is unresolved controversy surrounding the use of dietary supplements, particularly during specific treatment, and whether they affect the efficacy of treatment.

Antioxidants

Free radicals are highly reactive chemical compounds that can damage cells. They are created when an atom or molecule wins or loses an electron. Free radicals are formed naturally in the body and play an important role in many cell processes. At high concentrations, free radicals can be dangerous to the body and can damage all major components of cells, including DNA, proteins, and cell membranes. DNA damage can play a role in the formation of cancer and other diseases.

Antioxidants are chemical compounds that interact with free radicals and neutralize them, which prevents them from causing damage. There are two types: endogenous (produced by the body) and exogenous (from outside).

There are endogenous enzymatic defense systems against oxidation: superoxide dismutase, glutathione peroxidase, and catalase; when these enzymatic systems fail or are exceeded, an overproduction of superoxide ions and hydrogen peroxide is produced, which is not totally detoxified giving rise to the highly toxic hydroxyl radical (–OH).

Exogenous antioxidants come mainly from food—fruits, vegetables, and cereals (Table 23.1). There are, in turn, food antioxidants we find as food supplements; they are beta-carotene, lycopene, and vitamins A, C, and E (alpha-tocopherol). Selenium, zinc, and copper are part of the molecular structure of some of the antioxidant enzymes. Polyphenols such as flavonoids, quercetin, and resveratrol, are other important antioxidants.

Several *in vitro* and animal studies have shown that the presence of higher concentrations of exogenous antioxidants prevents the damage produced by free radicals that has been associated with the presence of cancer. For this reason, researchers have studied whether the use of dietary antioxidant supplements can help decrease cancer risk in humans. To date, in addition to numerous observational studies, a number of randomized controlled clinical trials (RCTs) have been published with variable results.

TABLE 23.1

Antioxidant Sources

Vitamin		Food Source
Vitamin E	Most important sources	Vegetable oils, cold-pressed seed oils, wheat germ, corn germ, almonds, hazelnuts, sunflower, soybeans, walnuts, peanuts
	Other significant sources	Fresh potatoes, avocado, celery, cabbage, fruits, chicken, fish
Vitamin C	Fruits	Lemon, sweet lemon (lime), orange, cashew, guava, mango, kiwi, papaya, blackberry, pineapple
	Vegetables	Tomato, leafy green vegetables (spinach, parsley, radish leaves), cabbage, cauliflower, broccoli, lettuce
Carotenoids	Beta-carotene	Yellow and orange vegetables and fruits, dark green vegetables
	Alpha-carotene	Carrot
	Lycopene	Tomato
	Lutein and zeaxanthin	Dark green leafy vegetables, broccoli
	Beta-criptoxantina	Citric fruits

Vitamin C

Vitamin C is a water-soluble vitamin, also known as ascorbic acid. It is stored in the body for only a short time and is eliminated in small amounts through the urine. It is an essential nutrient that in normal physiological concentrations has oxidation-reduction (redox) functions.

Since the 1970s, high doses of vitamin C have been studied for the treatment of cancer patients. In laboratory studies, it was reported that high doses of vitamin C have oxidation-reduction properties and that they decrease cell proliferation in prostate, pancreatic, liver, colon, mesothelioma, and neuroblastoma cell lines. In two studies of high-dose vitamin C in cancer patients, improved quality of life and decreased cancer-related side effects were reported. In fact, some human studies observed that high doses of vitamin C in cancer patients improved physical, mental, and emotional functioning, as well as symptoms of fatigue, nausea and vomiting, pain, and loss of appetite. Two prospective studies found that the intake of vitamin C is inversely associated with breast cancer incidences in certain subgroups. In the Nurses' Health Study, premenopausal women with a family history of breast cancer who consumed an average of 205 mg/day of vitamin C from their daily diet had 63% lower risk of developing breast cancer than those who consumed an average of 70 mg/day. In the Swedish Mammography Cohort, overweight women who consumed an average of 110 mg/day of vitamin C had a 39% lower risk of breast cancer compared to overweight women who consumed an average of 31 mg/day.

The most recent prospective cohort studies have found no association between dietary and/or supplemental vitamin C intake and breast cancer. In some human studies, it was observed that high doses of vitamin C administered intravenously in cancer patients improved the quality of life and physical, mental, and emotional functioning, as well as symptoms of fatigue, nausea and vomiting, pain, and loss of appetite.

Vitamin C is approved as a food supplement. The U.S. Food and Drug Administration (FDA) has not approved the use of high-dose vitamin C IV to treat cancer or other conditions.

Vitamin A: Retinol

Vitamin A is used to improve immune system function. It is also used to speed up the healing process and promote visual health (Table 23.2). The recommended daily intake is 700 micrograms (2310 international units) (Table 23.3).

Studies of vitamin A show no effect on the risk of cancer. While vitamin A has been found to reduce the growth of breast cancer cells *in vitro*, most epidemiological studies have failed to establish an association between retinol intake and breast cancer risk in women; however, a large prospective study found that a higher intake of vitamin A reduces the risk of breast cancer in premenopausal women with a family history of breast cancer.

Blood levels of retinol reflect the intake of preformed vitamin A, as well as provitamin A carotenoids such as beta-carotene. Although one case-control study established a relationship between higher levels of retinol and antioxidants in the blood and reduced risk of breast cancer, two prospective studies did not

TABLE 23.2

Deficit and Vitamins

Deficient Vitamin	Symptoms/Signs	Toxicity
A	Dry skin, dry eyes and blindness in advanced cases due to the loss of visual pigments	Exceeding the ability to store the vitamin can lead to poisoning.
E	People who cannot absorb high-fat diets leading to fat metabolism disorders.	In very high doses, it antagonizes the use of other fat-soluble vitamins.
C	Scurvy, defective formation and maintenance of collagen, increased susceptibility to infections, bleeding gums, and loose teeth	Diarrhea and gastrointestinal discomfort may cause kidney stones.

TABLE 23.3

Recommended Daily Requirements (RDRs)

Vitamins	RDRs for Men	RDRs for Women
A	5000 UI	4000 UI
E	10 mg	8 mg
C	60 mg	60 mg

observe any significant association between blood retinol level and subsequent risk of developing breast cancer.

Beta-Carotene

Beta-Carotene May Decrease Risk of Some Forms of Cancer

Beta-carotene is considered safe when it is consumed in food (Table 23.1) as part of a balanced diet. However, high doses of supplements can cause the skin to turn yellow or orange, and can cause increased damage to the body from free radicals.

As pointed out with antioxidants and cancer, there is a higher incidence among smokers, beta-carotene intake, and lung cancer, which would prohibit the intake of this antioxidant in patients with these characteristics.

In people diagnosed with cancer, diets rich in vegetables and fruits that contain the full range of carotenoids (not just beta-carotene) have been linked to a decrease in cancer recurrence. There is no evidence that supplements have contributed to the protective effect; more studies are needed.

Vitamin E: Alpha-Tocopherol

Vitamin E is a fat-soluble vitamin located in the cell membrane, important in the development of diseases related to oxidative processes, such as cardiovascular disease, cancer, diabetes, infections, rheumatic and neurological processes, pancreatitis, and aging.

Vitamin E can help to protect cell membranes against the damaging effects of free radicals, which can contribute to the

development of chronic diseases such as cancer. Vitamin E can also block the formation of nitrosamines, which are carcinogens formed in the stomach from nitrites consumed in the diet. It can also protect against the development of cancers by enhancing immune function (Table 23.2). In the body, it acts as an antioxidant, helping to protect cells against damage caused by free radicals, the compounds formed when the body converts the food we eat into energy. People are also exposed to the free radicals present in the environment through cigarette smoke, air pollution, and ultraviolet solar radiation.

Additionally, the body needs vitamin E to stimulate the immune system so that it can fight the bacteria and viruses that invade it. It helps to dilate blood vessels and prevent blood clots from forming inside them.

The use of vitamin E has been suggested as a possible therapy for the prevention or treatment of breast cancer. Published studies have included measurement of vitamin E levels, laboratory experiments, and population studies, but the result is not conclusive, and no conclusion can be reached at this time.

The Women's Health Study reported there is no reduction in the development of cancer with daily intake of natural sources of vitamin E. Previously, there have been other laboratory, population, and human studies that examined whether vitamin E is beneficial for the prevention of various cancers, including prostate, colon, and stomach cancers. More research is needed.

To conclude, there is no reliable scientific evidence as to whether vitamin E is effective as a treatment for any specific type of cancer. Caution is suggested in people undergoing chemotherapy or radiation treatments because the use of high-dose antioxidants may reduce the anticancer effects of these therapies. This area remains controversial, and studies have yielded variable results. High doses of vitamin E may also cause pain in cancer patients. Currently, we cannot be certain that taking this antioxidant is absolutely beneficial.

Minerals

Selenium

Selenium is a micro-mineral or trace element, essential for good health but only in small amounts. Selenium is incorporated into proteins forming selenoproteins, considered antioxidant enzymes. It helps to prevent cell damage caused by free radicals, contributes to the regulation of the thyroid gland, and plays an important role in our immune systems, among other functions. There are two important reserves of selenium in our organism. One comes from dietary selenium (selenomethionine) and the other from the liver, through selenium present in a liver enzyme (glutathione peroxidase). Vegetable foods, such as vegetables, are the most common sources of selenium in the diet. The amount of selenium present in vegetables that are consumed depends on the amount of mineral that was present in the soil where the plant grew.

Selenium prevents cell damage caused by the oxidation of free radicals, meaning it prevents cell aging and the appearance of chronic disease such as cancer and heart disease. It is fundamental for the correct functioning of the immune system, since it increases the production of white blood cells. It intervenes in the proper functioning of the thyroid gland, as it is an essential element for the development of normal growth and metabolism due to its role in the regulation of thyroid hormones. There are at least 25 selenoproteins identified with different functions, most with antioxidant functions.

Shamberger and Clark's ecological studies in Finland and in the United States showed that breast cancer incidence correlated inversely with exposure to selenium. But these studies do not allow us to draw definitive conclusions. In three prospective studies by Coates, Knekt, and Overvad, it was observed that the risk of breast cancer was higher in people with a very low plasma level. We must be aware that Finland is a country with one of the lowest levels of selenium, and these findings may suggest that women with an extremely low level of selenium have a higher risk of developing breast cancer. In the review carried out on antioxidant micronutrients and cancer by Garland in four of the five studies evaluated, a plasma level of selenium was found to be lower in cancer patients than in controls.

Zinc

For a long time, zinc has been known for playing a vital role in human health. The excess of zinc, or a lack of it, can cause cell death. There is a great deal of evidence about zinc's connection to disease states including neurodegeneration, inflammation, diabetes, and cancer.

Zinc levels in cells are controlled by protein molecules called zinc transporters. These are moved through the cell to ensure the correct levels are maintained. Zinc is found in cells throughout the body. It helps the immune system to fight against bacteria and viruses that invade the body. The body also needs zinc to make proteins and DNA, the genetic material present in cells. During pregnancy, infancy, and childhood, the body requires zinc to grow and develop well. Zinc also promotes wound healing and the normal functioning of the sense of taste and smell.

Studies have observed that menopausal women with breast cancer have lower zinc concentrations in the erythrocyte compartment, which may constitute a new prognostic biomarker and possible therapeutic target of breast cancer. The highest levels of intracellular zinc and ZIP7 transporter were found in breast cancers that were resistant to tamoxifen. CK2 was also known to be more common in cancers that favor cell growth. The discovery that CK2 opens ZIP7 suggests that drugs that block the release of zinc may also block the development of cancer. Early results from clinical trials of CK2 inhibitors suggest they are doing well. The concentration of zinc in breast cancer tissues is higher than in normal breast tissues. However, the mechanisms involved and the relationship with the zinc transporters are still unknown. With a zinc supplementation dietary treatment, mRNA expression of ZnT-1 in established human breast cancer is elevated by 24% and is almost two times higher than in the basal diet.

Magnesium

Magnesium is an essential mineral as it is involved in more than 300 enzymatic reactions. It participates in the metabolism of food components, in the transformation of complex nutrients into their elemental units, and in the synthesis of numerous organic products.

In order to develop all the functions in which this mineral is involved, an intake range of 150–500 mg/day is established as acceptable for the healthy adult population. Magnesium is mainly found in nuts and seeds—sunflower, sesame, almonds, pistachio, hazelnuts, and walnuts. Among cereals, it is found in wheat germ, yeast, millet, rice, and wheat. It can also be found in dairy products, fruits, and legumes (Table 23.4).

Magnesium is distributed in our body outside and inside the cells. Extracellular magnesium is involved in nerve and muscle transmission and in the proper functioning of the heart muscle (heart), and it plays a major role in muscle relaxation. Intracellular magnesium is part of the bone matrix. For athletes, magnesium is a key mineral because it plays, in balance with calcium, an important role in muscle function, relaxation, and muscle contraction.

Magnesium deficiency is carcinogenic, and in the case of solid tumors, a high level of magnesium supplementation inhibits carcinogenesis. The deficiency of carcinogenesis and magnesium increases the permeability of the plasma membrane and fluidity.

Anghileri proposed that changes in cell membranes are the main triggers of the cell transformation that leads to cancer. When they used induced cancer cells, they found there was much less magnesium binding to the phospholipids of the cancer cell membrane compared to normal cell membranes. It has been suggested that magnesium deficiency may lead to carcinogenesis by increasing membrane permeability. Magnesium-deficient cell membranes appear to have a smoother surface than normal membranes and a decreased membrane viscosity, analogous to cell changes in human leukemia.

TABLE 23.4

Minerals

Mineral	For	It Is In	Observations
Zinc	Growth, infections, cell reproduction, skin	Fish, meat, seafood, wholemeal bread, cereal, legumes, and eggs	10–15 milligrams per day
Sodium	Water control in tissues, heart rate		Excess affects the kidneys, heart, and blood pressure (increases); no more than 1600 milligrams a day
Magnesium	Neuromuscular irritability; conservation of the bone system; muscular-energy system; anorexia, nausea, tremors, vomiting, weakness, arrhythmia with personality alteration	Vegetables, nuts, green vegetables, soy, milk, bread, whole grain cereal, hard water	Between 200 and 400 milligrams per day
Selenium	Slows skin aging (antioxidant)	Seafood, liver, kidneys, meats, vegetables	55–70 micrograms per day
Copper	Anemia	Nuts, wheat, cocoa, fish	1.5–3 milligrams per day

There is a drastic change in the ionic flow of the external and internal cell membranes (increased amount of calcium and niacin, low levels of magnesium and potassium) in both damaged cancer membranes and magnesium deficiency.

It has been found that the main salts (Pb) are more leukemogenic when they are given to magnesium-deficient rats than when they are given to magnesium-sufficient rats, suggesting that magnesium has a protective effect.

There are no conclusive studies recommending use for breast cancer patients. A relationship has been observed between bone metastases and estrogens and magnesium.

Phytochemicals

Polyphenols

Polyphenols are compounds biosynthesized by plants in their fruits, leaves, stems, roots, seeds, or other parts. The main structural characteristic of polyphenols is to have one or more hydroxyl (–OH) groups attached to one or more benzene rings. Although they are primarily known for their antioxidant properties, most polyphenols also have other biological activities that are potentially beneficial for health. Polyphenols, which generally account for most of the antioxidant activity of fruits and vegetables, are classified into flavonoids (of which several thousand have been described in the plant kingdom) and nonflavonoids (for which several hundred have been described).

These compounds have vasodilator effects; they are able to improve the lipid profile and attenuate the oxidation of low-density lipoproteins (LDLs). They present clear anti-inflammatory effects, and these compounds are in turn capable of modulating the processes of apoptosis in the vascular endothelium.

A growing number of natural substances have been identified as modulators of the carcinogenesis process; among them are flavonoids that have been shown to have antimutagenic, anticarcinogenic, and antiproliferative action.

Among the numerous phenomena that occur during the carcinogenic process and offer an option for modulation by external factors are the formation of carcinogenic metabolites, which are formed by the action of cytosolic and microsomic enzymes. *In vivo* and *in vitro* studies have shown that flavonoids can modulate this enzyme activity. *In vitro* studies confirmed the protective role of quercetin, which exerts inhibitory effects against cancer cells in humans, in the colon, in the mammary and ovarian glands, in the gastrointestinal region, and in leukemia.

A possible explanation for these anticancer effects could be the increase that some flavonoids produce in the intracellular concentrations of glutathione through the regulation of the expression of the limiting enzyme in its synthesis. Additionally, the breast cancer effect could be due to its potent ability to inhibit aromatase activity, thereby preventing the conversion of androgens into estrogens.

There are studies supporting the antioxidant power of some flavonoids, such as resveratrol or green tea, in relation to cancer. We must continue to study this effect in order to reach a firmer conclusion.

Omega-3

Essential fatty acids are those fatty acids necessary for certain functions the body cannot synthesize, which must be obtained through diet. These are polyunsaturated fatty acids with all double bonds in cis position. The only two essential fatty acids for humans are α-linolenic ($18:3\omega$-3) and linolenic ($18:2\omega$-6). If these are supplied, the human body can synthesize the rest of the fatty acids it needs.

Both diet and biosynthesis provide most of the fatty acids required by the human organism, and excess protein and carbohydrates easily become fatty acids that are stored in the form of triglycerides. However, many mammals, including humans, are unable to synthesize certain polyunsaturated fatty acids with double bonds near the methyl end of the molecule. In humans, it is essential to ingest a dietary precursor for two series of fatty acids, the linoleic acid series (ω-6) and the linolenic acid series (ω-3 series).

Essential fatty acids are found mainly in oils, fish, seeds, and nuts, such as sunflower seeds, flax seeds, nuts, and olive or cod oils. The diet of animals for consumption may also cause them to contain large amounts of these fatty acids, for example, meat from pigs fed acorns or hens fed algae and fishmeal that lay eggs with higher amounts of these fatty acids. Certain foods are artificially enriched with omega-3, such as milk, soy milk, eggs, and so on.

It has been shown experimentally that the consumption of large amounts of omega-3 considerably increases the time of blood coagulation, which explains why in communities that consume many foods with omega-3, the incidence of cardiovascular disease is lower. Another study concluded that dietary intake of fatty acids ω-3 modestly reduces the course of coronary arteriosclerosis in humans.

Omega-3 fatty acids are a good source of lignans, compounds that may have a mild estrogenic effect. When a weak substance similar to estrogen takes the place of the body's natural strong estrogen in a breast cell's estrogen receptor, the weak substance may act as a relative antiestrogen. By acting this way, lignans may help fight the type of breast cancer that depends on estrogen to grow. However, research conducted so far to determine whether omega-3 fatty acids influence breast cancer risk has not been conclusive. A study in rats showed that a diet enriched with DHA induced a reduction in breast tumors, with a 60% increase in plasma levels of the tumor-suppressing protein BRCA1. It was observed that in animals receiving diets enriched with omega-3 fatty acids, there was an increase in the efficacy of the drugs doxorubicin and mitomycin C65, which are used to inhibit tumor growth. In addition, an increase in the inhibitory effect of the drug tamoxifen was observed in estrogen-dependent models, which would allow the potential use of omega-3 as an adjuvant to standard chemotherapy to be considered.

Conclusions

The oncology patient may be vulnerable due to the psychological effect of the diagnosis and the complexity of the treatments received. Dietary advice for the treatment of symptoms should be a fundamental pillar of care, which can help to improve the nutritional status and quality of life of these people.

Although in the rest of the population a balanced diet and adequate food intake are sufficient to provide the necessary vitamins and minerals, this is not always possible in this group. Multivitamin supplements (whose vitamin and mineral content is within the recommended amounts) may be useful in achieving a sufficient supply of micronutrients in cancer patients.

The use of these supplements with the sole purpose of preventing oncological diseases lacks evidence. Water-soluble vitamins in the general population can be safely administered, as the risk of toxicity is low. However, beta-carotene supplementation should be discouraged, especially in those at high risk of lung cancer (smokers or those who have had contact with asbestos).

In cancer patients on active treatment, an assessment of the benefits and risks of dietary supplementation should be made, taking into account possible interactions with the antineoplastic treatment they are receiving.

In the absence of consistent evidence, the advice on antioxidant supplementation during treatment should be preceded by a thorough evaluation of the advantages and disadvantages. The first step would be to evaluate the safety of the preparation and consult the possible interactions described between the nutritional supplement and the treatment the patient is receiving. There are databases that provide us with this information: Natural Medicines comprehensive database (http://www.naturaldatabase.com; http://www.naturalstandard.com), Natural Standard or Memorial Sloan Kettering Cancer Center (https://www.mskcc.org/cancer-care/treatments/symptom-management/integrative-medicine/herbs/search). It is important to bear in mind that although an interaction may not have been described, its existence cannot be ruled out.

In general, it should be recommended to avoid the use of supplements with high doses of antioxidants in patients under active treatment with radiotherapy or with any chemotherapeutic drug whose mechanism of action involves the generation of free radicals. Possible interactions should be minimized by separating supplementation and therapy as much as possible. In patients undergoing treatment with radiotherapy, which is usually administered continuously for a relatively short time, it should be taken into account that the effect lasts until several weeks after completion of its application, so antioxidant supplements should not be initiated until this period has elapsed.

In the case of chemotherapy, it is more complicated to establish a recommendation. Chemotherapy cycles are usually given every 2–3 weeks for longer periods. For most chemotherapeutic agents, their duration of action is unknown, so it is not possible to establish a time at which the administration of antioxidants can be considered safe. For this reason, it is recommended not to use them for the entire duration of chemotherapy. Finally, the intention of the treatment—curative or palliative—must always be taken to account.

BIBLIOGRAPHY

Staff MOF, Speaker BA. Magnesium Deficiency and Cancer. *Dr Sircus.* 2016; published online March 2. http://drsircus.com/magnesium/magnesium-is-basic-to-cancer-treatment/.

Alimentos que contienen ácidos grasos omega 3. http://www.Breastcancer.org. www.breastcancer.org/es/consejos/nutricion/reducir_riesgo/alimentos/omega3.

Anghileri LJ. Magnesium, calcium and cancer. *Magnes res.* 2009;22(4):247–55.

Anghileri LJ, Collery P, Coudoux P, Durlach J. Experimental relationships between magnesium and cancer. *Magnesium Bull.* 1981;3(1):1–5.

Avello M, Suwalsky M. Radicales libres, antioxidantes naturales y mecanismos de protección. *Atenea Concepc.* 2006;161–72.

Belanger CF, Hennekens CH, Rosner B, Speizer FE. The nurses' health study. *Am J Nurs.* 1978;78(6):1039–40.

Betacaroteno. www.Breastcancer.org. http://www.breastcancer.org/es/consejos/nutricion/suplementos/conocidos/betacaroteno

Beta-caroteno. MedlinePlus suplement.

Cha J, Roomi MW, Ivanov V, Kalinovsky T, Niedzwiecki A, Rath M. Ascorbate supplementation inhibits growth and metastasis of B16FO melanoma and 4T1 breast cancer cells in vitamin C-deficient mice. *Int J Oncol.* 2013;42:55–64.

Ching S, Ingram D, Hahnel R, Beilby J, Rossi E. Serum levels of micronutrients, antioxidants and total antioxidant status predict risk of breast cancer in a case control study. *J Nutr.* 2002;132:303–6.

Chio IIC, Tuveson DA. ROS in cancer: The burning question. *Trends Mol Med* 2017; published online April 17. DOI:10.1016/j.molmed.2017.03.004.

Clark LC, Graham GF, Crounse RG, Grimson R, Hulka B, Shy CM. Plasma selenium and skin neoplasms: A case-control study. *Nutr Cancer.* 1984;6:13–21.

Coates RJ, Weiss NS, Daling JR, Morris JS, Labbe RF. Serum levels of selenium and retinol and the subsequent risk of cancer. *Am J Epidemiol.* 1988;128:515–23.

Colditz GA, Manson JE, Hankinson SE. The Nurses' Health Study: 20-year contribution to the understanding of health among women. *J Women's Health* 1997;6(1):49–62.

Dorgan JF, Sowell A, Swanson CA et al. Relationships of serum carotenoids, retinol, alpha-tocopherol, and selenium with breast cancer risk: Results from a prospective study in Columbia, Missouri (United States). *Cancer Causes Control CCC.* 1998;9:89–97.

Dou QP. Molecular mechanisms of green tea polyphenols. *Nutr Cancer.* 2009;61:827.

Effects of gallium chloride oral administration on transplanted C3HBA mammary adenocarcinoma: Ga, Mg, Ca and Fe concentration and anatomopathological characteristics. https://www.researchgate.net/publication/19362254_Effects_of_gallium_chloride_oral_administration_on_transplanted_C3HBA_mammary_adenocarcinoma_Ga_Mg_Ca_and_Fe_concentration_and_anatomopathological_characteristics.

Garland M, Morris JS, Stampfer MJ et al. Prospective study of toenail selenium levels and cancer among women. *J Natl Cancer Inst.* 1995;87:497–505.

Gomez LS, Zancan P, Marcondes MC et al. Resveratrol decreases breast cancer cell viability and glucose metabolism by inhibiting 6-phosphofructo-1-kinase. *Biochimie.* 2013;95:1336–43.

Grasas omega-3: buenas para su corazón: MedlinePlus enciclopedia médica. https://medlineplus.gov/spanish/ency/patientinstructions/000767.htm.

Guirado Blanco O. Ácidos grasos omega-6 y omega-3 de la dieta y carcinogénesis mamaria: Bases moleculares y celulares. *Medicentro Electrónica*. 2015;19:132–41.

Gutiérrez VRJ. Daño oxidativo, radicales libres y antioxidantes. *Rev Cuba Med Mil*. 2002;31:126–33.

Harris HR, Bergkvist L, Wolk A. Vitamin C intake and breast cancer mortality in a cohort of Swedish women. *Br J Cancer*. 2013;109:257–64.

Jeurnink SM, Ros MM, Leenders M et al. Plasma carotenoids, vitamin C, retinol and tocopherols levels and pancreatic cancer risk within the European Prospective Investigation into Cancer and Nutrition: A nested case-control study: Plasma micronutrients and pancreatic cancer risk. *Int J Cancer*. 2015;136:E665–676.

Knekt P, Aromaa A, Maatela J et al. Serum selenium and subsequent risk of cancer among Finnish men and women. *J Natl Cancer Inst*. 1990;82:864–8.

Larsson SC, Holmberg L, Wolk A. Fruit and vegetable consumption in relation to ovarian cancer incidence: The Swedish Mammography Cohort. *Br J Cancer*. 2004;90(11):2167–70.

Lee IM, Cook NR, Manson JE et al. β-Carotene supplementation and incidence of cancer and cardiovascular disease: The Women's Health Study. *J Natl Cancer Inst*. 1999;91(24):2102–6.

Lee IM, Cook NR, Gaziano JM et al. Vitamin E in the primary prevention of cardiovascular disease and cancer: The Women's Health Study: A randomized controlled trial. *JAMA*. 2005;294(1):56–65.

Magnesio en la dieta: MedlinePlus enciclopedia médica. https://medlineplus.gov/spanish/ency/article/002423.htm.

Mansara P, Ketkar M, Deshpande R, Chaudhary A, Shinde K, Kaul-Ghanekar R. Improved antioxidant status by omega-3 fatty acid supplementation in breast cancer patients undergoing chemotherapy: A case series. *J Med Case Reports*. 2015;9:148.

Maruthanila VL, Elancheran R, Kunnumakkara AB, Kabilan S, Kotoky J. Recent development of targeted approaches for the treatment of breast cancer. *Breast Cancer Tokyo Jpn*. 2017;24:191–219.

Office of Dietary Supplements: Vitamina E. https://ods.od.nih.gov/factsheets/VitaminE-DatosEnEspanol/.

Overvad K. Selenium and cancer. *Bibl Nutr Dieta*. 1998;141–9.

Press M. La vitamina E en la dieta protege contra muchos tipos de cáncer pero el uso en suplementos no tiene beneficios. *Med. Press*. 2012; published online April 23. http://www.medical press.es/la-vitamina-e-en-la-dieta-protege-contra-muchos-tipos-de-cancer-pero-el-uso-en-suplementos-no-tiene-beneficios/.

Selenio en la dieta: MedlinePlus enciclopedia médica. https://medlineplus.gov/spanish/ency/article/002414.htm (accessed April 27, 2017).

Semba RD. The role of vitamin A and related retinoids in immune function. *Nutr Rev*. 1998;56:S38–48.

Shamberger RJ, Frost DV. Possible protective effect of selenium against human cancer. *Can Med Assoc J*. 1969;100:682.

Shivappa N, Harris H, Wolk A, Hebert JR. Association between inflammatory potential of diet and mortality among women in the Swedish Mammography Cohort. *Eur J Nutr*. 2016;55(5):1891–1900.

Srivastava S, Somasagara RR, Hegde M et al. Quercetin, a natural flavonoid interacts with DNA, arrests cell cycle and causes tumor regression by activating mitochondrial pathway of apoptosis. *Sci Rep*. 2016;6:24049.

Steinmetz KA, Kushi LH, Bostick RM et al. Vegetables, fruit, and colon cancer in the Iowa women's health study. *Am J Epidemiol* 1994;139(1):1–15.

Sun D, Zhang L, Wang Y et al. Regulation of zinc transporters by dietary zinc supplement in breast cancer. *Mol Biol Rep*. 2007;34:241–7.

Thiébaut ACM, Chajès V, Gerber M et al. Dietary intakes of omega-6 and omega-3 polyunsaturated fatty acids and the risk of breast cancer. *Int J Cancer*. 2009;124:924–31.

Triana GEB, Saldaña Bernabeu A, Saldaña García L. El estrés oxidativo y los antioxidantes en la prevención del cáncer. *Rev Habanera Cienc Médicas*. 2013;12:187–96.

Tukiendorf A. *Magnesium Intake and Hepatic Cancer*. 2007:155–70.

Valenzuela BR, Bascuñan GK, Chamorro MR, Valenzuela BA. Ácidos grasos omega-3 y cáncer, una alternativa nutricional para su prevención y tratamiento. *Rev Chil Nutr*. 2011;38:219–26.

Vitamin A. www.Breastcancer.org. http://www.breastcancer.org/es/consejos/nutricion/suplementos/conocidos/vit_a

Vitamina E. http://www.Breastcancer.org. www.breastcancer.org/es/consejos/nutricion/suplementos/conocidos/vit_e.

Zhang S, Hunter DJ, Forman MR et al. Dietary carotenoids and vitamins A, C, and E and risk of breast cancer. *J Natl Cancer Inst*. 1999;91:547–56.

24

Introduction to Vascular Complications in Oncology Patients

Emilce Insua Nipoti

Introduction

Vascular complications in oncological patients are usually serious and may entail a higher morbidity/mortality associated with the neoplastic process. Complications due to vascular obstruction in advanced neoplasias can cause syndromes with complex therapeutic approaches (such as the Budd-Chiari or superior vena cava syndromes), as well as complications derived from chemotherapy due to cardiac, renal, or spinal cytotoxic effects, or from long-term radiotherapy-induced vascular lesions. However, the vascular pathology most often associated with neoplastic pathology is the venous thromboembolic disease, in which deep vein thrombosis may occur weeks or months prior to detection of the underlying neoplasia. Chemotherapy and antineoplastic hormone therapy have been associated with thrombotic and hemorrhagic cerebrovascular events. Some studies have found a larger incidence of cerebrovascular events with cisplatin, whereas tamoxifen is related with an increased risk of arterial and venous thromboembolism.

Secondary *Budd-Chiari syndrome* is a rare condition caused by occlusion of the suprahepatic veins due to tumoral thrombosis or compression, characterized by the insidious or acute occurrence of painful hepatomegaly, jaundice, ascites, splenomegaly, venous collateral circulation, and edema of the extremities. The most common oncological etiology is hepatocellular carcinoma, followed by renal carcinoma, adrenal gland carcinoma, nephroblastoma, or Wilms tumor and leiomyosarcoma. The diagnosis is confirmed by the clinic on analysis of ascites characterized by high protein content, except in acute forms and imaging studies (abdominal ultrasound, computed tomography [CT] scans, and magnetic resonance imaging [MRI]). Morbidity and mortality are usually associated with the evolution of liver failure and basic neoplastic pathology [1].

Superior vena cava syndrome (SVCS) is caused by obstruction of the superior vena cava through intraluminal occlusion, extrinsic compression, and/or neoplastic invasion. The most commonly involved tumor is lung cancer (80%), followed by mediastinal nodal metastasis, and hematological neoplasia. Symptoms usually appear in an insidious manner, being characterized by dyspnea, cyanosis, and head and neck edema with collateral circulation due to vein distention in the neck and chest. The most common radiographic alterations are widening of the upper mediastinum and the presence of pleural effusion. Imaging methods such as CT and MRI provide more information for the diagnosis. The prognosis of patients with SVCS is closely related to the prognosis of the underlying disease [2].

As a serious complication in long-term lymphedema, the so-called *Stewart-Treves syndrome* or *angiosarcoma* that develops over an extremity previously affected with lymphedema becomes particularly significant. The time elapsed between the development of the lymphedema and the angiosarcoma diagnosis is 8–10 years on average; long-term patient follow-up is therefore very important. The evolution of angiosarcoma is aggressive, with fast locoregional growth, a tendency to early and remote metastasis, and high mortality [3].

There are other cardiovascular complications caused by the progression of neoplastic disease or associated with chemotherapy and/or radiotherapy, such as *radiation-induced vasculopathy* with early stenosis of coronary arteries, calcification of the ascending aorta, and involvement of intra-/extracranial vessels with increased incidence of carotid stenosis after cervical radiotherapy. Vasculopathy of intracranial vessels (postradiation moyamoya syndrome) has also been described in children. Cavernous malformations and aneurysms with a higher risk of presenting cranial hemorrhage have also been described after cranial radiotherapy.

Acute renal failure in oncological patients has a multifactorial origin; the most common causes are those related to chemotherapy due to the risk of nephrotoxicity, since the kidney is one of the main routes for cytostatic elimination, and complications derived from the neoplastic process itself. The treatment of acute renal failure is usually conservative, although it may require hemodialysis, for which it might be necessary to assess the risks and benefits of the different vascular accesses [4].

Cerebrovascular complications show a high incidence and a great impact on the morbidity/mortality of patients with cancer. They may represent the first manifestation of an oncological disease, but they can also be related to treatment neurotoxicity (chemo- and radiotherapy). The incidence of cerebrovascular diseases is probably similar in patients with cancer and the general population, but in the former it is possible to identify the specific causes of a stroke, such as those related to the tumor itself (tumor compression or infiltration, tumor embolism, intratumoral hemorrhage, tumoral aneurysm rupture), those originating in complications from chemotherapy treatments (nonbacterial thrombotic endocarditis, cerebral intravascular coagulation, vein thrombosis, thrombocytopenia), or those associated with radiotherapy (late vasculopathy) or vascular lesion due to surgery. The most common causes of cerebrovascular disease seem to be different in patients with hematological and solid neoplasias. In patients with hematological neoplasia (especially leukemia), cerebral hemorrhage is more common than ischemic stroke, its etiology being more usual than septic stroke and disseminated intravascular coagulation. In patients with solid neoplasia, ischemic cerebral stroke caused by nonbacterial thrombotic endocarditis and disseminated intravascular coagulation is more common [5].

In Spain and in other developed countries, an increase in the incidence of new cancer cases is observed, but with a decrease in mortality; these survival achievements may condition the appearance of complications associated with the survival of oncological patients, such as *secondary lymphedema,* which has a great impact on patients' quality of life since it may occur several years after oncological diagnosis and treatment.

Most carcinomas use lymphatic vessels for local and remote dissemination, so the lymphatic system may be affected in oncological patients due to either locoregional progression of the tumor or oncological treatment (surgery, chemo- and radiotherapy).

In developed countries, the main cause of lymphedema is that secondary to neoplasias due to surgical resection or lymphatic invasion. The most common is that related to breast cancer treatments. The incidence of lymphedema secondary to neoplasia treatment increases with survival. About 20% of breast cancer patients who have undergone a mastectomy with axillary clearance and radiotherapy will develop lymphedema of the upper extremities at 6 months, 36% at 1 year, and 54% at 36 months. In the case of conservative resections and sentinel node (SN) ablation, this incidence decreases to 5%–17% [6].

Neoplastic secondary lymphedema of the lower extremities has an incidence of 17%–41% in association with the treatment of carcinoma of the uterus, 36% for carcinoma of the vulva, 5% for carcinoma of the ovary, and 23%–80% for carcinoma of prostate, lymphoma, and melanoma [7].

The diagnosis of secondary lymphedema is mainly clinical (by taking the case history and physical examination), being the early diagnosis of lymphostasis; the correction of predisposing factors derived from oncological treatments (immobility of the extremity, associated surgical and vascular complications, radiodermatitis, scars, etc.) is of great importance [8].

Cancer-related secondary lymphedema of the extremities typically affects the proximal region of the extremity, with the possibility of spreading to all of it, including toes and fingers. Measuring the circumference and analyzing the volume of the extremities are a few methods used to assess the seriousness of lymphedema; it is of great importance to do these before performing any oncological therapy for the early detection and treatment of lymphostasis [9]. The survival of oncological patients conditions an increase in secondary lymphedema, an insidious and chronic disease that significantly affects patients' quality of life and may be potentially disabling [10].

It is important to diagnose and treat the edema when mild to prevent its evolution. Women with mild lymphedema are three times more likely to suffer moderate or serious lymphedema than women without this condition [9].

Sentinel Node Biopsy

The best results are obtained with prevention, using conservative oncological techniques like *Sentinel Node (SN) biopsy,* which has significantly reduced the incidence of postmastectomy lymphedema, and the establishment of early diagnosis and treatment protocols in preclinical manifestation phases (phase 0).

Several studies have proven that lymphedema is more common in patients with axillary node dissection and clearance (20% incidence) than in those with SN biopsy (5%–17% incidence), with most of them mild, depending on the threshold of the diagnosis and the duration of the follow-up [9,11].

Aside from the lymphatic pathways of the extremities, which are described in Chapter 25, the main node chains that can be affected in more common neoplasias are as follows:

- Head and neck node chains
- Axillary and pectoral (supraclavicular, infraclavicular, axillary, and internal mammary) node chains
- Inguinal and iliac-lumbar node chains
- Epicolic and mesocolic nodes
- Peribronchial, subpleural, mediastinal nodes

Metastatic nodal involvement is the most significant prognostic factor in malignant tumors because it means disease spread.

The concept of SN *biopsy* is based on the fact that the lymphatic drainage of malignant tumors follows an orderly, predictable pattern toward a certain node region. The location and selective biopsy of this first node allows us to assess the locoregional extension of the neoplastic disease and its TNM classification. Until recent years, the only valid method to confirm this involvement was lymphadenectomy, but since early detection programs are becoming increasingly more common, most tumors are diagnosed without the presence of node involvement, so lymphadenectomy does not provide any benefit.

Selective Sentinel Node Biopsy

The histological study of SNs by *selective sentinel node biopsy (SSNB)* allows the physician to choose the most appropriate type of surgery for each patient. Clinical value lies in its predictive value since it is accepted that, if negative, the other nodes are also negative, and therefore, it is not necessary to remove them [12].

The technique consists of performing an isotopic lymphogammagraphy, usually 24 hours before surgery, by peri- or intratumoral injection of a colloid radiotracer marked with technetium 99, and assessment of the uptake at the level of the main drainage nodes. Lymphoscintigraphy can also provide information about the tumor's lymphatic drainage pattern.

Once located, the skin is marked over the SN with indelible ink to guide the surgical approach and perform the intraoperative biopsy of the marked node. If positive, a lymphadenectomy will be performed during the same surgery; if negative, nodes will not be cleared, and the physician will wait for the final report. If node metastasis or micrometastasis is confirmed, postponed lymphadenectomy is indicated.

About 20% of patients with primary skin melanoma have nodal metastasis, which reduces survival. When the SN is negative, the incidence of relapse and metastasis is lower.

Contraindications to performing SSNB are pregnancy, chemotherapy, radiotherapy or long previous mammary surgery, inflammatory carcinoma, multicentric tumor or greater than 5 cm, or clinically (or by ultrasound) pathological axilla confirmed by puncture with fine needle; positive node involvement is indicative of lymphadenectomy, although there is some controversy about this indication in advanced tumors.

SSNB reduces surgical mortality and complications of lymphadenectomy in breast and vulva cancers. (There is metastasis of the inguinal lymph nodes in about 20%–35% of patients with tumors clinically limited to the vulva.)

The advantages of SSNB include reduction of surgical morbidity/mortality and of complications associated with lymphadenectomy, like decrease in dehiscence of the suture, seromas, wound infections, vascular-nervous lesions, pain and immobility of the extremity, and reduction of the incidence of secondary lymphedema (from 36%–54% to 5%–17%) [13], with a resulting decrease in the risk of angiosarcoma of lymphatic origin.

SSNB is a fully validated technique for the treatment of breast cancer and melanoma [14–16].

REFERENCES

1. Liu FY, Wang MQ, Duan F, Fan QS, Song P, Wang Y. Hepatocellular carcinoma associated with Budd-Chiari syndrome: Imaging features and transcatheter arterial chemoembolization. *BMC Gastroenterol.* 2013 Jun 24;13:105.
2. Varona Porres D, Andreu Soriano J, Pallisa Núñez E, Persiva Morenza O, Roque Pérez A. Actualización: Patología vascular torácica en pacientes oncológicos. *Radiología.* 2011;53(4):335–48.
3. Sánchez Medina MT, Acosta A, Vilarb J, Fernández- Palaciosa J. Carta científico-clínica: Angiosarcoma en linfedema crónico (síndrome de Stewart-Treves). *Actas Dermosifiliogr.* 2012;103:545–7.
4. Lavilla FJ, Martín S, García Fernández N et al. Fracaso renal agudo en el paciente oncológico. Análisis clínico y pronóstico. *Rev Electron Biomed/Electron J Biomed.* 2004;3:9–14.
5. Bushnell CD and Goldstein LB. Risk of ischemic stroke with tamoxifen treatment for breast cancer: A meta-analysis. *Neurology.* 2004;63:1230–3.
6. DiSipio T, Rye S, Newman B, Rye S, Hayes S. Incidence of unilateral arm lymphoedema after breast cancer: A systematic review and meta-analysis. *Lancet Oncol.* 2013 May;14(6): 500–15.
7. Beesley V, Janda M, Eakin E et al. Lymphedema after gynecological cancer treatment: Prevalence, correlates and supportive care needs. *Cancer.* 2007;109(12):2607–14.
8. Vogelfang D. Edemas de los miembros inferiores. In: *Medicina Estética y Antienvejecimiento Fernandez.* Tresguerres JAF, Insua Nipoti E, Castaño Cambara P, Tejero Garcia P. Editorial Médica Panamericana, 2nd Ed. 2018. p. 275–82.
9. Norman SA, Localio AR, Potashnik SL, Torpey HAS, Kallan MJ, Weber AL. Lymphedema in breast cancer survivor: Incidence, degree, time course, treatment and symptoms. *J Clin Oncol.* 2009;27:390–7.
10. Alonso Álvarez B, García Montes I. Linfedema y discapacidad. In: *Guía de práctica clínica: Orientación diagnóstica y terapéutica del linfedema.* © 2017 Capítulo Español de Flebología y Linfología, pp.133–34.
11. Hayes SC, Janda M, Cornish B, Battistutta D, Newman B. Lymphedema following breast cancer: Incidence, risk factors and effect on upper body function. *J Clin Oncol.* 2008;26:3536–42.
12. Wright MJ. *Surgical Treatment of Breast Cancer.* 2014. http://emedicine.medscape.com/article/1276001-overview
13. Giuliano AE, Ballman K, McCall L et al. Locoregional recurrence after sentinel lymph node dissection with or without axillary dissection in patients with sentinel lymph node metastases: Long-term follow-up from the American College of Surgeons Oncology Group (Alliance) ACOSOG Z0011 Randomized Trial. *Ann Surg.* 2016;264:413–20.
14. Mc Gregor JM and Sasieni P. EDITORIAL: Sentinel node biopsy in cutaneous melanoma: Time for consensus to better inform patient choice. *Br J Dermatol.* 2015;172:552–4. http://onlinelibrary.wiley.com/doi/10.1111/bjd.13666/epdf
15. Lyman GH, Somerfield MR, Bosserman LD, Perkins CL, Weaver DL, Giuliano AE. Sentinel lymph node biopsy for patients with early-stage breast cancer: American Society of Clinical Oncology Clinical Practice guideline update. *J Clin Oncol.* 2017;35(5):561–4.
16. Youssef MM, Cameron D, Pucher PH, Olsen S, Ferguson D. The significance of sentinel lymph node micrometastasis in breast cancer: Comparing outcomes with and without axillary clearance. *Breast.* 2016;30:101–4.

25

Anatomy of Lymphatic Drainage of the Limbs

José Luis Ciucci and Andrea Lourdes Mendoza

Introduction

Most carcinomas use lymphatic vessels for local and remote dissemination, so the lymphatic system (LS) may be affected in oncological patients due to either locoregional progression of the tumor or oncological treatment (surgery, chemo- and radiotherapy); for this reason, it is essential to have thorough anatomical knowledge of lymph flows and nodal centers.

In developed countries, the main cause of lymphedema is that secondary to neoplasias due to surgical resection or lymphatic invasion. The most common overall is that related to breast cancer treatments involving the upper limbs, although in the lower limbs the most common is that related to melanoma or uterus, vulva, ovarian, or prostate cancer.

Metastatic nodal involvement is the most significant prognostic factor in malignant tumors because it means disease spread. The concept of the sentinel node (SN) is based on the fact that the lymphatic drainage of malignant tumors follows an orderly, predictable pattern toward a certain node region. The location and selective biopsy of this first node decreases the morbidity of nodal clearance if negative, and if positive, allows assessment of the locoregional extension of the neoplastic disease and its TNM classification.

Superficial Lymph Flows of the Upper Limb

1. *Forearm*: There are four superficial lymph flows in the forearm.

• Two anterior	Anterointernal or anterior ulnar surface
	Anteroexternal or anterior radial surface
• Two posterior	Posterointernal or posterior ulnar
	Posteroexternal or posterior radial

There are a few lymphatic vessels in the palm of the hand and many in the back of the hand.

Lymphatic vessels go up the fingers, through the back of the hand, and to the posterior region of the forearm, embracing it near the middle third of this region, going through the ulnar and radial edges, and arriving to its anterior face, where they drain into the anterointernal and anteroexternal lymph flows.

No nodes have been found along the pathway of these lymph flows.

Each lymph flow is independent because each one drains into a certain region of the hand and forearm.

When arriving at the elbow region, they will become part of the bicipital and tricipital lymph flows.

2. *Arm*: There are six lymph flows in the arm.

• Three anterior or bicipital	Medial anterior or bicipital
	Anterointernal or basilic
	Anteroexternal or cephalic
• Three posterior or tricipital	Internal tricipital
	Medial tricipital
	External tricipital

The medial bicipital flow, made of 7–12 lymphatic vessels, is the most important in the upper limb, going over the fleshy part of the biceps and draining lymph into the axillary nodes, mainly in the external mammary nodal group.

The basilic lymph flow, made of two or three lymphatic vessels, is very short and shadows the basilic vein, quickly becoming deeper as it follows the humeral flow.

The cephalic or external bicipital lymph flow is the anterior derivative flow of the upper limb. It shadows the cephalic vein throughout its pathway and drains lymph into the transverse cervical flow.

Posterior or tricipital flows have fewer lymphatic vessels than anterior flows, which can be divided into internal, medial, and external, each one made of one or two lymphatic vessels. The first two take lymph to the axilla, whereas the external flow, described by Caplan in 1982 in Buenos Aires, goes through the deltoid-triceps area, draining through the triangle of round muscles into the posterior scapular flow. This is the posterior extra-axillary derivative flow (Figures 25.1 and 25.2).

Superficial Node Chains

The superficial ulnar chain is an ulnar subepitrochlear group in the elbow. It is found on the upper third of the forearm, at the level of the superficial ulnar vein, below the epitrochlea, which is made of one to two (subepitrochlear) nodes. It takes lymph preferably from the little finger, and its efferents drain into the basilic chain.

The basilic chain is the most important superficial chain of the upper limb, constituting the epitrochlear group. This node chain, which is made of one to three (supraepitrochlear) nodes, shadows the basilic vein. It receives lymphatic drainage from the

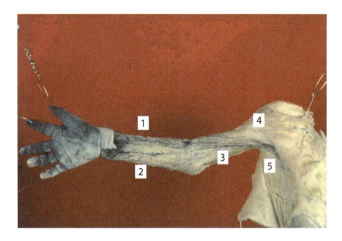

FIGURE 25.1   (1) Anterior superficial radial flow. (4) External bicipital (cephalic) flow. (2) Anterior superficial ulnar flow. (6) Axillary nodes. (3) Medial bicipital flow.

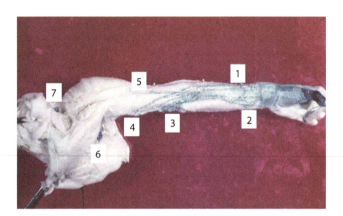

FIGURE 25.2   (1) Posterior superficial radial flow. (5) External bicipital (cephalic) flow. (2) Anterior superficial radial flow. (6) Axillary nodes. (3) Upper internal bicipital (basilic) flow. (7) Transverse cervical nodal group. (4) Medial bicipital flow (as described by Caplan).

middle, ring, and little fingers, the anterointernal and posterointernal regions of the hand, and the forearm.

The cephalic chain is named as such because it is in the pathway of the cephalic vein. It is almost constant and made by nodes that can be found in different areas:

- In the middle third of the arm, at the level of the external bicipital canal (brachial-bicipital nodes)
- One single node in the upper third of the arm, between the deltoid and biceps muscles (deltoid-bicipital)
- One single node (deltoid-pectoral) between the deltoid and the pectoralis major muscles, at the level of the deltoid-pectoral area
- One to three nodes in the deltoid-pectoral area, at the subclavicular level (subclavicular nodes)

It takes lymph from the fingers, usually through one single lymphatic vessel, as well as from the skin regions of the forearm and the arm.

Subclavicular nodes also receive lymphatic drainage from the scapulohumeral joint and the deltoid region.

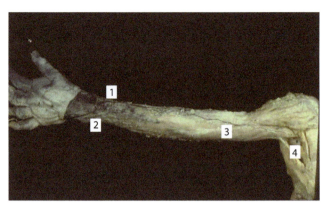

FIGURE 25.3   (1) Posterior superficial radial flow. (4) Scapular nodes. (2) Posterior superficial ulnar flow. (3) Medial tricipital flow. Extra-axillary (or Caplan's) derivative flow.

In general, nodes cannot be felt; therefore, if they can, lymphatic drainage must be suspended and the patient should be referred to a doctor for analysis, except in the case of a pathological node that has become chronically palpable (infarcted node) (Figure 25.3).

Axillary Node Chains

Axillary nodes are at the center of lymphatic drainage of the upper limb and the anterolateral and posterolateral regions of the thoracic wall, including the mammary gland.

There are three vertical node chains:

- External mammary chain
- Upper thoracic chain
- Subscapular chain

There is also a horizontal node chain:

- Axillary vein chain

See Figure 25.4.

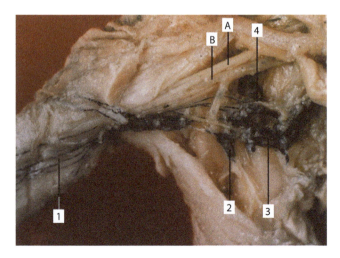

FIGURE 25.4   (1) Anterior bicipital flow. (4) Upper thoracic chain. (2) Subscapular chain. (A) Brachial plexus. (3) External mammary chain. (B) Axillary vein.

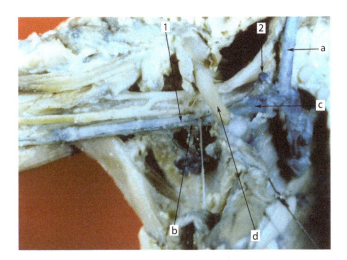

FIGURE 25.5 (1) Radial-humeral-cervical flow. (b) Axillary vein. (2) Node of the internal jugular chain. (c) Subclavian vein. (a) Internal jugular vein. (d) Clavicle (as described by Ciucci).

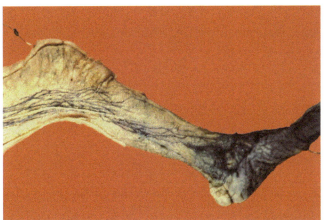

FIGURE 25.6 Anterointernal or tibial great saphenous lymph flow.

Extra-Axillary Derivative Flows

The cephalic flow was described by Mascagni: After going through the deltoid-pectoral area together with the cephalic vein, the lymphatic vessel passes by the clavicle and enters the supra-clavicular region, where nodes are stationed in the transverse cervical chain.

The deltoid-triceps flow or posterior superficial flow was described by Caplan (1969): Lymphatic vessels go through the deltoid-pectoral area of the back arm, where nodes (lower scapular nodes) are stationed at the level of the triangle of the round teres major and minor muscles and the long part of the triceps, going on from there toward the parietal vessels.

The deep radial-humeral-cervical derivative flow was described by Ciucci (1988): This flow is made of one single lymphatic vessel that originates in the superficial radial flow, goes through the aponeurosis, and continues along the humeral flow. It keeps going up along the axillary vein, without stationing nodes, and behind the clavicle to drain lymph in a node of the internal jugular chain.

See Figure 25.5.

Superficial Lymph Flows of the Lower Limb

Superficial lymph flows of the lower limb can be classified into three groups:

1. Lower or tibial saphenous lymph flows (foot and leg)
2. Middle or popliteal saphenous lymph flows (knee)
3. Upper or femoral saphenous lymph flows (thigh)

Lower or Tibial Saphenous Lymph Flows

The *anterointernal or tibial great saphenous lymph flow* goes from the toes, along the internal marginal vein to the projecting soleus ring, toward the great popliteal saphenous flow. This flow originates in the toes, in the skin of the back, the sole and joints of the foot, and then goes up the internal premalleolar region,

where it is closely related with the great saphenous vein and the internal saphenous nerve. It goes through the inner leg, fanning out to include the largest area for the lymphatic drainage until reaching the projecting soleus ring, when all lymph flows come together again with the great saphenous vein and the internal saphenous nerve.

The *posteroexternal or posterior saphenous lymph flow* comprises two lymphatic vessels originating in the lymph capillaries of the fourth and fifth toes, proceeding through the sole and back of the foot, along the external dorsal vein, and then proceeding through the external retromalleolar region, closely related with the posteroexternal saphenous vein and the external saphenous nerve. It shadows this vein throughout its pathway until draining lymph into the superficial popliteal node.

See Figures 25.6 and 25.7.

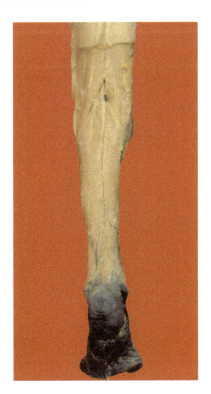

FIGURE 25.7 Posteroexternal or popliteal saphenous lymph flow.

Middle or Saphenous Popliteal Lymph Flows

These can be classified as follows:

- Great saphenous popliteal lymph flow
- Posterior saphenous popliteal lymph flow

The *great saphenous popliteal lymph flow* is the continuation of the tibial great saphenous flow from the projecting soleus ring to the projecting third adductor ring, where it forms the femoral great saphenous flow. It is made of eight to ten lymphatic vessels that meet in the inner knee, together with the great saphenous vein and the internal saphenous nerve. It is highly important in phlebology and plastic and traumatological surgery due to the fact that the lesions that may occur could interrupt drainage of the tibial great saphenous flow.

The *posterior saphenous popliteal lymph flow* is made of one to two lymphatic vessels, efferents of the superficial popliteal node that follow the junction of the posteroexternal saphenous vein and drain into the deep popliteal nodes (Figure 25.8).

Upper or Femoral Saphenous Lymph Flows

Lymph flows of the thigh can be divided into two anterior flows and two posterior flows.

The *anterointernal or femoral great saphenous flow* comprises 8–15 lymphatic vessels; it is the continuation of the great saphenous popliteal flow, shadowing the great saphenous vein. It fans out in the inner thigh and ends up in the lower inguinal nodes.

The *anteroexternal or femoral small saphenous flow* comprises three to seven lymphatic vessels, originating in the outer

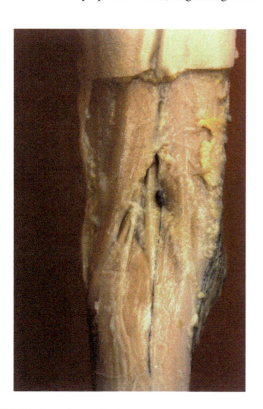

FIGURE 25.8 Posterior popliteal saphenous lymph flow; superficial popliteal node.

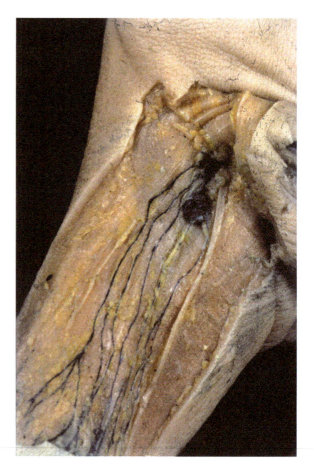

FIGURE 25.9 Anterointernal or femoral great saphenous superficial flow.

knee and following the accessory or dorsal saphenous vein of the thigh to drain lymph in the lower inguinal nodes.

The *posterointernal femoral lymph flow* comprises five to eight lymphatic vessels; it originates in the back skin of the thigh, covers it from the back, and goes through the inner thigh to reach the upper inguinal nodes.

The *posteroexternal femoral lymph flow* comprises 7–15 lymphatic vessels; it originates in the back skin of the thigh, covers it from the outer part to reach the anterior thigh, and thus drains lymph into the upper inguinal nodes (Figure 25.9).

Superficial Nodal Centers of the Lower Limb

The most important superficial nodal centers of the lower limb are as follows:

- Inguinal nodal group
- Superficial popliteal nodes

Inguinal Nodal Group

Consisting of 15–20 lymph nodes, this is the most important superficial nodal group of the lower limb and can be classified into three upper groups and two lower groups:

1. Upper outer or superficial iliac circumflex group
2. Upper middle or subcutaneous abdominal group

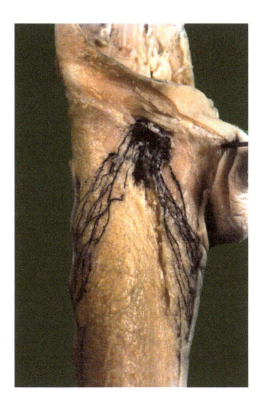

FIGURE 25.10 Posterointernal femoral lymph flow and posteroexternal femoral lymph flow; inguinal nodes.

3. Upper inner or external pudendal group
4. Lower outer or anterior saphenous group
5. Lower inner or great saphenous group

See Figure 25.10.

Posteroexternal Saphenous or Upper Popliteal Node

This nodal center, comprising one to three lymph nodes, is located at the level of the popliteal fossa and receives the lymphatic vessels of the leg's posteroexternal or posterior saphenous flow, leaning on the greater sciatic nerve. Efferent lymph flows stem from these lymph nodes toward deep popliteal nodes.

Derivative Flows of the Lower Limb

Although the lower limb does not have derivative flows of its own, like the upper limb, we can consider that external genitalia "lend" it their contralateral flows, which will behave as derivative flows.

These contralateral flows of external genitalia are as follows:

1. Suprapubic flow
2. Perineal flow

They activate when there is an inguinal node block generating retrograde hypertension and thus causing lymphatic reflux through these two flows toward the contralateral limb.

The lymphatic system of the lower limb has communicating lymph flows that connect those in the same aponeurotic stratum (superficial-to-superficial and deep-to-deep), and piercing lymph flows that connect those from different aponeurotic strata (superficial-to-deep and deep-to-superficial). These are true safety valves in case of lymphatic hypertension, the knowledge of which is essential for manual lymphatic drainage therapy.

BIBLIOGRAPHY

Aubry (según Poirier P. et Charpy A.). *Traité d'Anatomie Humaine*. París: Masson Editeurs; 1902;2:1257–58.

Bardeleben K et al. Atlas der topographischen Anatomie. Pl. 14, Jena. 1908.

Bartels P. Das Lymphgefassystem. *Jena*. 1908;1:161–4.

Bartels P. Das Lymphgefassystem. *Jena*. 1908;4:188–95.

Baum H. Die Lymphgefabe der metacarpo und metatarso-phalangelalenke des Menschen. *Anat Anz*. 1929;67:301–18.

Caplan I. *Anatomía quirúrgica de los Linfáticos de la Mama. Día Médico (Nro. Especial 41° aniversario)*. Buenos Aires, 1969:2183.

Caplan I. Le Systeme Lymphatique du Pouce. Memoires du Laboratoire D'Anatomie de la Faculté de Médécine de París. 1977.

Caplan I. *Drenaje linfático del miembro superior*. En LEDUC A. y col. Traitment physique de Íoedeme du bras. 2nd ed. París: Masson, 1991.

Ciucci JL. Grandes corrientes linfáticas del miembro superior. *Tesis de Doctorado*. Universidad Nacional de Buenos Aires, 1988.

Ciucci JL. Anatomía del Drenaje Linfático del Miembro Superior. En Memorias del Symposium Zyma sobre Linfedema. *V Congreso de la Sociedad Panamericana de Flebología y Linfología*. Buenos Aires, Mayo de;1992:17–32.

Ciucci JL. Morfología del Sistema Linfático. *IV Reunión Internacional de Linfología*. S'Agaró (España), 27 y 28 de Octubre de 1995:29–43.

Ciucci JL. Investigación Anatómica del Drenaje Linfático del Miembro superior. Su importancia en la patología traumatológica. *XXXIII Congreso Argentino de Ortopedia y Traumatología Asociación Argentina de Ortopedia y Traumatología*. Buenos Aires, 2000.

Ciucci JL. *Linfedema del miembro superior postratamiento del cáncer de mama*. 1ra edición. ISBN 987-21801-0-5, Ed. Nayarit, Octubre 2004:21–37.

Ciucci JL. *Linfedema de los miembros inferiores*. 1ra edición. ISBN 978-987-21801-4-0, Ed. Nayarit, Febrero 2009:21–39.

Ciucci JL. *Tratamiento físico del edema. Drenaje linfático manual*. 1ra. Edición. ISBN 978-987-28471-0-4. Agosto, 2012:9–21.

Ciucci JL, Zalazar J, Marcovecchio L. El sistema linfático de la glándula mamaria en relación con las indicaciones quirúrgicas actuales. Premio Avelino Gutiérrez. Academia Nacional de Medicina. Buenos Aires, 1993.

Coget J. et al. L'Anatomie et physiologie du lymphatique. *Les Oedemes des Members Inférieurs. Artéres et Veines*. 1984;Mar–Apr:133–4.

Echeverri AJ. Note sur les lymphatiques du membre superieur. *Ann Anat Pathol*. 1935;12:319–20.

Gerota D. Zur technik der Lymphgefassinjektion. Eine nue Injektionsmasse der Lymphagefasse. Polychrome injection. *Anat Anz., 12; 216 Y Vehr Anat Ges*. 1896:151–52.

Grossmann F. Ueber die Axillarem Lymphdrussen. *Inaug. C. Vogt Editeures. Dissert*, Berlin, 1896.

Jamain A. *Tratado Elemental de Anatomía Descriptiva y de Preparaciones anatómicas.* Madrid, 1874:441–2.

Kubik ST. The possible drainage ways of lymphatic territories after alterations of peripherical collectors after lymphadenectomy. *Folia Angiologica* 1980;XXVIII 7/8:228–37.

Latorre J, Maeso J. Anatomía, Fisiología y Fisiopatología del Sistema Linfático. En: *Linfedema.* Edika-Med. S.A. (Edic.) Barcelona: Médicas, 1991.

Mascagni P. *Varoum Lymphaticorum corporis humanin descriptio et iconographia.* Pl. 32, Siena: 1787.

Poirier P, Charpy A, Delmare G. *Traité d'Anatomie Humaine.* París: Masson Editeurs, 1902;I:1257–58.

Rouviere H. *Anatomie des lymphatiques de l'homme.* París: Masson Editeurs, 1932.

Sappey P. *Traité d'Anatomie Descriptive.* París: Angéiologie, Delahaye et Lacrosnier Editeurs, 1874:800–9.

Sappey P. *Description et iconographie des vaisseaux lymphatiques.* París, 1888;2:788–95.

Savariaud J. Ganglion aberrant du pli du coude. *Bull. Et Mém de la Soc Anat de París,* 1912;14:141–4.

Severanu G. Die Topographie der Lymphgefasse der finger nebst Bermerkungen zur Technik der Lymphgefasse. Inyektionen mit Polychromen Massen. *Anat. Anz.,* 1906;29(Sup):275–6.

Testud L. *Tratado de Anatomía Humana.* 2ª ed. Barcelona: Salvat Editorial;1894;6:478–9.

Tillaux P. *Tratado de Anatomía Topográfica.* Barcelona: Espasa Ed., 1880: 513.

Verdelet Adenítis sus-épitrochléen chez les indigénes de nos colonies. *J.de Med.* De Bordeaux. París: 1920:441.

Verge Brian F. Lymphatiques des muscles de la main et de l'avant bras. *Annales D'Anatomie Pathologique et Normale. París.* 1929;VI:1129–31.

Verge Brian F. Note sur les lymphatiques cutanés de membre inférieur. Ann d'Anat. Norm Méd-Chir., París. 1930;T. VII, 4:503–4.

26

Prevention and Treatment of Secondary Lymphedema of Extremities, Early Diagnosis of Lymphostasis, and Postsurgical Prevention and Conservative Treatment of Lymphedema

Ángela Río and Paloma Domingo

Prevention: Early Diagnosis of Lymphostasis

Access to information, knowledge, disclosure, and the presence of specialized professionals are the basic tools to properly prevent lymphedema. This prevention is based on three fundamental pillars: information (understanding the pathology, educational programs, early diagnosis, etc.), early physical therapy, and exercise.

For secondary lymphedema, knowing its etiology or main risk factors (extension of surgery, lymphadenectomy, radiotherapy, and obesity) should be enough to prevent it. The reality is that patients undergoing surgery for several types of cancer sometimes get little information about the risk of developing lymphedema and how to prevent it, and they later must face multiple physical, psychological, and social barriers [1]. There are some controllable risk factors that could be avoided by following simple guidelines. Health personnel need to be more aware about prevention and early diagnosis of lymphedema. See Figure 26.1. A study by Forner-Cordero et al. [2] claimed that only about 25% of patients who underwent surgery for breast cancer had received any type of information after surgery. Based on the results obtained by Lam et al. [3], three-fifths of surveyed patients with a history of cancer said they had not been warned about the risk of developing lymphedema, and half of the participants were not satisfied with their first consultation about their lymphedema.

Other authors (e.g., Ferro and Pérez [4]) discuss the deficiencies in quantity and quality, in anticipation and integration, and in the reporting processes of information to oncology patients.

Based on the study by Arenillas [5], only 59% of medical staff believe that lymphedema prevention is practiced at the hospital where they work, 31% openly state that it is not being performed, and 10% do not know.

Also, research is lacking on preventive advice or educational programs for patients with risk factors for lymphedema. Precautions are mainly based on physiological principles (e.g., avoiding excessive heat or infections). In our opinion, we do not believe that the use of standardized rules presented in a "list-of-prohibitions" format is appropriate for the prevention of lymphedema. When conveying information on how to prevent lymphedema, this must involve active listening, being verbal, personalized information adapted to each patient and presented in a simple language and creating a privacy environment where patients feel comfortable to express and ask anything they

need. The presence of a relative may be convenient for them to become aware of the potential limitations in daily activities [6,7]. Prohibitions will be as few as possible and recommendations will be provided in a positive tone.

There are different medical tests to assess the morphology and functioning of the lymphatic system, the study of which is hard due to its structural and anatomical characteristics. Some tests, performed before breast cancer surgery, may be useful to assess patients' initial state and determine potential risk groups; if performed in postsurgery phases, they may help detect infraclinical lymphedema and therefore enable setup of an early prevention program:

- *Bioimpedance* (BI) or multiple-frequency bioelectrical impedance analysis (MFBIA) is based on the opposition of cells, tissues, or body fluids to the flow of an electric current, and measures total and segmental body water, enabling estimation of fat-free body mass and fat mass. Some advantages include its low cost, ease of transportation, harmless nature, and low interobserver variability.

- BI is used for early detection of lymphedema and has been validated in Australia and the United States for this end [8]; several studies have proven to be highly reliable to predict lymphedema, enabling its diagnosis up to 4 months before the disease shows any clinical signs [9].

- Bioimpedance, together with perimetry, enables the early diagnosis of lymphedema and, consequently, makes its prevention easier [10].

- *Near-infrared fluorescence* (NIRF) is an emerging imaging tool in the field of lymphology. The subcutaneous injection of a marker like Indocyanine Green (ICG) with a special PDE camera enables real-time visualization of the structure of the superficial lymphatic network, the ganglia, and the lymphangion activity, but not the deep pathways. This qualitative method does not exclude lymphogammagraphy, the use of which for early detection of lymphedema is based on the observation of delayed uptake, downward reflux, or even complete absence of opacification in more advanced stages [11]. Furthermore, according to Jean Paul Belgrado

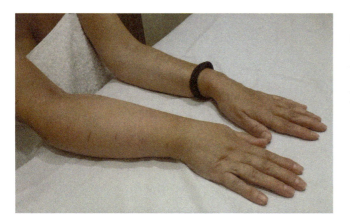

FIGURE 26.1   Upper limb secondary lymphedema.

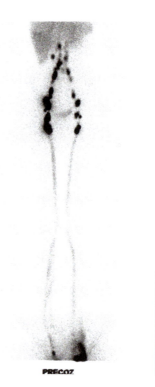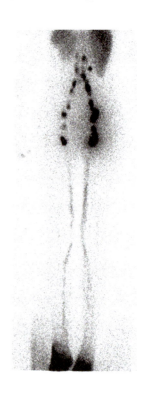

PRECOZ

FIGURE 26.2   Lymphography.

from the Free University of Brussels, NIRF could help physical therapists improve hand movements since it offers the opportunity to assess manual lymphatic drainage methods with real-time feedback. Another study, also by Belgrado et al., [12] presented at the 26th World Congress of Lymphology (2017) and titled "Early Detection of BCRL: Interest of Near-Infrared Fluorescence Imaging," shows promising results as a sensitive tool to detect the imminent risk of developing secondary lymphedema. This technique is currently used for the preoperative location of functioning lymphatic vessels to perform lymphovenous anastomosis.

- *Lymphoscintigraphy, indirect isotope lymphography, or lymphogammagraphy* is a diagnostic method that provides gammagraphic images for the functional examination of the lymphatic system. It is a physiological method to determine the extension and type of surgery, locate the sentinel node, and study the lymphatic network and the lymphedema by subcutaneously injecting a radiopharmaceutical, usually Tc99. It is a very useful test to diagnose and guide physical therapy in difficult cases, especially proximal *or starting lymphedemas,* and to assess the lymphatic function of the contralateral extremity [13]. It also tests the adsorption and evacuation capabilities of the lymphatic system. Under certain conditions, it may determine the rate of adsorption, which is very interesting from a therapeutic perspective [14]. In their study, "Protocol of lymphedema prevention after breast cancer surgery," Cestari et al. suggest a prevention protocol in which all patients are studied using lymphogammagraphy and, if positive (backflow), even in the absence of a clinical lymphedema, a standard sleeve is preventively prescribed for domestic chores and flying. See Figure 26.2.

- *Magnetic resonance lymphangiography* (MRL) with or without contrast. MRL's advantage over lymphography is that it can highlight static signals of structures full of slow-motion fluid, like lymphatic vessels. It shows the exact depth of the lymphatic vessel and vein. It is a safe technique to study the lymphatic system and plan its surgery [15–17].

The study by Ferguson et al. [18], conducted between 2005 and 2014 in 632 patients at risk of developing post–breast cancer lymphedema and which included 3041 measurements, concluded that there was not a statistically significant relationship between volume increase in said extremities and blood extraction, the application of injections, or plane flights. These results are important to help redesign proper prevention strategies, which are partially determined by the information perceived and assimilated by the patient. Preventive protocols have been created, justified by a decrease in the occurrence rate of lymphedema after early physical therapy in post–breast cancer patients, but they are currently not being properly conducted. According to Torres et al. [19], early physical therapy (manual lymphatic drainage, scar massage, stretching, progressively active shoulder exercises) and a guideline educational program prevent lymphedema in patients who have undergone breast cancer surgery. Around 7% of patients using a prevention program based on early physical therapy developed lymphedema versus 25% who only used an educational program as prevention. Likewise, Castro-Sánchez et al. [20] obtained positive results from the functional assessment and evaluation of the extremity volume on the operated side after preventive treatment of secondary lymphedema with an elastic containment garment and manual lymphatic drainage.

The prevention-related aspect due to physical exercise is particularly interesting. In the review by McNeely et al. [21], early postoperative exercise is claimed to help prevent lymphedema, as long as it is carefully performed by a specialized professional, and to benefit the functionality of the shoulder joint in women after breast cancer, helping to prevent axillary retraction, cording (superficial lymphatic thrombosis or axillary web syndrome), decreased muscle strength and other factors/

complications that can develop the appearance of lymphedema. Furthermore, early supervised exercise, as well as progressive resistance training, does not increase the risk of lymphedema in any case, but can even prevent it and improve patients' quality of life [22]. Even if resistance training is of moderate intensity, not only is it safe, but it has a beneficial impact on body composition, bone health, muscle strength, physical function, and quality of life [23]. According to the systematic review by Baumann et al. [24], progressive strength training, together with dynamic exercises (physical therapy), is safe and helps prevent or even decrease lymphedema if it already exists.

Treatment

The treatment of choice for lymphedema is usually conservative; if this fails, a pharmacological or surgical treatment can be performed, which should be started as early as possible.

Conservative Treatment

Conservative treatment uses decongestive physical therapy of the lymphedema or complex decongestive therapy (CDT), which consists of a set of four measures used simultaneously to reduce the volume of the extremity, favoring the functioning of the lymphatic system, caring for the skin to prevent infections, and improving the quality of tissues by reducing and softening fibrosis. These four measures are:

- Manual lymphatic drainage
- Compression/containment measures
- Exercise
- Skin care

The treatment with CDT is performed in two phases: (1) an intensive or shock phase and (2) a maintenance phase. The first phase involves daily treatment for 2–3 weeks with manual lymphatic drainage, compression bandages (for about 20 hours, removing them only for cleaning and to apply different therapies), myolymphokinetic exercises, and skin care aimed at fully reducing every aspect of the lymphedema. The maintenance phase begins at the end of the first, and its purpose is to keep and optimize the results obtained. Once an optimal reduction of volume has been achieved, the bandage will be replaced with a containment garment (sleeve/sock). Manual lymphatic drainage treatments are spread progressively further apart, continuing with patient guidance and education about exercising and skin care, and offering them advice and recommendations for their daily lives [25].

Manual Lymphatic Drainage

This very gentle skin massage technique stimulates lymph flow in order to decrease the consistency and volume of the edema [26]. It is also used to treat scars and improve the amplitude of movement. Torres et al. [19] recommend it to prevent lymphedema through the activation of alternative drainage

pathways in an immediate postoperative setting. Manual lymphatic drainage also helps improve the mobility of the affected extremity [22].

Compression and Containment Garments

The use of elastic compression and containment garments is essential to treat lymphedema, being one of the most significant therapies for volume reduction and later maintenance. It is usually performed with multilayer bandaging [27], especially during the intensive phase of treatment, when more compression than containment is needed. Based on the material (elastic, inelastic, adhesive, cohesive), the size of the bandages, and the number of layers, several options of compression bandages exist, which can be applied in different ways (circular, semibraiding, braiding). See Figure 26.3.

The decision to use one or the other depends on the state of the lymphedema, the choice of the therapist, the purpose of the bandage, the clinical characteristics of the lymphedema, and the patient and material availability. The first layer of multilayer compression bandaging is applied with an inelastic bandage, and the rest with bandages of little elasticity. A double-containment bandage is currently used as well, the first layer being made of inelastic material and the rest of long-elasticity material [14]. The physical therapist must choose at each time, adapting the most appropriate type of bandaging to each patient. The use of bandages is essential to maintain the volume reduction reached, especially after the manual lymphatic drainage treatment.

Later, during the maintenance phase, containment instead of compression is used, which is achieved by using different types of garments, either standard or customized (sleeves, socks, gloves, etc.), knitted with flat or circular stitches [28]. Compression/containment garments generate a pressure gradient in which distal pressure is higher than that applied on the proximal part, favoring the flow of the lymphatic transport. Furthermore, garments protect against extrinsic and intrinsic trauma caused by interstitial pressure tightening the skin. It is recommended to use the garments for all activities (especially while exercising or performing vigorous tasks) for up to 20 hours a day and change them when deterioration of elasticity is noticed (around every 3–6 months) or when less pressure is

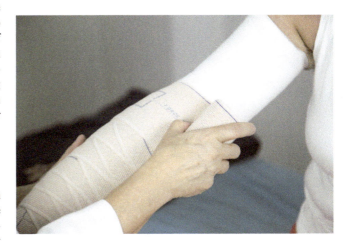

FIGURE 26.3 Herringbone bandage.

perceived (the garment's usual pressure varies between 30 and 60 mm Hg). Bertelli et al. [29] found a statistically significant reduction of edema in patients wearing these garments for 6 consecutive hours a day. The time of use is not currently unanimous, with the recommendation being between 12 and 24 hours. Its use has little contraindications (peripheral arteriopathies or ulcerations), and sometimes they are even recommended as prevention [30]. Treatment adherence and compliance are hard for patients because wearing these garments is uncomfortable, antiaesthetic, and expensive. Patient education is therefore key to ensure their compliance and adherence to treatment [31–33].

Exercise

For years, it has been discussed whether exercising may be a risk factor or a risk-reducing factor. Exercising increases blood flow and blood pressure, therefore increasing the production of lymph in the exercised area, generating volume changes by muscle contraction and stretching (muscle pump), increasing physiological lymphatic drainage, and stimulating and improving lymph flow. For this purpose, different authors describe the synergic, beneficial effect of reducing the volume of lymphedema by actively exercising and using low-elasticity compression mechanisms thanks to the changes they cause in lymphatic drainage [34]. See Figure 26.4.

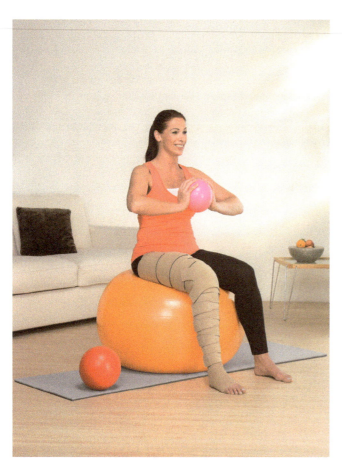

FIGURE 26.4 CircAid compression bandaging (by courtesy of medi GmbH).

According to Lane et al. [35], based on the patient profile and the location of the lymphedema, the changes caused by exercising on lymphatic drainage show a physiological variation. Myolymphokinetic exercises, which try to stimulate the lymph flow of the affected extremity toward the trunk, are the most recommended, and, if performed correctly, they reduce the risk of developing lymphedema. Exercises allowing a gain in range of movement and strength, besides improving physiological lymphatic drainage thanks to the pumping effect that muscle contractions cause on lymph vessels, result in a better functioning when performing daily activities [36].

For George et al. [37], it is appropriate and advisable to exercise with a moderate-to-vigorous intensity for 150 minutes a week, or at least 20 minutes a day for 5 days a week.

Regarding resistance exercises, there has been controversy about their prescription. Some benefits have been observed in patients with lymphedema or at risk of suffering it as long as it is properly performed, because it increases muscle volume and, in consequence, the pumping effect and functionality of the extremity [38]. In the reviews by Stuiver et al. [22] and Baumann et al. [24], it is confirmed that said exercise is advisable and effective after breast cancer treatments, it does not increase the risk of developing lymphedema but can even prevent it, and it may be practiced in a safe and beneficial manner.

Skin Care

Due to volume increase of lymphedema during its evolution, tissues tend to suffer more infections because of immunological deficit and skin tightening, among other causes. For this reason, it is necessary to pay special attention to skin hygiene, cleaning, and hydration. Nowicki and Siviour [39] recommend to regularly apply moisturizing creams to replace the skin's sebum, secreted in normal conditions, ensuring skin's humidity retention and nutrition, which are reduced in lymphedema [40].

According to some authors, besides CDT, conservative treatments include pressotherapy, diet, and psychological support.

Pressotherapy is another physical therapy that may be helpful; however, the evidence is currently controversial since the latest studies claim that it is neither effective nor advisable to treat secondary lymphedema [41].

Regarding diet, although modification is encouraged in clinical practice, more evidence is needed to support its benefits. According to Arenillas [5], there are very few professionals who consider diet as a factor to take into account in the treatment of lymphedema, most considering it unimportant. Some physicians admit they do not know if patients should follow some kind of preventive or therapeutic diet for lymphedema.

Patients with lymphedema, particularly women, have shown significant psychiatric social-, sexual-, and functional-related morbidity and deterioration, so psychological support must be a part of their treatment [42]. For this purpose, relaxation techniques, social support strategies, and techniques to facilitate the expression of emotions and feelings are used [43]. In the study by Arenillas [5], more than half of doctors state that patients with breast cancer receive psychological support. Emotional problems significantly reduce the quality of life of patients with lymphedema, so they must be properly addressed [44].

These days, aside from CDT, we have the *Godoy method*, a new way to approach lymphedema.

Global Lymphatic Therapy: Godoy Method

It is made of different techniques or forms of therapy that, based on the pathology, can be used in isolation or combined [45].

The therapies involved in the *Godoy method* are:

- Cervical lymphatic therapy (CLT)
- Manual lymphatic therapy (MLT)
- Mechanical lymphatic therapy (McLT)
- Compression/containment therapies
- Skin therapies
- Patient education to maintain results

As was the case with CDT, it is performed in two phases: an intensive or shock phase and a maintenance phase. Intensive treatment (or shock therapy) allows a volume reduction of about 10% a day and about 40%–50% in a week. In grades I and II, it is possible to almost completely eliminate the edema in 95% of patients in 1–6 weeks. The treatment is ambulatory, but sometimes patients must remain in the clinic for several hours a day.

Cervical Lymphatic Therapy or Cervical Stimulation

This maneuver is performed in the supraclavicular fossa, near the base of the neck, and can be used in isolation, especially in congenital lymphedema [34,46,47].

Manual Lymphatic Therapy

The difference with other drainage techniques is the use of linear and compression maneuvers to stimulate the production of lymph and the mobilization of macromolecules [48]. See Figure 26.5.

Mechanical Lymphatic Therapy

For mechanical drainage, the Drs. Godoy have developed different devices that enable the performance of passive exercises of the upper and lower extremities, which favor the formation of lymph and the mobilization of macromolecules [49,50]. For optimal results, patients must remain focused and perform their exercises for several hours, between 2 and 6–8 hours. The amount of time will depend on the stage of the lymphedema, and therefore its volume and consistency.

Compression Containment

During the first (intensive) phase of treatment, compression garments made of cotton and polyester (*grosgrain*) are used to help decrease the volume and fibrosis of the edema [51]. During this phase, patients must wear the compression garment all day and night, adjusting and adapting it as necessary. This is an extremely important part of the therapy and requires patient commitment.

Concerning skin care and active exercises, the Godoy method follows the same guidelines as CDT.

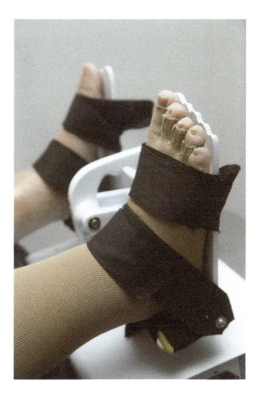

FIGURE 26.5 Lower limb passive exercise using the patented device of Godoy.

Pharmacological Treatment

The controversy about the use of drugs for lymphedema is remarkable. For many years, the use of diuretics in these patients has been recommended, but recently it has been proven that they are not appropriate since they mobilize the fluid component of lymphedema (water) and leave macromolecules stuck in the extracellular space, which entails a later rebound effect, increasing the volume of the extremity again. Additionally, there are known adverse effects caused by diuretics in the body, such as hypotension, dehydration, or electrolyte imbalance [43,52].

According to Casley-Smith, Morgan, and Piller [53], the use of benzopyrones was very extensive in patients with lymphedema, mainly in Australia. They may be plant extracts, or semisynthetic or completely synthetic preparations [54]. As reviewed by Badger et al. [55], these have now stopped being prescribed since the scientific evidence has not been able to prove their benefits regarding volume control, pain, or discomfort of the extremities due to lymphedema.

A recent pilot study by Rockson et al. [56] suggests an NSAID (ketoprofen) as a potential support for the lymphatic system by improving volume and consistency of lymphedema and generating other positive histopathological and plasma changes.

REFERENCES

1. Río-González A, Molina-Rueda F, Palacios-Ceña D, Alguacil-Diego IM. Living with lymphoedema—The perspective of cancer patients: A qualitative study. *Supportive Care Cancer.* 2018;26(6):2005–13.
2. Cordero IF, Garrido DM, Langa JM. *Necesidad de información para la prevención del linfedema posmastectomía.* Rehabilitación, 2003;37(3):141–4.

3. Lam R, Wallace A, Burbidge B, Franks P, Moffatt C. Experiences of patients with lymphoedema. *J Lymphoedema.* 2006;1(1):16–21.

4. Ferro T and Pérez JP. *Necesidades de información en el cáncer de mama y de atención en la supervivencia.* Federación Española de Cáncer de Mama, 2013.

5. Arenillas Pérez M. *Linfedema: Prevención y calidad de vida.* 2008.

6. Godoy JM and Godoy MF. *Câncer de mama e linfedema de membro superior.* Sao Jose do Rio Preto, SP, *Brasil.* 2005. ISBN - 85 - 903670-2-9

7. Sebastián J, Bueno M, Mateos N. *Apoyo emocional y calidad de vida en mujeres con cáncer de mama.* Madrid: Ministerio De Trabajo y Asuntos Sociales. Instituto De La Mujer, 2002.

8. Arlan S and Biffaud JC. Effect de la chirugie axilar sur le système lymphatique. *Kinésithér Scient.* 2012;537:09–18.

9. Cornish BH, Chapman M, Thomas BJ, Ward LC, Bunce H, Hirst C. Early diagnosis of lymphedema in postsurgery breast cancer patients. *Ann New York Acad Sci.* 2000;904:571–5.

10. Shah C, Arthur DW, Wazer D, Khan A, Ridner S, Vicini F. The impact of early detection and intervention of breast cancer-related lymphedema: A systematic review. *Cancer Med.* 2016;5(6):1154–62.

11. Giacalone G, Belgrado JP, Bourgeois P, Bracale R, Moranine J. A new dynamic imaging tool to study lymphoedema and associated treatment. *The Eur J Lymphol.* 2011;22(62).

12. Belgrado JP, Vandermeeren L, Vankerckhove S, Valsamis JB, Hertens D, Beier B, Etbaz S, Carly B, Liebens F. Early detection of secondary lymphedema after ancer treatments. *The European Journal of Lymphology.* 2017;29(76):15.

13. Vignes S, Coupé M, Baulieu F, Vaillant L. Limb lymphedema: Diagnosis, explorations, complications. French Lymphology Society, *J Mal Vasc.* 2009;34(5):314–22.

14. Ferrandez JC, Serin D. *Rééducation cáncer du sein. Les explorations du sistéme lymphatique.* Ed: Masson, 2006:81–95.

15. Liu N, Zhang Y. Magnetic Resonance Lymphangiography for the Study of Lymphatic System in Lymphedema. *J Reconstruction Microsurg.* 2016;32(1):66–71.

16. Cellina M, Oliva G, Menozzi A, Soresina M, Martinenghi C, Gibelli D. Non-contrast Magnetic Resonance Lymphangiography: An emerging technique for the study of lymphedema. *Clin Imaging.* 2018;12(53):126–33.

17. Zeltzer A, Brussaard C, Koning M, De Baerdemaeker R, Hendrickx B, Hamdi M, de Mey J. MR lymphography in patients with upper limb lymphedema: The GPS for feasibility and surgical planning for lympho-venous bypass. *J Clin Oncol: Off J Am Soc Clin Oncol.* 2018;118(3):407–15.

18. Ferguson C, Swaroop M, Horick N et al. Impact of ipsilateral blood draws, injections, blood pressure measurements, and air travel on the risk of lymphedema for patients treated for breast cancer. *J Clin Oncol: Off J Am Soc Clin Oncol.* 2016;34(7):691–8.

19. Torres Lacomba M, Yuste Sánchez MJ, Zapico Goni A, Prieto Merino D, Mayoral del Moral O, Cerezo Téllez E, Minayo Mogollon E. Effectiveness of early physiotherapy to prevent lymphoedema after surgery for breast cancer: Randomised, single blinded, clinical trial. *Br Med J.* 2010;340:b5396.

20. Castro-Sánchez A, Moreno-Lorenzo C, Matarán-Peñarrocha G, Aguilar-Ferrándiz M, Almagro-Céspedes I, Anaya-Ojeda J. Prevención del linfedema tras cirugía de cáncer de mama mediante ortesis elástica de contención y drenaje linfático manual: Ensayo clínico aleatorizado. *Medicina Clínica.* 2011;137(5):204–7.

21. McNeely M, Peddle CJ, Yurick J, Dayes I, John R. Conservative and dietary interventions for cancer-related lymphedema. *Cancer.* 2011;117(6):1136–48.

22. Stuiver M, Tusscher MR, Agasi-Idenburg CS, Lucas C, Aaronson N, Bossuyt PM. Conservative interventions for preventing clinically detectable upper-limb lymphoedema in patients who are at risk of developing lymphoedema after breast cancer therapy. *Cochranedatabase Syst Rev.* 2015;4.

23. Simonavice E, Kim JS, Panton L. Effects of resistance exercise in women with or at risk for breast cancer-related lymphedema. *Suppor Care Cancer.* 2017;25(1):9–15.

24. Baumann FT, Reike A, Hallek M, Wiskemann J, Reimer V. Does exercise have a preventive effect on secondary lymphedema in breast cancer patients following local treatment-a systematic review. *Breast Care (Basel).* 2018;13(5):380–5. doi:10.1159/000487428

25. ISL International Society of Lymphology. The diagnosis and treatment of peripheral lymphedema: 2013 Consensus document of The International Society of Lymphology. *Lymphology.* 2009;46(1):1–11.

26. Devoogdt N, Van Kampen M, Geraerts I, Coremans T, Christiaens M. Different physical treatment modalities for lymphoedema developing after axillary lymph node dissection for breast cancer: A review. *Eur J Obstet Gynecol Reprod Biol.* 2010;149(1):3–9.

27. Badger C, Peacock JL, Mortimer PS. A randomized, controlled, parallel-group clinical trial comparing multilayer bandaging followed by hosiery versus hosiery alone in the treatment of patients with lymphedema of the limb. *Cancer.* 2000;88(12):2832–7.

28. Hornsby R. The use of compression to treat lymphoedema. *Professional Nursing.* 1995;11(2):127–8.

29. Bertelli G, Venturini M, Forno G, Macchiavello F, Dini D. An analysis of prognostic factors in response to conservative treatment of postmastectomy lymphedema. *Surg, Gynecol Obstet.* 1992;175(5):455–60.

30. Benadiba C, Álvarez B, Manada M, Cobo M, Hernández M. Tratamiento con prendas de presión. *Rehabilitación.* 2010;44:58–62.

31. Casley-Smith, Judith R, Casley-Smith, John R. Modern treatment of lymphoedema I. Complex physical therapy: The first 200 Australian limbs. *Australas J Dermatol.* 1992;33(2): 61–8.

32. Földi E, Földi M, Weissleder H. Conservative treatment of lymphoedema of the limbs. *Angiology.* 1985;36(3):171–80.

33. Preston NJ, Seers K, Mortimer PS. Physical therapies for reducing and controlling lymphoedema of the limbs. *Cochrane Database Syst Revi.* 2004;4.

34. Godoy MF, Pereira MR, Oliani A, de Godoy JM. Synergic effect of compression therapy and controlled active exercises using a facilitating device in the treatment of arm lymphedema. *Int J Med Sci.* 2012;9(4):280–4.

35. Lane KN, Dolan L, Worsley D, McKenzie DC. Upper extremity lymphatic function at rest and during exercise in breast cancer survivors with and without lymphedema compared with healthy controls. *J Appl Physiol.* 2007;103(3):917–25.

36. Box RC, Reul-Hirche HM, Bullock-Saxton J, Furnival CM. Physiotherapy after breast cancer surgery: Results of a randomised controlled study to minimize lymphoedema. *Breast Cancer Res Treat.* 2002;75(1):51–64.

37. George SM, Irwin M, Matthews CE et al. Beyond recreational physical activity: Examining occupational and household activity, transportation activity, and sedentary behavior in relation to postmenopausal breast cancer risk. *Am J Public Health.* 2010;100(11):2288–95.

38. Sagen A, Karesen R, Skaane P, Risberg MA. Validity for the simplified water displacement instrument to measure arm lymphedema as a result of breast cancer surgery. *Arch Phys Med Rehabil.* 2009;90(5):803–9.

39. Nowicki J and Siviour A. Best practice skin care management in lymphoedema. *Wound Practice, Res: J Aust Wound Manag Assoc.* 2013;21(2):61.

40. Woods ME. *Lymphoedema Care.* John Wiley & Sons, 2008.

41. Shao Y, Qi K, Zhou QH, Zhong DS. Intermittent pneumatic compression pump for breast cancer-related lymphedema: A systematic review and meta-analysis of randomized controlled trials. *Oncol Res Treat.* 2014;37(4):170–4.

42. Dorval M, Maunsell E, Deschenes L, Brisson J, Masse B. Long-term quality of life after breast cancer: Comparison of 8-year survivors with population controls. *J Clin Oncol: Off J Am Soc Clin Oncol.* 1998;16(2):487–94.

43. Robles JI. Linfedema: Una patología olvidada. *Psicooncología.* 2006;3(1):71.

44. Kwan W, Jackson J, Weir LM, Dingee C, McGregor G, Olivotto IA. Chronic arm morbidity after curative breast cancer treatment: Prevalence and impact on quality of life. *J Clin Oncol: Off J Am Soc Clin Oncol.* 2002;20(20):4242–48.

45. Godoy JM and Guerreiro de Godoy F. Godoy & Godoy technique in the treatment of lymphedema for under-privileged populations. *Int J Med Sci.* 2010;7(2):68–71.

46. Godoy JM. Godoy & Godoy technique of cervical stimulation in the reduction of edema of the face after cancer treatment. *The Q J Med.* 2008a;101:325–6.

47. Godoy JM, Pereira de GA, Dias T, Guerreiro MF. The Godoy & Godoy cervical stimulation technique in the treatment of primary congenital lymphedema. *Pediat Rep.* 2008b;4(3):2.

48. Pererira JM, Lozzi AJ, Ferreira W, Guerreiro MF. New method to assess manual lymph drainage using lymphoscintigraphy. *Nuclear Medicine Review.* 2012;15(2):75–7.

49. Bordin A, Guerreiro Godoy MF, Pereira de Godoy JM. Mechanical lymphatic drainage in the treatment of arm lymphedema. *Indian J Cancer.* 2009;46:4–337.

50. Libanore D, Buzato E, Barufi E, Guimarães T, Matias de Carvalho EM. Bioimpedance assessment of edema in patients with mastectomy-related lymphedema treated by mechanical lymph drainage using the RAGodoy® device. *J Phlebol Lymphol.* 2011;4:31–3.

51. de Godoy JM, Lopes Pinto R, Pereira de Godoy AC, de Fátima Guerreiro Godoy M. Synergistic effect of adjustments of elastic stockings to maintain reduction in leg volume after mechanical lymph drainage. *Int J Vasc Med.* 2014;2014:640189. doi:10.1155/2014/640189

52. Ojeda J, Peñarrocha G, Lorenzo C, Labraca N, Martínez I, Martínez A. Fisioterapia en el linfedema tras cáncer de mama y reconstrucción mamaria. *Fisioterapia.* 2009;31(2):65–71.

53. Casley-Smith JR, Morgan RG, Piller NB. Treatment of lymphedema of the arms and legs with 5, 6–benzo-[alpha]-pyrone. *New England J Med.* 1993;329(16):1158–63.

54. Ramelet A. Pharmacologic aspects of a phlebotropic drug in CVI-associated edema. *Angiology.* 2000;51(1):19–23.

55. Badger C, Preston NJ, Seers K, Mortimer PS. Benzopyrones for reducing and controlling lymphoedema of the limbs. *Cochrane Database Syst Rev.* 2004;(2):CD003140. doi:10.1002/14651858.CD003140.pub2

56. Rockson S, Tian W, Jiang X et al. Pilot studies demonstrate the potential benefits of antiinflammatory therapy in human lymphedema. *J. Clin Investig Insight.* 2018;3(20).

27

Prevention and Treatment of Venous Thromboembolism

Agustin Arroyo Bielsa

Introduction

It may be asked why the discussion of venous thromboembolic disease (VTED) requires its own chapter. However, despite the close interrelationship and the epidemiological data that are analyzed later, the reality is that patients still need to be educated about the importance of VTED in cancer.

In October 2018, the results of a survey mainly conducted in oncology patients of five European countries were published [1]. The survey was commissioned by the European Cancer Patient Coalition and conducted by the Quality Health organization of the United Kingdom. This patient awareness study had three primary objectives:

1. Establish the level of concern of cancer patients about VTED.
2. Learn when oncology patients start becoming aware of VTED risks.
3. Ascertain informational gaps in the oncological path and look for ways to improve the degree of awareness in patients.

The survey was taken by 1344 subjects, with great predominance of patients with breast cancer (46%). For this and presumably other factors, the survey was particularly answered by women (75%). Most patients (72%), at the time of completing the survey, confessed to having no knowledge that cancer entails an increased risk of VTED compared with the population without cancer; and a quarter of those who did know knew because they had already suffered a thromboembolic episode.

Another interesting fact is that one-third of surveyed patients were using anticoagulants, but only 40% of these admitted they were told about their potential adverse effects.

Patients with better knowledge and more awareness in general were those suffering some type of hematologic cancer.

The survey analyzed many data, based on which it established a series of recommendations for clinicians and oncological organizations to try harder to ensure that patients with cancer know they have an increased risk of VTED, and about the role of some specific factors like surgery, chemotherapy, radiotherapy, central venous catheter, and so on. Verbal information is as important as providing patients with written documents and ways to obtain information online.

Epidemiology

Many epidemiological data support the position outlined. Twenty percent of oncology patients experienced venous thromboembolic events. This is because patients with cancer are four to eight times more at risk of developing a VTED event than patients without cancer [2–4]. VTED incidence in oncological populations is 4%–20%, and it is possible that the risk of VTED in patients with cancer has increased in the last two decades.

However, detection methods have considerably improved (helical computed tomography). There is greater diagnostic awareness among doctors treating oncology patients. Their survival and quality of life have clearly increased thanks to highly developed palliative care programs. Likewise, as we see later, new treatments have emerged that may be thrombogenic.

Several etiopathogenic factors explain the relationship between cancer and increased risk of VTED. On the one hand, to generalize, tumor cells produce tissue factor, a transmembrane glycoprotein that binds to factor VII and activates factors IX and X, generating thrombin and fibrin. On the other hand, we have the cancer procoagulant factor, a cysteine protease that can activate factor X independently from factor VII. Other elements to take into account are the existence of adhesion molecules, inflammatory cytokines, and angiogenic factors.

The risk of suffering an episode of VTED in patients with cancer is not stable, varying throughout the entire oncological process (Figure 27.1). At the time of diagnosis, the risk has increased compared with the general population. However, if the patient needs hospitalization, said risk notably increases during the following 3–6 months (together with many other associated risk factors: surgery, immobilization, infections, etc.) or during treatments like chemotherapy. The risk decreases to similar levels in patients without cancer when remission is achieved through proper treatments. Relapse, disease progression, and occurrence of metastasis significantly increase the risk again [5,6].

VTED plays a very important role in the morbidity/mortality of cancer patients (Figure 27.2). Naturally, the progression of the oncological disease is the fundamental cause of mortality in these patients (71%); however, VTED is in second place (9%), together with any cause of infectious origin [2,6]. That is to say, 1 out of 10 cancer patients die because of a venous thromboembolic complication. Most importantly, 60% of deaths due to pulmonary thromboembolism (PTE) occur when the patient had a localized oncological or low-tumor–burden disease. In other words, these deaths can be avoided. Furthermore, VTED is

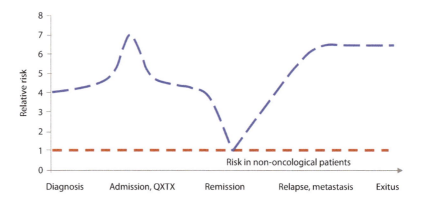

FIGURE 27.1 Relative risk of VTED in oncology patients throughout time.

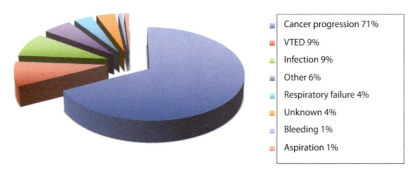

Cancer progression 71%
VTED 9%
Infection 9%
Other 6%
Respiratory failure 4%
Unknown 4%
Bleeding 1%
Aspiration 1%

FIGURE 27.2 Morbidity/mortality of oncology patients.

associated with an increase in early mortality in patients undergoing chemotherapy.

VTED in oncology patients versus patients without cancer is usually characterized by a higher morbidity/mortality, higher recurrence rates, and a larger number of hemorrhagic complications.

Risk Factors

In patients with cancer, three types of VTED risk factors can be distinguished: (1) Patient-dependent risk factors, (2) cancer-dependent risk factors, and (3) treatment-dependent risk factors.

Patient-Dependent Risk Factors

Table 27.1 presents patient-dependent risk factors. Within the section of analytical alterations, the following should be noted:

> Platelet count greater than 350,000/mm^3
> White blood cell count greater than 11,000/mm^3
> Hemoglobin less than 10 gr/dL
> *Other*: Tissue factor in tumor cells, circulating tissue factor, P-selectin, C-reactive protein (PCR)

Race may be another factor to take into account, since a larger incidence of VTED has been documented in African American versus Asian oncology patients.

Cancer-Dependent Risk Factors

As seen in Figure 27.1, and taking into account the natural curve of cancer evolution, the first 3–6 months have the higher incidence of VTED.

Location and histology are important, and in this sense, we can place pancreatic cancer as first in the list by far. Brain, lung, ovarian, kidney, stomach, esophageal, bone, and liver cancers, lymphoma, and myeloma are also classified as high-risk cancers. Breast cancer, prostate cancer, and melanoma may be considered low-risk cancers. And in the middle we place uterine cancer, bladder cancer, colon cancer, and leukemia.

Of course, the stage of the disease and the presence of metastasis increase the risk of VTED in most tumors.

Other factors associated with cancer may have an influence, like the existence or absence of compression of the adjacent venous structures.

Treatment-Dependent Risk Factors

Several treatment modalities applied to patients with cancer may increase the risk of suffering a thromboembolic event: chemotherapy, radiotherapy, surgery, placement of a central venous catheter (CVC), hormone therapy, erythropoietic agents, and antiangiogenic agents [7]. Transfusions or simple hospitalizations are other factors to take into account. Patients undergoing chemotherapy are 2–6.5 times more likely to suffer a thromboembolic event.

Aflibercept (Zaltrap), an antiangiogenic used in colorectal cancer, increases the risk of vein and arterial thrombosis, and bleeding. However, bevacizumab (Avastin), a monoclonal antibody with a similar indication, can increase arterial complications and bleeding, but this is not clear in the case of vein thrombosis. Tamoxifen and raloxifene clearly increase the risk of VTED (especially in the first 2 years) above aromatase inhibitors like anastrozole and letrozole. The androgenic block and

TABLE 27.1

Patient-Dependent Risk Factors for Venous Thromboembolic Disease (VTED) in Patients with Cancer

Patient-Dependent Risk Factors

Advanced age

Obesity

General health

Comorbidities: Infection, kidney failure, respiratory disease, etc.

Tobacco

Immobilization

History of VTED

Hereditary mutations

Analytical alterations

Race

TABLE 27.2

Wells Criteria for Deep Venous Thrombosis

Clinical Aspects	Score
Active cancer	1
Prior immobilization	1
Greater than 3 days of immobilization or surgery 4 weeks before	1
Edema	1
Edema + heat	1
Rhizomelic edema	1
Collateral circulation	1
Localized pain	1
Probability of alternative diagnosis	−2
Final score	
Low probability	0
Medium probability	1–2
High probability	3 or more

TABLE 27.3

Wells Criteria for Pulmonary Thromboembolism (PTE)

Clinical Aspects	Score
PTE as more probable diagnosis	3
Suspicion of deep venous thrombosis (DVT)	3
Tachycardia (>100 beats/min)	1.5
Surgery or immobilization 1 month before	1.5
History of PTE or DVT	1.5
Hemoptysis	1
Active cancer	1
Final score	
Low probability	0–1
Medium probability	2–6
High probability	7 or more

TABLE 27.4

Geneva Score Revised for Pulmonary Thromboembolism (PTE)

Clinical Aspects	Score
Age older than 65 years	1
History of PTE or deep vein thrombosis	3
Surgery with general anesthesia or LL fracture 1 month before	2
Active or cured cancer in the last year	2
Unilateral pain in leg	3
Hemoptysis	2
Tachycardia (75–94 beats/min)	3
Tachycardia (>95 beats/min)	5
Pain upon palpation and unilateral edema in leg	4
Final score	
Low probability	0–1
Medium probability	2–6
High probability	7 or more

estramustine also increase the risk of VTED, especially in the long term (from the second year).

Diagnosis

The purpose of this chapter is not to review the clinical aspects of deep venous thrombosis (DVT) but to remind about the role of the main tools of the diagnostic algorithm. Table 27.2 shows Wells criteria for DVT in which each item has a score of one, subtracting two points from the total if there is a probable alternative diagnosis. Although the presence of so many items with the word "edema" might seem confusing, it must be made clear that if a patient develops rhizomelic edema with flogotic signs in the extremity, it must be scored three points. A final score of one to two points will be considered middle probability, and three or more points, high probability. This differentiation is important, as can be seen in the diagnostic algorithm, particularly concerning the role of the D-dimer. Figure 27.3 clearly shows that D-dimer is not a routine test because it loses value, and unnecessary resources are overused.

Regarding PTE diagnosis, two tests must be noted: Wells criteria for PTE (Table 27.3) and the Geneva score revised for PTE (Table 27.4). They both share similar items, such as hemoptysis, suspicion of DVT, active cancer, history of VTED, and so on; however, the Geneva score is a little more complete, including aspects like age or giving more importance to aspects like tachycardia. It is easier to reach a high level of diagnostic probability with the Geneva score.

Prophylaxis

In this section about VTED prophylaxis in patients with cancer, four scenarios will be analyzed: surgery, hospitalization due to acute process, central venous catheter, and outpatients undergoing chemotherapy treatment.

Venous Thromboembolic Disease Prophylaxis in Surgery

In general, we can say that any patient with cancer undergoing surgery will receive VTED prophylaxis. This will begin in the preoperative setting, have a duration of 7–10 days, and last 1 month in the following cases: pelvic or abdominal surgery, obesity, subjects older than 65 years, comorbidity, and advanced state of neoplasia.

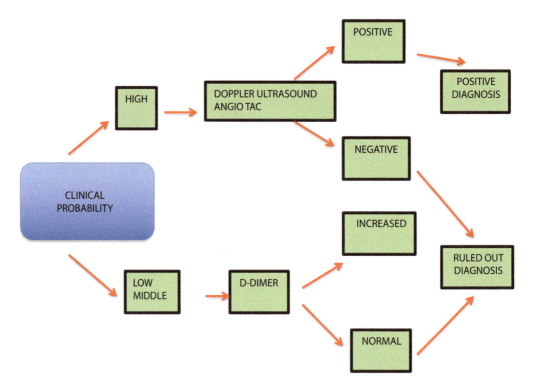

FIGURE 27.3 Diagnostic algorithm of deep venous thrombosis.

Venous Thromboembolic Disease Prophylaxis in Hospitalization Due to Acute Process

Based on the analysis of several existing studies, we must conclude that VTED prophylaxis is certainly necessary in patients with cancer when they are hospitalized due to some acute, nonsurgical process. In the ARTEMIS study [8], which included 849 patients, 15.4% with cancer, two groups were compared, one receiving fondaparinux as prophylaxis and the other, placebo. There was a significant difference ($p = .029$) in venous thromboembolic events between the fondaparinux group (5.6%) and the placebo group (10.5%). This meant a 47% decrease in relative risk, and no differences were found regarding hemorrhagic complications. In the MEDENOX study [9] that compared one group receiving enoxaparin as prophylaxis and a placebo group, findings were similar: 5.5% of VTED in the enoxaparin group versus 14.9% in the placebo group, and a risk reduction of 63%. Likewise, no hemorrhagic differences were found. The same can be said about the PREVENT study [10], which included 3706 patients (5.1% with cancer). In this case, dalteparin was compared with placebo. Risk reduction was of 44% for the prophylaxis group, and again, no hemorrhagic complications were found.

Patients lying in bed in their homes must receive the same kind of prophylaxis. However, being admitted to chemotherapy is not reason enough to receive prophylaxis; other risk factors must be considered, and aspects like the ability to walk must be insisted upon.

Venous Thromboembolic Disease Prophylaxis in Those with Central Venous Catheter

The incidence of symptomatic VTED in patients that carry a CVC varies based on each case; although it is between 0.3% and 20%, it is usually considered a low incidence, so VTED thromboprophylaxis

is not considered a routine procedure just for this indication. The performance of refined techniques by expert hands using the least amount possible of thrombogenic materials is the most significant aspect. The least thrombogenic entrance is usually through the right subclavian vein, placing the tip of the catheter at the junction of the superior vena cava and the right atrium.

Venous Thromboembolic Disease Prophylaxis in Outpatients Undergoing Chemotherapy Treatment

Although this is a controversial scenario, routine thromboprophylaxis is not usually considered necessary. Risk patients must be detected and classified based on chemotherapy and type of cancer. For this purpose, we have Khorana's predictive model [11]. According to Table 27.5, if the final score is 0, we are talking about a low-risk category; between 1 and 2, middle risk; and 3 or more, high risk. Based on the study analyses, it is usually deduced that low-molecular-weight heparins (LMWHs) reduce the incidence of VTED during chemotherapy, but with low repercussion [12]. However, if we focus on studies about high-risk patients, like CONKO 004 [13] or FRAGEM [14], in cases of advanced pancreatic cancer, the benefits of thromboprophylaxis with LMWHs during chemotherapy are clearly significant and clinically relevant.

In summary, we can say that guidelines do not recommend routine thromboprophylaxis in outpatients undergoing chemotherapy, saving it instead for high-risk cancers in patients with low risk of bleeding [15–18].

Treatment

In the treatment of VTED episodes in patients with cancer, LMWHs play a remarkable role both in the immediate phase

TABLE 27.5

Khorana's Predictive Model

Characteristics of the Patient	Score
Cancer location:	
Very high risk: Stomach, pancreas	2
High risk: Lung, lymphoma, gynecological, germinal, bladder	1
Pre-QxTx platelets ≥350,000/mL	1
Hemoglobin <10 gr/dL or use of erythropoietin	1
Pre-QxTx WBC ≥11,000/mL	1
BMI ≥35	1

of the first 5–10 days (many studies and meta-analyses confirm that the pharmacokinetics of LMWHs is more predictable, and at least as efficient and safe as unfractionated heparin), in lengthy treatments, and in secondary prophylaxis. This is because the treatment with antivitamin K anticoagulants (AVK ACO) has some disadvantages: it requires frequent dose adjustments; there are many drug-drug interactions; toxicities secondary to chemotherapy (basically thrombopenia) are handled worse; malabsorption and tumor cachexia syndromes mean significant variations of intake; and due to common and necessary invasive procedures, patients are forced to interrupt their treatment.

Furthermore, the probability of VTED recurrence is lower with LMWHs than with AVK ACO, with similar hemorrhagic complications. In this regard, five randomized studies about LMWHs versus AVK ACO can be emphasized. All of them show a clear tendency toward LMWHs, although two (CANTHANOX, OCENOX), which have small samples, did not reach statistical significance [19,20]. The CLOT and LITE studies, with larger samples, have a $p < .05$ regarding recurrence [21,22]. A fifth study called CATCH, which included 900 patients recruited and assigned to two groups, reached a $p = .07$ [23]. All studies are based on a 100% therapeutic dose of LMWHs, except CLOT, which uses a 75% dose from the first month of treatment.

However, there is not such scientific clarity regarding treatment duration. We can ensure a minimum of 3 months, and extend it to 6 months if risk factors, like active cancer, persist. But beyond 6 months, guidelines recommend a prolonged treatment with LMWHs if there is active cancer and low risk of bleeding [24].

In 2016, CHEST published an update of the VTED treatment guide; the previous guide was from 2012 [25]. Although there is a clear preference for the new direct-acting ACO (ACOD) versus AVK ACO for the prolonged treatment of VTED in patients without cancer, LMWHs are still preferred for cancer patients. For those patients who cannot be treated with anticoagulants, CHEST 2016 introduces for the first time the role of aspirin as secondary prophylaxis.

In any case, the decision concerning prolonged treatments for these patients must be individualized. Thus, we consider active, progressive or metastatic cancer, chemotherapy, or the persistence of the thrombus as factors to maintain coagulation; and we have to consider these alongside factors involving a higher risk of bleeding, like previous hemorrhages, severe thrombopenia, subjects older than 65 years, and fragile patients.

The mortality risk due to bleeding is doubled in patients with cancer. The risk of bleeding is influenced by factors like anticoagulation, thrombopenia, surgery and invasive procedures, the presence of highly vascularized tumors or that invade large vessels, and so on.

Regarding the accumulated incidence of VTED during anticoagulant treatments, patients with cancer have 3.2 times more chance of recurrence than patients without cancer [26]. Different models intended to stratify the risk of VTED recurrence in patients with cancer have many similar items, like gender, location of the VTED episode, and posttreatment levels of D-dimer [27].

The first step to treat VTED recurrence is to differentiate it from postthrombotic sequelae. If the recurrence is confirmed, we must check what anticoagulant treatment the patient was receiving (and if it was the right one) and assess a potential progression of the tumor disease, aside from ruling out a potential heparin-induced thrombopenia. If the patient was receiving AVK ACO or ACOD, we must change it to LMWHs. If the patient was already taking LMWHs, we will increase the dose in 25% for a month (in many cases with anti-Xa activity control). Other—more controversial—actions would be to add aspirin to the treatment or modify chemotherapy.

Management of Incidental Pulmonary Embolism

There should be special mention of those patients presenting with an unexpected diagnosis of pulmonary embolism (PE). This diagnosis represents about 50% of VTED episodes in patients with cancer. When compared with the classic symptomatic PE, we can say that it has the same recurrence, the same mortality, and the same risk of bleeding; therefore, it requires the same treatment. Only in those cases of asymptomatic incidental PE, with negative LL Doppler ultrasounds for DVT, can we use a different treatment and base our therapeutic decision on clinical monitoring and serial ultrasounds [28].

Central Venous Catheter–Related Thrombosis

Since patients with cancer often have CVCs, this is a situation that deserves to be studied individually. We have already discussed some aspects in the prophylaxis chapter, and, in general, we concluded that routine VTED prophylaxis is not necessary in CVC carriers. If not clinical, the search for thrombosis is not necessary either.

There is a series of catheter-related factors that make thrombosis more common: a peripheral over a central catheter; femoral over jugular, and jugular over subclavian; the left side over the right side; the more caliber and number of lights, the more probabilities; and more common in occurrence during the first week after insertion (and, in this regard, practice and expertise of the professional are important).

Other factors depend on cancer itself or the patient characteristics. Therefore, CVC thrombosis is more frequent in metastatic cancer, chemotherapy, thoracic radiotherapy, erythropoietic stimulants, catheter infection, thrombophilia, and so on.

Once vein thrombosis in a CVC carrier has been diagnosed, the treatment is anticoagulation; it can only be removed if the light is thrombosed, if the catheter is infected, if the catheter is not being used, or if it is not evolving properly despite the anticoagulant treatment. If the catheter is removed, LMWHs must be maintained for at least 3 months. If the patient cannot take anticoagulants, the placement of a cava filter is not justified. If the catheter is not removed, the patient will stay on anticoagulants while carrying it.

REFERENCES

1. European Cancer Patient Coalition. Cancer-associated thrombosis awareness survey: Results report; October 2018. https://thrombosisuk.org/downloads/ECPC_2018_Cancer_associated_thrombosis_awareness_survey_report.pdf

2. Khorana AA, Francis CW, Culakova E, Kuderer NM, Lyman GH. Thromboembolism is a leading cause of death in cancer patients receiving outpatient chemotherapy. *J Thromb Haemost.* 2007 Mar;5(3):632–4.

3. Bloom JW, Vanderschoot JP, Oostindier MJ, Osanto S, van der Meer FJ, Rosendaal FR. Incidence of venous thrombosis in a large cohort of 66,329 cancer patients: Results of a record linkage study. *J Thromb Haemost.* 2006;4(3):529–35.

4. Otten HM, Mathijssen J, ten Cate H, Soesan M, Inghels M, Richel DJ, Prins MH. Symptomatic venous thromboembolism in cancer patients treated with chemotherapy: An underestimated phenomenon. *Arch Intern Med.* 2004 Jan 26;164(2):190–4.

5. Lyman GH. Venous thromboembolism in the patient with cancer: Focus on burden of disease and benefits of thromboprophylaxis. *Cancer.* 2011 Apr 1;117(7):1334–49.

6. II Consenso SEOM sobre la ETEV en pacientes con cáncer. http://www.seom.org/seomcms/images/stories/recursos/II_Consenso_SEOM_enf_tromboembolica_cancer.pdf

7. Hisada Y, Geddings JE, Ay C, Mackman N. Venous thrombosis and cancer: From mouse models to clinical trials. *J Thromb Haemost.* 2015 Aug;13(8):1372–82.

8. Cohen AT, Davidson BL, Gallus AS, Lassen MR, Prins MH, Tomkowski W, Turpie AG, Egberts JF, Lensing AW; ARTEMIS Investigators. Efficacy and safety of fondaparinux for the prevention of venous thromboembolism in older acute medical patients: Randomised placebo controlled trial. *BMJ.* 2006 Feb 11;332(7537):325–9.

9. Turpie AG. Thrombosis prophylaxis in the acutely ill medical patient: Insights from the prophylaxis in MEDical patients with ENOXaparin (MEDENOX) trial. *Am J Cardiol.* 2000 Dec 28;86(12B):48M–52M.

10. Leizorovicz A, Cohen AT, Turpie AG, Olsson CG, Vaitkus PT, Goldhaber SZ; PREVENT Medical Thromboprophylaxis Study Group. Randomized, placebo-controlled trial of dalteparin for the prevention of venous thromboembolism in acutely ill medical patients. *Circulation.* 2004 Aug 17;110(7):874–9.

11. Khorana AA, Kuderer NM, Culakova E, Lyman GH, Francis CW. Development and validation of a predictive model for chemotherapy-associated thrombosis. *Blood.* 2008;111(10):4902–7.

12. A. Falanga, M. Marchetti. Oncology; In: Key NS, Makris M, O'Shaughnessy D, Lillicrap D. *Practical Hemostasis and Thrombosis.* 2nd ed. Wiley-Blackwell, 2011.

13. Pelzer U, Opitz B, Deutschinoff G et al. Efficacy of prophylactic low-molecular weight heparin for ambulatory patients with advanced pancreatic cancer: Outcomes from the CONKO-004 Trial. *J Clin Oncol.* 2015 Jun 20;33(18):2028–34.

14. Maraveyas A, Waters J, Roy R et al. Gemcitabine versus gemcitabine plus dalteparin thromboprophylaxis in pancreatic cancer. *Eur J Cancer.* 2012 Jun;48(9):1283–92.

15. Mandala M, Clerici M, Corradino I, Vitalini C, Colombini S, Torri V, De Pascale A, Marsoni S. Incidence risk factors and clinical implications of venous thromboembolism in cancer patients treated within the context of phase I studies: The "SENDO experience". *Ann Oncol.* 2012 Jun;23(6):1416–21.

16. Farge D, Debourdeau P, Beckers M et al. International clinical practice guidelines for the treatment and prophylaxis of venous thromboembolism in patients with cancer. *J Thromb Haemost.* 2013 Jan;11(1):56–70.

17. Lyman GH, Bohlke K, Khorana AA et al.; American Society of Clinical Oncology. Venous thromboembolism prophylaxis and treatment in patients with cancer: American Society of Clinical Oncology Clinical Practice Guideline Update 2014. *J Clin Oncol.* 2015 Feb 20;33(6):654–6.

18. Muñoz AJ, Viñolas N, Cubedo R, Isla D. SEOM guidelines on thrombosis in cancer patients. *Clin Transl Oncol.* 2011 Aug;13(8):592–6.

19. Meyer G, Marjanovic Z, Valcke J, Lorcerie B, Gruel Y, Solal-Celigny P, Le Maignan C, Extra JM, Cottu P, Farge D. Comparison of low-molecular-weight heparin and warfarin for the secondary prevention of venous thromboembolism in patients with cancer: A randomized controlled study. *Arch Intern Med.* 2002 Aug 12-26;162(15):1729–35.

20. Deitcher SR, Kessler CM, Merli G, Rigas JR, Lyons RM, Fareed J; ONCENOX Investigators. Secondary prevention of venous thromboembolic events in patients with active cancer: Enoxaparin alone versus initial enoxaparin followed by warfarin for a 180–day period. *Clin Appl Thromb Hemost.* 2006 Oct;12(4):389–96.

21. Lee AY, Levine MN, Baker RI, Bowden C, Kakkar AK, Prins M, Rickles FR, Julian JA, Haley S, Kovacs MJ, Gent M; Randomized Comparison of Low-Molecular-Weight Heparin versus Oral Anticoagulant Therapy for the Prevention of Recurrent Venous Thromboembolism in Patients with Cancer (CLOT) Investigators. Low-molecular-weight heparin versus a coumarin for the prevention of recurrent venous thromboembolism in patients with cancer. *N Engl J Med.* 2003 Jul 10;349(2):146–53.

22. Hull RD, Pineo GF, Brant RF, Mah AF, Burke N, Dear R, Wong T, Cook R, Solymoss S, Poon MC, Raskob G; LITE Trial Investigators. Long-term low-molecular-weight heparin versus usual care in proximal-vein thrombosis patients with cancer. *Am J Med.* 2006 Dec;119(12):1062–72.

23. Lee AY, Kamphuisen PW, Meyer G, Bauersachs R, Janas MS, Jarner MF, Khorana AA; CATCH Investigators. Tinzaparin vs warfarin for treatment of acute venous thromboembolism in patients with active cancer: A Randomized Clinical Trial. *JAMA.* 2015 Aug 18;314(7):677–86.

24. Noble SII, Shelley MD, Coles B, Williams SM, Wilcock A, Johnson MJ; Association for Palliative Medicine for Great Britain and Ireland. Management of venous thromboembolism in patients with advanced cancer: A systematic review and meta-analysis. *Lancet Oncol.* 2008 Jun;9(6):577–84.

25. Kearon C, Akl EA, Ornelas J et al. Antithrombotic Therapy for VTE Disease: CHEST Guideline and Expert Panel Report. *Chest.* 2016 Feb;149(2):315–52.

26. Prandoni P, Piccioli A, Pagnan A. Recurrent thromboembolism in cancer patients: Incidence and risk factors. *Semin Thromb Hemost.* 2003 Dec;29(Suppl 1):3–8.

27. Kyrle PA. Predicting recurrent venous thromboembolism in cancer: Is it possible? *Thromb Res.* 2014 May; 133 Suppl 2:S17–22.

28. Di Nisio M, Lee AY, Carrier M, Liebman HA, Khorana AA; Subcommittee on Haemostasis and Malignancy. Diagnosis and treatment of incidental venous thromboembolism in cancer patients: Guidance from the SSC of the ISTH. *J Thromb Haemost.* 2015 May;13(5):880–3.

28

Cosmetic-Medical Treatments

M. Lourdes Mourelle and B. N. Díaz

Cosmetic Care of the Skin (M.L. Mourelle)

The increase in the incidence of cancers in the population has multiplied efforts for the development of new therapeutic agents and with them greater survival of the patients. Cancer treatments improve but are not without side effects, some of which limit the patient's quality of life, both during therapy and years after its cessation. One of the aspects that both therapists and patients value is the care of the skin and physical appearance to improve the side effects and sequelae in the skin and its annexes.

No one now doubts that the improvement of the cancer patient's well-being and self-esteem contributes positively to their recovery. A study by Titeca on quality of life (QoL), comparing patients with cosmetic care versus others who did not receive treatment, shows a statistically significant difference between the cosmetic group and the control group in two areas of QoL, mood state and self-perception of the disease [1]. Another study [2] compared two groups of patients treated for breast cancer, in which the control group did not receive any treatment, and the control group received aesthetic treatment for side effects of therapy on the skin. The alterations treated were hand-foot syndrome, nail damage, edema, xerosis, rash, and radiodermatitis, and the aesthetics treatments were manicure and pedicure with antiflakiness cream, massage, emollient oil, and nourishing and lenitive emulsion. The health-related quality of life (HRQoL) questionnaire was applied before and after 28 days of treatment, twice a week. The study concluded that there was a significant difference between both groups; the treated patients perceived that the symptoms of the indicated disorders improved, and distress was also reduced.

The changes that occur in the skin of cancer patients undergoing chemotherapy and radiotherapy vary according to the type of therapeutic agent used. Nails and hair can be affected (with paronychia and alopecia, among other alterations), as well as the skin, where pruritus, xerosis, folliculitis (skin rash), hyperpigmentation, and hand and foot erythema (palmar-plantar erythrodysesthesia) can occur. In addition, the skin becomes more sensitive to allergens, more prone to infection, and also more sensitive to ultraviolet (UV) radiation [3]. The skin, in addition to being a mechanical barrier, has important immune functions, with cells and chemicals coordinated to exercise defensive functions. If this function is altered, problems may appear not only locally but also remotely, since the cutaneous immune system works in connection with the rest of the body.

These skin manifestations have a great impact on the quality of life of the cancer patient, and that is why it is necessary to address them from a professional point of view. For this, it is essential to treat the symptoms with cosmetics and dermocosmetics for skin care, but also with a camouflage effect, so that adverse effects can be minimized, and the patient's self-esteem is enhanced.

More Frequent Skin Disorders

There are differences between the skin manifestations and reactions caused by chemotherapy and by radiotherapy. With chemotherapy, xerosis, skin rash, and hand-foot erythema mainly occur; in radiotherapy, a series of symptoms are produced, grouped under the name of radiodermatitis. Different adverse reactions are also seen with targeted treatments and immunotherapy; thus, acneiform eruptions are more frequent in patients treated with epidermal growth factor receptor and mitogen-activated protein kinase inhibitors; BRAF inhibitors frequently produce secondary skin tumors (squamous cell carcinoma and keratoacanthomas), changes in preexisting pigmentary lesions, and hand-foot reactions. Immune checkpoint inhibitors (ICIs) produce maculopapular rash, and eczema-like or psoriatic lesions, lichenoid dermatitis, xerosis, and pruritus. Mucositis and oral hyperkeratotic lesions are also observed. Furthermore, targeted treatments and endocrine therapy frequently produce late alopecia, and targeted therapies can also damage the nail plate, with paronychia and periungual pyogenic granuloma distinct from chemotherapy-induced lesions. Delayed nail growth, onycholysis, and brittle nails may also occur [4].

Mucosal disorders: Oral mucositis is quite frequent and manifests with redness in the mouth with a burning sensation. It can be very painful and therefore prevents normal food intake, sometimes making necessary treatment with powerful anti-inflammatory drugs.

The endobuccal epithelium is especially sensitive to the cytotoxic effect of chemotherapy. Mucositis corresponds to inflammatory phenomena induced by chemotherapy, by radiotherapy, and to a lesser extent, by targeted therapy that develops in the entire mucosa of the digestive tract, from the mouth to the anus.

Clinically, chemotherapy-induced mucositis appears after the first or first cycles (inflammatory ulcerations varying from limited to diffuse, on the ventral and lateral sides of the tongue, base of the mouth, soft palate, or mucosa of the cheek); if radiation therapy is associated, it affects more areas and can be complicated by pain, which will limit feeding and even speech.

These chemotherapy-induced lesions can occur with induced but more limited therapies, in the form of aphthoid ulcerations [5].

Xerostomia (endo-oral dryness) has also been observed after radiotherapy, with frequent sequelae such as dysgeusia (modification of the sense of taste) and mucous pigmentation.

Cutaneous xerosis: Cutaneous xerosis, or extremely dry skin, consists of an increase in the dryness of the skin and/or mucosa, which in certain cases can be very intense. It is one of the most frequent side effects of systemic therapies that appears several weeks after treatment. When aggravated, it can be complicated by secondary *Staphylococcus aureus* or herpes simplex infections [6]. Generally, it is a simple cutaneous dryness, mainly in the extremities and trunk, which manifests itself with fine scales and sometimes rough skin, a feeling of tightness, and sometimes pain. Sometimes it is accompanied by skin inflammation, eczematiform, and more or less intense itching.

With epidermal growth factor receptor inhibitors (EGFRIs), cracked eczema can occur in the lower extremities or as painful fissures in the toes or heels. Sometimes, less frequently, they present a form of ichthyosis [7].

Skin rash: This is one of the most frequent manifestations and follows a chronological pattern with peaks of severity during the first 2 weeks of chemotherapy [8]. It manifests with papules and pustules, intense itching, pain, and sometimes spontaneous bleeding from the lesions [4]. Some studies indicate that it may appear in 43%–85% of patients treated with EGFRIs [9]. However, the lesions tend to fade after a few weeks or months. It is located in all areas where the sebaceous glands are abundant, such as the face and scalp, the trunk (presternal and interscapular area), and much less frequently in the limbs. The impact on the quality of life is very high. It should be borne in mind that although it may look like an acneiform rash, it is not, since there are no obstructive lesions characteristic of acne, such as microcysts and comedones, and it is not common for acne to have a burning sensation, itching, and pain [5].

Toxic erythema in chemotherapy: This term was proposed by Bolognia in 2008 in order to group together the clinical manifestations induced by chemotherapy. It comprises a set of skin reactions that are sometimes described separately or by other names (e.g., chemotherapy-related bilateral dermatitis associated with eccrine squamous syringometaplasia [CBDESS] or, to a lesser extent, symmetrical drug-related intertriginous and flexural rash [SDRIFE]) and clinically characterized by painful erythematous, violaceous, and/or edematous plaques of the hands, feet, and intertriginous regions that may have a dusky appearance and develop bullae with subsequent erosions [10]. Many of these symptoms are associated with other skin disorders such as erythrodysesthesia, acral erythema, hand-foot syndrome, toxic erythema of the palms and soles, eccrine squamous syringometaplasia, epidermal dysmaturation, and neutrophilic eccrine hidradenitis [11–13]. It is usually a toxic, nonimmunoallergic mechanism and, therefore, dose dependent and with an often similar histological pattern [5].

Cutaneous itching: The itchy skin can be a consequence of dry skin or due to the involvement of internal organs (e.g., in the case of jaundice or kidney dysfunction). It can be accompanied by itching and be generalized [14].

Ulcerations: These manifest as a loss of continuity of the skin that affects the deepest layers, dermis and hypodermis, with little tendency to spontaneous repair. They may be due to the tumor itself, but very often they are associated with chemotherapy treatment with EGFRIs, angiogenesis inhibitors, platelet-derived growth factor receptor (PDGFR) inhibitors, and so on [15].

Dermatitis: This can be many and varied—related to the tumor or as a consequence of chemotherapy treatments, scaly or blistering dermatitis, with atrophies, and even with increased hair [16].

Hand-foot syndrome: This is a specific clinical manifestation of cancer treatments and occurs both in chemotherapy treatments and in targeted therapies, although in the first case they are more diffuse, and with targeted therapies they appear earlier and are more localized [5]; it is also called acral erythema or Burgdorf syndrome. It presents as an extensive inflammatory erythema on the palms of the hands and soles of the feet (usually bilateral), sometimes with edema and varying degrees of desquamation, hyperkeratosis, or blisters. It has a great impact on the QoL of the patient, so it may be necessary to reduce the dose and even stop treatment [17].

Lymphedema: This usually affects the extremities (arms and legs) and is generally a consequence of the surgical removal of lymph nodes or radiotherapy treatments in the area. It can appear immediately or years after the end of treatment [18].

Alopecia and changes in the amount of hair: The most notable alteration is alopecia, which is due to chemotherapy treatment that causes toxicity in hair that is in its active growth phase (anagen). In the studies by Naveed et al., it is highlighted that in a large percentage of patients suffering from alopecia, this is related to an anagen effluvium and in a lower percentage with a telogen effluvium. Due to the psychological impact, patients consider this the main burden of the disease, sometimes constituting a stigma, because through this alteration, the disease is shown to others. Rarely, hirsutism or hypertrichosis can occur [16].

Nail disorders: Different alterations can occur, mainly color alterations (melanonychia and leukonychia), followed by nail ridging, onycholysis, Beau lines, paronychia, brittle nail, and nail infection.

Other changes resulting from chemotherapy: There are a set of alterations that can be dermatoses or facial imperfections but that all affect personal self-image to a great extent.

- *Hyperpigmentations*: These appear mainly in the acral areas but can also be generalized [16]. They usually disappear once the treatment is finished; they are often accentuated by sun exposure, so it is convenient to use a sunscreen.
- *Photosensitivity*: The skin is sensitive to sun exposure, so specific protectors will be applied. The sensitivity is induced by ultraviolet A (UVA) light, and it is more of a phototoxicity than a photoallergy. Aggravation of preexisting dermatoses (e.g., subacute lupus) or the phenomenon of UV recall (or reappearance of an erythema) may occur after the injection of certain chemotherapeutic substances, in which an erythema reappears in the area that had previously been irradiated [19].
- *Vascular disorders*: There can be vasculitis-like lesions, periorbital edema, and flushing, among other reactions [16].

Radiodermatitis: As a side effect of radiotherapy treatments, multiple skin reactions occur that have been grouped under the term *radiodermatitis*. It is produced by the aggression that radiotherapy inflicts on the cutaneous barrier, diminishing the regenerative capacity of the skin cells; there is damage to blood vessels and therefore to the nutritional supply necessary for skin regeneration.

The main manifestations during the acute phase are erythema, which appears in the first weeks; dry desquamation, due to a reduction in the mitotic capacity of the germ layer of the epidermis, with itching and peeling; moist desquamation (a complication of the previous stages), due not only to damage to the basal layer of the epidermis, but also to damage to the vessels of the dermis; and ulceration and necrosis, which rarely occur, but can occur due to reirradiation, usually 6 weeks or 2 months after irradiation if the connective tissue has been damaged. Reepithelialization develops from 6 to 8 weeks from the undamaged cells. As a side effect, hyperpigmentation, reduction or suppression of sebaceous and sweat glands, and hair removal can occur, due to the high sensitivity of anagen follicles to radiation [20].

In the subacute phase (6 months to 1 year after completing radiotherapy), hyperpigmentation and hypopigmentation, telangiectasias, skin atrophy, or ulcerations appear. In the chronic phase (1–5 years later) the most common manifestations are atrophy, dermal fibrosis, telangiectasias, and permanent skin depilation. In the final phase (which begins 5 years later) there is a high risk of developing skin cancer [20].

Other alterations: Other facial alterations or imperfections that affect personal self-image are as follows [21]:

- Hypersensitivity to certain cosmetics, with a tendency to redden
- Color changes, vascular or brown spots
- Alteration of the pores, which become more evident
- Presence of facial telangiectasias
- Flaccidity increases (cheekbones accentuate and eyes sink)
- Sallow tone and loss of luminosity

All these alterations not only cause discomfort to the patient but also contribute to modifying the patient's perception of his or her own body and body image, which is why an approach to cosmetic care from different points of view—medical, psychological, and aesthetic—is necessary.

Dermocosmetics for the Care of the Cancer Patient (M.L. Mourelle)

When providing care to the cancer patient, it is necessary to distinguish the different phases, since the cosmetic products (and aesthetic care) that can be applied will vary in each of them. Thus, in the phases prior to chemotherapy and/or radiotherapy, there are fewer limitations, since it is a matter of preparing the skin to minimize side effects, but during the treatment itself, the actions and cosmetics will be limited. Once medical treatment is finished, the objective is to aid recovery of the skin and its adnexa in the shortest possible time.

There is little scientific evidence on the use of cosmetics in caring for the skin of the cancer patient. Most of the guidelines of the cancer treatment centers indicate that moisturize and emollience are necessary. The treatment must always be personalized and adapted to each specific case.

Cosmetics are products aimed at improving the structure, morphology, and appearance of skin, with the assistance of excipients and active ingredients adapted to different skin types (normal, oily, combination, sensitive, etc.). Cosmeceuticals, although a term not officially recognized, are defined as "cosmetic products with biologically active ingredients purporting to have medical or drug-like benefits" [22].

Three main groups of skincare cosmetics can be established: cleansers, moisturizing and maintenance products, and sunscreens. In addition, hair cleansers (shampoos) and cosmetics are used to repair the hair structure and to maintain the scalp. For nails, emollient products are used; for the maintenance of the nail plate and, in postoncological care, toxic-free decorative cosmetics could be included.

There are no specific active ingredients for caring for the skin of the cancer patient; those that repair the skin barrier will be used, respecting the natural cycle of epidermal renewal, with little or no toxicity, and of high quality and purity.

Oils and Butters

Vegetable oils and butters provide numerous properties to the skin, since they have a good affinity for the skin and have a protective, emollient, and regenerative action. They are therefore the active ingredients of choice in skin care to alleviate many of the cutaneous symptoms resulting from oncological treatments, such as xerosis, flaking, and irritation. They must be selected from those of adequate purity, and in the case of oils, those derived from first cold pressing will be preferred so that they retain all their active compounds (unsaturated fatty acids, vitamin E, etc.). The most used are murumuru butter, shea, cocoa, mango, kokum; olive, borage, jojoba, argan, babassu, baobab, macadamia, kukui, and so on. Rose hip oil is also used for its regenerative potential, especially indicated to improve healing.

The oils rich in polyunsaturated fatty acids (PUFAs) are of great interest, since it has been shown that their lack can cause skin dryness, flaking, and eczema, and they are also related to the health of the immune system of the epidermis. They are abundant in the oil of flax, evening primrose, hemp, pumpkin, safflower, borage, black cumin, sunflower, and so on [23]. Sacha Inchi (*Plukenetia volubilis*) seed oil is also used in regenerative cosmetics for its richness in PUFAs, tocopherols, and phytosterols, and its antioxidant capacity [24].

Other oily active ingredients of interest are unsaponifiables, which contain carotenoids (precursors of vitamin A), tocopherols (such as vitamin E), and phytosterols; an example is avocado unsaponifiables [23].

Antioxidants

These are essential to protect cell membranes from lipid peroxidation and capture free radicals that decrease the antioxidant defenses of the skin. It should be remembered that with chemotherapy and radiotherapy treatments, many free radicals are generated, so once the therapy is finished, it is necessary to bring the skin back to its natural balance.

The most used antioxidants are superoxide dismutase, our skin's natural enzyme that needs the presence of selenium and zinc, which can be provided through the diet but also as an active ingredient in cosmetics. Glutathione, which is generated from the amino acids cysteine, glutamic acid, and glycine, also has free antiradical action, which also requires the presence of selenium and zinc; its topical use to prevent radiodermatitis has therefore been studied [25]. Other antioxidants of interest are *N*-acetylcysteine, lipoic acid, and grapefruit seed extracts and lycopene from tomato [26].

Vitamins

There are numerous studies showing the role of various vitamins in skin health.

Vitamin A and its precursor beta-carotene: This is involved in the maintenance, repair, and formation of new epidermal cells, regulating epidermal keratinization; additionally, in its acidic form (retinoic acid), together with vitamin C, it has been shown to intervene in the synthesis of collagen [27]. However, retinoic acid, due to its irritance, cannot be used in formulations for the skin of the cancer patient, since it would increase irritation, further weakening the skin barrier.

Vitamins of group B: These contribute to a greater or lesser extent to maintaining the health of the skin and hair; they are also coenzymes in energy production. They are water soluble and quite stable, penetrating through the stratum corneum, and are frequently used for the production of cellular energy and to improve the protection of the skin barrier.

Vitamin B3 (niacinamide) is perhaps the most studied to treat skin inflammation and erythrosis, calming irritation. The advantages of niacinamide are its anti-inflammatory effects due to inhibition of proinflammatory factors, as well as its ability to increase the expression of serine palmitoyltransferase as the key enzyme for ceramide synthesis [28]. Therefore, studies have been carried out to evaluate the protective effect of cosmetic preparations with 4% niacinamide during radiotherapy, obtaining a significant improvement in symptoms [29].

Vitamin B5 or D-panthenol acts like a moisturizer, improving stratum corneum hydration, reducing transepidermal water loss and maintaining skin softness and elasticity. Activation of fibroblast proliferation, which is of relevance in wound healing, has been observed both *in vitro* and *in vivo* with dexpanthenol. Accelerated reepithelization in wound healing, monitored by means of the transepidermal water loss as an indicator of the intact epidermal barrier function, has also been seen. Dexpanthenol has been shown to have an anti-inflammatory effect on experimental UV-induced erythema. The stimulation of epithelization and granulation and the mitigation of itching were the most prominent effects of formulations containing dexpanthenol; they also improved the symptoms of skin irritation, such as dryness of the skin, roughness, scaling, pruritus, erythema, and erosion/fissures, over 3–4 weeks [30]. A study of colloid gel versus dexpanthenol demonstrated the clear clinical benefit of a hydroactive colloid gel over an oil-in-water (O/W) emulsion containing 5% dexpanthenol for the prevention of radiotherapy-induced moist desquamation [31].

Vitamin B6 (pyridoxine pure crystalline powder or pyridoxine hydrochloride forms) acts as a coenzyme in amino acid metabolism and maintains healthy skin; it also controls oily skin. A review by Chen et al. concluded that, although there is insufficient scientific evidence, vitamin B6 in doses of more than 400 mg may improve some of the manifestations of hand-foot syndrome [32]. According to the metabolism of pyridoxine, it could be converted into pyridoxal phosphate in red blood cells.

Pyridoxal has also been discovered to be a potent antagonist of P2X purinergic receptor, which accelerates repair of the skin barrier and prevents epithelial hyperplasia [33].

Biotin, vitamin B7, is involved in important metabolic pathways, such as gluconeogenesis, fatty acid synthesis, and amino acid catabolism, and as a cofactor in the transfer of CO_2 groups to various target macromolecules, while pyridoxal participates in regeneration of tetrahydrofolate and in glutathione biosynthesis. Both vitamins play important roles in energy metabolism. Further progress in biotin function investigation has revealed its epigenetic properties and a role in cell signaling and in defense against reactive oxygen species [34]. In a study carried out by these authors, using a PAMAM G3 dendrimer with measured linkages of nine biotin molecules and ten molecules of pyridoxal-phosphate (BC-PAMAM), they manage to reduce inflammation in HaCaT keratinocytes, which opens an interesting perspective for the treatment of skin inflammation.

Vitamin C or ascorbic acid: Along with vitamin E, this has been shown to be able to neutralize free radicals. Furthermore, it is essential for the synthesis of collagen fibers and plays a protective role for the skin against the erythema produced by the aggression of UV light [35]. For topical use, it is used in the forms of magnesium ascorbyl phosphate, magnesium ascorbyl palmitate, and magnesium ascorbyl tetraisopalmitate, which are more soluble and stable and more easily penetrate the skin.

Vitamin D (cholecalciferol, ergocalciferol): Among other actions, this intervenes in the differentiation of keratinocytes. The European Cosmetics Directive explicitly bans the use of vitamin D2 (ergocalciferol) and vitamin D3 (cholecalciferol); however, calcitriol is used topically to control the proliferation of keratinocytes in psoriasis. Calcitriol also participates in the proper maintenance of the calcium gradients in the skin and stimulates the formation of antimicrobially effective peptides such as defensins and cathelicidins. The effect of these peptides is particularly interesting in the context of inflammatory processes in neurodermatitis cases. Additionally, calcitriol prolongs self-protection of the skin during exposure to UVB radiation as it stimulates the heat shock proteins [36,37]. However, a study by Nasser et al. in which treatment with calcitriol ointment is compared with an O/W emulsion in patients undergoing radiotherapy, concludes that topical vitamin D ointment is not superior to Aqua cream for prevention of radiation-induced dermatitis in women treated with adjuvant radiation for breast cancer [38].

Vitamin E (α-tocopherol): This is known for its antioxidant capacity, its ability to counteract free radicals and protect cells against photoaging caused by UV light. In addition, when applied to the skin, it reduces erythema, swelling, lipid peroxidation, and DNA damage [39]. In cosmetics it is applied in the form of esters (mainly tocopherol acetate); when associated with vitamin C (in the form of ascorbyl phosphate) its protective effect on the skin against damage caused by UV radiation is enhanced. Moreover, vitamin E acetate, as well as sodium ascorbyl phosphate, have been shown to be bioconverted to the vitamins E and C, and thus to significantly improve photoprotection of sunscreens against free radical formation in viable epidermal layers [39]. Analogues can also protect healthy skin against the aggression of radiotherapy treatments [40].

Hydrophilic Film-Forming Substances

Among the most widely used hydrophilic film-forming compounds in cosmetics is hyaluronic acid. Hyaluronic acid (HA) is a major constituent of the extracellular matrix of the skin. It has demonstrated remarkable rheological, viscoelastic, and hygroscopic properties that are relevant to wound healing [41]. Several studies demonstrated that hyaluronic acid creams can considerably reduce the intensity and duration of unwanted reactions during radiotherapy [42,43].

Thermal Springs Waters

Its use as an anti-inflammatory has been endorsed by numerous clinical studies. They are generally mineral-medicinal waters (or natural minerals in their most common denomination) of low or medium mineralization, rich in selenium, zinc, magnesium, among other minerals and trace elements [44].

Clays

Clays have antiphlogistic properties and have been used in therapy since time immemorial. The best-known clays are bentonites, a type of smectite, and kaolin, a kaolinite compound. Kaolin can be applied to skin lesions, with calming effects, as long as it is kept moist, applying a gauze moistened in thermal water interposed between the affected area and the clay plaster. Otherwise, drying is more difficult to remove and can cause discomfort. Green clay from France (Montmorillonite) is also used for its calming and bactericidal properties; in fact, there are experiences in thermal centers where a decrease in skin irritation caused by chemotherapy treatments has been observed, although more studies are needed to confirm these first impressions. For use in caring for cancer patients, these must be of high purity, with the guarantee that they do not have heavy metals that can be harmful [45].

Peloids

These are products made from a solid substrate, usually clays or mineral water sediments, mixed with a liquid substrate that is always mineral-medicinal, sea or salt lake water; they are also called thermal muds or thermal peloids. They are widely used in spas to treat various dermatological conditions, such as dermatitis, psoriasis, burns, and so on. There are few studies of its efficacy in the care of the disorders derived from cancer treatment, although there is some experience in spas that indicates they can be effective in calming itching and reducing erythrosis. Its use is endorsed by its applications in the aforementioned dermatological disorders [46,47].

Plant Extracts and Other Botanical Assets

Various plant extracts have calming and anti-inflammatory actions. The most studied and used are marshmallow (*Althaea oficinalis*), roman chamomille (*Anthemis nobilis*), marigold (*Calendula officinalis*), mallow (*Malva sylvestris*), and blackelder (*Sambucus nigra*). Others are used for their epithelializing and skin-regenerating properties, such as gotu kola (*Centella asiatica*), licorice (*Glycyrrhiza glabra*), milk thistle (*Silybum marianum*), jurema (*Mimosa tenuiflora*), and comfrey (*Symphytum officinale*) [23].

It is important to consider that, like oils and butters, when these types of extracts (or derived active substances) are used for the formulation of oncological skincare cosmetics, they must come from controlled organic cultures with the absence of pesticides or contaminants that can affect damaged skin.

The case of aloe (*Aloe vera*) is controversial, since despite the fact that its juice or gel has been considered a good pain reliever, anti-inflammatory, and healing aid [48], it has been observed that there are people in whom it has produced skin reactions, although Bosley et al. suggest that these reactions appeared to be associated with anthraquinone contaminants in the preparation [49]. Additionally, aloe gels form a "dry" film on the skin, which in some cases is not the most suitable, since emolliency is required (as in the case of skin flaked by the action of radiotherapy). Likewise, a recent study concludes that the administration of aloe gel to prevent oral mucositis is not more effective than the application of the nonactive gel base [50]. Another study by Hoopfer et al. draws similar conclusions in the use of aloe extract or cream to reduce symptoms or the severity of skin reactions after radiotherapy treatment [51]. The recommendations of the nursing guidelines for the management of radiodermatitis do not recommend them either, since it has not been shown to be more effective than creams with an external aqueous phase [52,53].

Regarding the prevention of radiotherapy injuries, in a review by Hall et al., several plants and botanical assets are cited as emergent radioprotectants, including curcumin (curcuma longa), as an antioxidant, anti-inflammatory, and antiproliferative; quininic acid (coffee, cocoa) as an antioxidant, decreasing DNA damage; lycopene (*Lycopersicon esculentum*), as antioxidant, peroxidation inhibitor, and free radical scavenger; rutin (a bioflavonoid from different plants and extracts as *Ruscus aculeatus* or *Prunus avium*) as an antioxidant; hemocyanin (*Rapana thomasiana*) as a radiomitigator; black tea extract (*Camellia sinensis*) as a free radical scavenger; silymarin (*Silybum marianum*) as an antiapoptotic agent, reducing DNA damage. This author also considers other emerging therapies as genistein (an antioxidant and anti-inflammatory), manganese superoxide dismutase-plasmid liposome (MnSOD-PL) gene therapy (an antioxidant, decreasing free radical production and inflammatory cytokine release), and caffeine (an antioxidant and anti-inflammatory) and tetrahydrobiopterin, an enzymatic cofactor involved in neurotransmitters and nitric oxide synthesis (for modulation of free radical-induced damage), among others [54]. Glutamine, a nonessential amino acid, widely studied for its potential beneficial effects in a number of pathologies associated with radiation toxicity including mucositis, dermatitis, and esophagitis, is cited in this same review.

Algae and Derivatives

Algae have been used since time immemorial for their important applications in health, both in food and in the preparation of drugs and cosmetics. Some algae compounds may be of interest in caring for the cancer patient, mainly those that have moisturizing, demulcent, and antioxidant properties. Among them are sulfated polysaccharides, fucoidan, and laminaran as antioxidants; astaxanthin and phlorotannins as anti-inflammatories; alginates and carrageenans as moisturizing and protective agents; fucoxanthin that promotes repair of the protein filaggrin, involved in the epidermal barrier; and micosporine-like amino acids (MMAAs) for their potential use in sunscreens. It is also worth mentioning ectoine (1,4,5,6-tetrahydro-2-methyl-4-pyrimidinecarboxylic acid), an osmoprotectant present in halophilic bacteria, which improves skin inflammation and is currently being investigated for the treatment of moderate atopic dermatitis [55].

There are already algae-based products on the market (e.g., INCI name *Ascophyllum nodosum* extract; *Asparagopsis armata* extract) to prevent radiodermatitis; some emulsions have been tested in this type of case, showing preventive activity and reducing itching and flaking symptoms [56].

Other Assets or Compounds of Interest

It is essential to mention the ingredients of sunscreens, keeping the skin away from the most harmful sun radiation. Sunscreens with physical filters are recommended, because they form a barrier on the epidermis that reflects radiation, and do not penetrate the skin. The most used are titanium dioxide and zinc oxide. We can also include so-called biological filters, which are antioxidants and free radical scavengers, among which are vitamin E and some of the botanical extracts mentioned earlier.

Among the moisturizing compounds, in addition to those mentioned, is urea, which is used in creams in concentrations of 5%–10% to improve and prevent cutaneous xerosis [3].

An asset of interest that has also been used in creams for the prevention and treatment of dermitis is β-glucan. β-Glucans are polysaccharides constructed of glucose monomers linked by β-glucosidic bonds, which mainly exist in cereals (barley and oat), yeast, mushrooms, and algae, with immunomodulatory properties, among others [57–59]. Emulsions containing β-glucan have been used to prevent radiodermatitis, with an increase in skin hydration and reduction of itching [56].

Another study where patients are prescribed moisturizers to prevent radiation-induced damage, with measurement of hydration using biometric techniques (corneometer), shows that in all cases it is possible to reduce the symptoms of skin toxicity. The products used included product A with pure vitamine E; product B with Omega-3,6,9; product C with natural triglycerides-phytosterols, product D with β-glucan and sodium hyaluronate, and product E with *Vitis vinifera* extract, the latter two being the most effective [60].

There are few studies on the use of growth factors, although some describe their effects on healing, which seems to be a promising area of research. In a multicenter prospective cohort study of 1172 patients undergoing radiotherapy for variable malignancies [61], an epidermal growth factor (EGF)–based cream was used to investigate the safety and effectiveness in the prevention of radiation dermatitis in patients with cancer. The cream contains 0.005% recombinant human EGF, with the presence of additional ingredients, such as ceramide, hyaluronic acid, Inca omega oil (*Plukenetia volubilis* seed oil), *Portulaca oleracea* extract, mango butter, and meadowfoam oil. The results suggest that a recombinant human EGF-based cream could be safely applied to prevent or alleviate radiation dermatitis. It may also be of interest to use copper peptides for improving wound contraction and epithelization [62].

Taking into account the important role that calcium plays in maintaining the epidermal barrier [63], products that contain calcium in their formulation may be appropriate, constituting a possible area of research; There are already patents on the market (Patent US8535904B2) that also include plant extracts. Other studies show that the use of sucralfate with Cu and Zn salts can delay the appearance of radiodermatitis, although more studies are needed that compare with the control group [64].

Dressing films are also of interest for both the prophylaxis and the treatment of radiotherapy-induced skin reactions. Silicone dressings are suitable for patients with fragile skin and do not cause tissue trauma during removal [65]; however, for patients with moist desquamation, it is important to minimize excess moisturizing and skin maceration, so another dressing was launched into the market to prevent this problem (Mepitel). Mepitel dressing is vapor permeable, and so allows excess moisture to evaporate through the dressing. It is therefore indicated for superficial wounds, where it promotes a moist healing environment. It is also used to protect fragile and sensitive skin from microbial contamination, fluid strikethrough, and other external contamination [66,67].

Another study on Mepilex Lite (a self-adhesive dressing consisting of a thin flexible sheet of absorbent hydrophilic polyurethane foam bonded to a water vapor–permeable polyurethane film backing layer) in radiation-induced erythema concluded that compared with aqueous cream, Mepilex Lite dressings did not significantly reduce the incidence of moist desquamation but did reduce the overall severity of skin reactions [68].

Calcium alginate dressings are also widely used in the management of severe bioradiation dermatitis and allow improved treatment tolerability and reduced treatment interruption [69].

Silver foam dressing, used in the treatment of burns and ulcers, has been shown to resist wound bacteria, promote wound healing, and shorten recovery time, effectively relieving the pain of patients [70,71]. When used in oncology, it has also been demonstrated as effective in reducing radiation dermatitis, apparently because of its antibacterial properties [72]. Nevertheless, another study by Aquino-Parsons concluded that silver leaf nylon dressing use did not demonstrate a decrease in the incidence of inframmammary moist desquamation but did decrease itching in the last week of radiation and 1 week after treatment completion [73].

Finally, it is necessary to mention medications for frequent topical use that, although not dermocosmetics, contain ingredients to reduce inflammation; this is the case with corticosteroid creams and Biafine, whose main asset is trolamine, one of the most used, but which has not been shown to be more effective than cosmetic creams [74].

Oncological Cosmetics and Cosmeceutical Formulation (M.L. Mourelle)

There are basic rules for the formulation of cosmetics and cosmeceuticals for the care of the cancer patient, which can be summarized as follows:

- Low number of ingredients in the formulation: this reduces the possibility of using potentially irritating ingredients.
- The excipients should be emollient due to the increased presence of dry and sensitive skin in this type of patient.

- The use of potentially irritating substances should be avoided (e.g., hydroxy acids, retinoids, the most common depigmenting agents, alcohol in high proportions, etc., are excluded).
- Known sensitizing agents and allergens, published in dermatological guidelines, should be excluded.
- Vasodilators and any type of skin sensory stimulants should also be excluded (with special caution for the use of essential oils).

Recommendations for Care of the Skin of the Cancer Patient (M.L. Mourelle)

Currently there is a broad consensus on the need for care of the skin of the cancer patient in the sense that it can improve the discomfort caused by the effects of cancer treatments on the skin and improve the QoL of patients. In a study carried out by Haley et al. [75], in which patients were offered three products to test (skin moisturizer, face moisturizer, and face wash), the tolerability of products specifically formulated for the care of the skin in cancer patients was high, even for patients with sensitive or rosacea skin and those who treat associated skin dryness, after 4 weeks of treatment. Furthermore, they considered that their QoL had improved [75]. Previously, the study from Titeca cited earlier on the impact of cosmetic care on the QoL of patients with breast cancer obtained similar results, concluding that at the end of treatment, patients who received cosmetic care remained more self-confident and were more optimistic [1].

In the scientific review and practical guide prepared by the Supportive Care Guidelines Group (SCGG) in 2006, the conclusion was that skin washing, including gentle washing with water alone with or without mild soap, should be permitted in patients receiving radiation therapy to prevent acute skin reaction. There is insufficient evidence to support or refute specific topical or oral agents for the prevention or management of acute skin reaction. In the expert opinion from the SCGG, the use of a plain, nonscented, lanolin-free hydrophilic cream may be helpful in preventing radiation skin reactions. In addition, a low-dose (i.e., 1%) corticosteroid cream may be beneficial in the reduction of itching and irritation [76]. In a survey conducted by this same author in 2018 among Canadian radiotherapy departments, it was concluded that there was great variability among guidelines and advice for caring for the skin of the cancer patient, and that although this advice is carried out interprofessionally, greater collaboration is needed; the approach to patient care should combine theory (e.g., moist wound healing), available evidence, and a conscious focus on minimizing patient stress to encourage a sense of normalcy and self-determination. Where there is little evidence, we should encourage informed patient preference with a "stress-reduction framework" that minimizes disruption to already established hygiene habits [77].

As indicated, it is convenient to differentiate between the different phases of treatment: before, during, and after cancer treatment. Table 28.1 summarizes the recommendations that, in all cases, should be personalized according to the specific situation of each patient and always under medical supervision and control.

As a general rule, the following are recommended:

- All the cosmetics used must have a pH related to the skin (pH = 5.5).
- Mild, emollient, and irritant-free (anionic) surfactants should be used, preferably with naturally occurring amphoteric surfactants (e.g., glycoside derivatives).
- Provide daily emollience and hydration with nontoxic and irritant-free products.
- Use sun protection (inorganic/physical filters) whenever necessary.
- The use of camouflage makeup (always with medical authorization and with high-quality products and free of potential allergens) may be recommended as it improves the patient's self-esteem and quality of life.
- Avoid rubbing the skin excessively; the use of exfoliants should be banned, and a cotton wipe (muslin type) should be used for skin cleansing. The same applies to the skin of the body, drying it "to touch," without rubbing.
- The use of depilatories is prohibited; if necessary, hair removal will be used with personal hair removal machines (mechanical hair removal by avulsion) and, in extraordinary cases, using the razor blade, applying abundant emollient and then epithelializing.
- Deodorant use is controversial; there are studies that indicate that deodorant can be irritating and others that there is no proof; the norm is prudence and proof of use [78].
- Avoid high or very low temperatures that can accentuate skin disorders (baths and showers will be lukewarm).

Aesthetics, Beauty, and Wellness Care (M.L. Mourelle)

As indicated in the previous sections, cosmetic care provides great benefits for improving the QoL of the cancer patient, and aesthetic care provided by qualified aestheticians also contributes to this well-being [2]. That is why it is of great value to present recommendations so that health professionals can guide their patients about the care that is allowed or, on the contrary, not recommended before, during, and after cancer treatment. Table 28.2 summarizes some recommendations of beauty and wellness care [21].

Cosmetic hair care: Approximately one and a half months after the last treatment cycle, hair begins to grow, although it does not do so uniformly in all areas. During this period, hair and wig coexist until the appearance adapts to the growth of the new hair. It is also important to take care of the scalp with the aforementioned treatments of hygiene and hydration. While the growth process lasts, it is advisable to rest from the wig for at least 8 hours a day so that the hair can grow healthier, and the use of the dryer and direct hair coloring products should be avoided.

From 3 months on, the hair should already have a moderate length. It would be time to propose color changes (always performed with a sensitivity test to avoid unexpected reactions).

TABLE 28.1

Dermocosmetic Care of Oncological Patient

Skin Disease / Side Effect	Dermocosmetic Care	References
Scars:	Emollients and moisturizers	Fabbrocini et al. [98]
• Eutrophic, hypertrophic, anesthetics	Hyaluronic acid, musk rose, and hypericum oil 1–2 times a day	
	Photoprotection (stick)	
	Corrective make-up for specific occasions	
• Keloid	Gel or silicone dressings	
Xerosis	Cleansing with no aggressive surfactants and foaming substances, acidic skin care system (pH 5.5)	Fabbrocini et al. [98]
	Avoid soaps	Bensadoun et al. [3]
	Avoid exfoliating products (hydroxy acids, benzoyl peroxide)	
	W/O emulsions with lipids and natural vegetable fats (karité, jojoba, avocado…), aloe, niacinamide, vitamin E	
	Emollients with urea 5%–10%	
	Avoid ointments (may lead to follicular occlusion and folliculitis)	Wohlrab et al. [29]
	Avoid products with petrolatum, paraffin, vaseline and silicones (cyclomethicone, dimethicone)	Pardo-Masferrer et al. [99]
Moist squamation	Hydrogels for low exudation	Bolderston et al. [76]
	Hydrocolloids, foam dressings and alginates	
	Hydrophilic vapor permeable dressing	McQuestion [53]
	Silver dressings	Spasić et al. [20]
Rash	Early treatment even for mild reaction	Burtness et al. [100]
	Cleansing products without astringent agents	Fabbrocini et al. [98]
	O/W emulsions with unsaponifiable substances: karité, jojoba, and olive, sesame, macadamia, and argan oils	
	Avoid: alcohol, topical retinoid and benzoyl peroxide	Segaert et al. [101]
	Photoprotection with nonocclusive excipients	Fabbrocini et al. [98]
	Nonocclusive make-up	Bensadoun et al. [3]
Radiodermatitis	The same as xerosis	Fabbrocini et al. [98]
	Combination of antioxidants (ubiquinone, seaweed extracts, red vine)	
	Hyaluronic acid aqueous creams and gels	Primavera et al. [42]
	Calendula officinalis cream	Kodiyan et al. [102]
	Photoprotection with nonocclusive excipients	Pommier et al. [103]
Ulceration and fissures	Creams and pastes based on vitamin E and zinc oxide	Fabbrocini et al. [98]
	Silver dressing	McQuestion [53]
Paronychia	Local antiseptics	Bensadoun et al. [3]
	Liquid bandage or glue for nail splitting	
Hand and foot syndrome	Urea or salicylic acid ointments	Bensadoun et al. [3]
Scalp and hair structural disorders	pH = 5.5 shampoo	Navarro [104]
	Avoid aggressive surfactants	
	Moisturizing creams and masks	

The most recommended would be the use of highlights, avoiding touching the hair base and the scalp. As hair grows, cuts should be made to clean and shape [21].

Other wellness techniques: The Society for Integrative Oncology working group to develop recommendations carried out a scientific review of the recommended techniques for managing pain and stress during the treatment of breast cancer. The study indicates that meditation techniques (especially mindfulness), yoga, and image relaxation are recommended to treat anxiety and mood swings. Yoga, massage, music therapy, and meditation are recommended for reducing stress, depression, and fatigue, and for improving QoL [79].

Patients often resort to complementary techniques without informing their medical team, and cancer survivors frequently seek traditional complementary and integrative medicine (TCIM). That is why professionals from around the world have discussed and presented recommendations on the integration of the various existing therapies to treat symptoms derived from

cancer at the International Congress on Integrative Medicine and Health in 2018; among the conclusions, they cite that it is necessary to collaborate in the search for safe and effective approaches to providing biologically based therapies within a supportive cancer care context [80].

Camouflage Cosmetics (M.L. Mourelle and B.N. Díaz)

Visible injuries derived from cancer treatment cause great emotional impact on patients. Various studies [81] show that the diseases that occur with visible dermatological injuries cause important psychological disorders in patients such as depression, low self-esteem, anguish, anger, shame, and social isolation, among others, making it necessary to treat cancer from a comprehensive perspective, with the clear objective to improve the QoL of patients. For this reason, in addition to the aforementioned

TABLE 28.2

Aesthetics, Beauty, and Wellness Care

Before Cancer Treatment

Techniques and Treatments to Avoid

Do not use tools and materials that erode the skin (files, sponges, towels, etc.).

Do not exfoliate the skin.

Do not apply ultraviolet radiation (natural or tanning lamps).

Do not undertake comprehensive hair removal.

Recommended Aesthetic Treatments

Objective:

Strengthen the skin: Hydrate, nourish, and regenerate.

Relax tensions.

Treatments:

Face hydration: From 3 to 4 months before medical treatment, avoid exfoliation or dermabrasion, use emollient and moisturizing cosmetics.

Body hydration: With emollient cosmetics and manual techniques, which can be combined with chromotherapy and relaxing music therapy.

Back and arm massage: To promote patient relaxation and, where appropriate, prepare the skin and muscles for surgical intervention.

Tired legs massage: A type of circulatory massage that will help alleviate the collateral effects of the disease on the body, activating venous return and reducing edema.

Massage and hydration of the scalp: This produces well-being and, before the imminent hair loss in case of chemotherapy, prepares the skin for the adaptation of the wig.

Relaxing massage: This has the goal of well-being, since it improves circulation, restores energy, and improves emotional well-being. It will be done with medical authorization.

Hand and foot treatments: With the aim of improving hydration and achieving well-being.

Micropigmentation: Corrective makeup can be performed, drawing the eyebrows and eyelashes that the patient will lose with chemotherapy, at least 2 months before medical treatment.

During Cancer Treatment

Techniques and Treatments to Avoid

Do not use waxing.

Do not use facial or body exfoliation (do not use AHA or enzymes; gommage is also contraindicated if the skin is very sensitive).

Do not use pure essential oils.

Do not clean skin with abrasive substances or equipment or electrotherapy techniques (iontophoresis, etc.).

Do not cut the cuticle of the nails in hand and foot care.

Do not use nail polishes; in any case, use natural and hypoallergenic cosmetic products.

Do not use dyes, perms, solvents, etc.

Do not use cosmetics with potentially irritating or sensitizing assets (both cleansing lotions and tonics will be mild).

Do not use products with direct hormonal activity in the affected organ (e.g., estrogen-like, such as *Salvia sclarea*).

Recommended Aesthetic Treatments

Objective:

Minimize and/or mitigate the effects on the skin of chemo and radiotherapy.

Treatments:

Facial treatments: These will adjust to the individual variations suffered during the healing process. Cosmetic products will be soothing (symphite, comfrey) and moisturizing (aloe), without parabens or alcohol. Peels and scrubs are generally discouraged at this stage. High quality clays (French green clay or kaolin) can be used to calm irritations due to their antiphlogistic properties.

Body hydration treatments: Anointing with creams and body oils very rich in nutrients and regenerators (rosehip oil, shea butter, grape seed oil) and soothing as aloe vera, chamomile, etc. Epithelizing and healing assets are also used such as: gotu kola, hypericum, eleutherococcus, etc. It may be necessary to use assets that improve microcirculation: ginkgo biloba, sweet clover, etc.

Back massage: Indicated to relieve tension, providing well-being and general relaxation. In some cases it may be convenient to perform manual lymphatic drainage, under medical supervision.

After Cancer Treatment

Techniques and Treatments to Avoid

Do not use products with alcohol.

Do not use aggressive treatments with peels or scrubs.

(Continued)

TABLE 28.2 (*Continued*)

Aesthetics, Beauty, and Wellness Care

Do not use very active or energetic massage on affected skin areas.

Recommended Aesthetic Treatments

Objective:

Repair the skin.

Treatment adapted to the needs of each person and case.

Treatments:

In addition to those mentioned in the previous phases, the following may be carried out:

Depigmentation treatments to remove stains: With laser or pulsed light, better than with chemical depigmentation agents that can irritate sensitive skin.

Treatments for flaccidity: Radiofrequency is the best option, along with manual techniques and regenerative cosmetics.

For sallow or dull skin: Pulsed light, laser or LED, along with regenerating cosmetics.

Treatments for telangiectasias: The best option is pulsed light.

Aesthetic Medicine techniques can be recommended to give volume.

Source: Adapted from Antepazo E, Mourelle ML. *Estética Reparadora. Especialización en cuidados postraumáticos y posquirúrgicos*, Estética & Wellness, Madrid; 2017:141–60.

skin care, training these patients in simple self-makeup techniques to disguise the lesions, through the use of so-called correction and camouflage makeup, can be of great help.

The study by Merial-Kieny et al. [82], which evaluated the tolerance and satisfaction of postchemotherapy corrective makeup in 90 patients, revealed a tolerance greater than 95% for the eyebrow pencil corrector and the contour corrector of lips. At the same time, an improvement in the QoL in general was found for 81.2% of the patients and self-esteem in 76.8%. This being the case, it can be understood why more and more professionals in the health-care field [83] are trained and advised on cosmetics, which will act as an aid throughout the oncological process.

Since ancient times, texts and iconographies confirm the use of makeup for various purposes. In this respect, concealer and camouflage makeups, understood as therapeutic resources, are used to highlight aesthetic features and disguise dermatological symptoms derived from treatments [84], becoming a wellness complementary therapy, improving self-esteem [85] and minimizing the psychosocial effects of cancer [86]. Scars, alopecia, dark circles, dyschromias, nail changes, and xerosis are some of the adverse effects secondary to oncological processes [5] that these preparations camouflage, trying to achieve greater luminosity and improving skin tone and radiance.

Composition

Concealer and camouflage makeups are decorative cosmetics with a high covering power that temporarily mask or conceal visible defects on the skin and provide greater luminosity. They consist of the following:

- Pigments of natural origin (inorganic or organic) or synthetic that modify the color of the skin. Their selection will be conditioned by functional, chemical, and technological parameters and also by safety factors [87], which in the case of cancer patients become a notable factor. International bodies regulating the manufacture and marketing of cosmetics, such as the European Commission (Regulation [EC]

No. 1223/2009 of the European Parliament and of the Council of November 30, 2009 on cosmetic products) and the U.S. Food and Drug Administration (Federal Food, Drug, and Cosmetic Act [FD&C Act] (Title 21: Food and Drugs. Chapter 9: Federal Food, Drug, and Cosmetic Act. Subchapter VI: Cosmetics. 21 USC 361: Adulterated cosmetics) authorize and condition the use of the different colorants, ensuring their safety. The market trend toward natural ingredients makes certification and control bodies such as ECOCERT and NATRUE [88] certify the use of natural pigments, thus minimizing possible allergies derived from synthetics.

- Active treatment substances with emollient and film-forming properties include beeswax (wax alba), castor oil; sun protection such as titanium dioxide; reparative agents such as vitamins A and E, rose hip, hydrolyzed wheat protein, pyrrolidine carboxylic acid sodium salt; and painkillers such as glycerin and aloe vera, among others.

- Aqueous and anhydrous excipients characterize various cosmetic forms such as solutions, gels, sticks, pencils, and loose or compact powders.

- Preservatives and correctors minimize the potential [85], as well as the comedogenicity, of the formula [83].

According to Dr. Oliver Jones (Royal Melbourne Institute of Technology), and Emeritus Professor Ben Selinger, AM (Australian National University), the scientific community considers the use of parabens in cosmetics to be safe; however, some companies have begun to replace them due to consumer demand, and hence the controversy concerning its use in dermocosmetics for the cancer patient. Therefore, more studies are needed to evaluate its effects in patients with altered or decreased skin barrier [89].

Pigments are insoluble in the medium in which they are applied and colored by dispersion, avoiding being mixed with the epicutaneous emulsion; for use in cancer patients, the inclusion of inorganic pigments in cosmetics should be carried out by means of vehicles that prevent their penetration, which will minimize possible allergies and toxicities, as long as the skin barrier and its immune function are not fully restored.

The natural, inorganic pigments (ferric oxides, titanium dioxide, zinc oxide, kaolin, gypsum, talc, sodium and sulfur silicate, etc.) that are more resistant to light and heat, although more opaque, or organic (charcoal, rice starch, carrot oil, beet powder, cochineal extract, etc.), cause various appreciable multicolor combinations [87].

Due to their multiple purposes, some white pigments stand out. Titanium dioxide, which is physiologically inert and desirable for both sensitive and oncological skin, is notable for its high covering power and for acting as a physical filter against solar radiation. Zinc oxide is useful due to its covering properties (which are greater the smaller the particle size, and less as it absorbs sebum and skin moisture), its use as a softener and antiseptic, in addition to its properties as a sunscreen. On the penetration of zinc oxide nanoparticles into the skin, the Scientific Committee on Consumer Safety (SCCS) of the European Commission reported in 2012 that a very small amount of zinc in soluble form can pass through the skin. However, there is great controversy, given that, due to its small size, it will be able to easily penetrate the airways when applying cosmetic sprays [90].

As for colored pigments, metallic oxides are common, among others, such as black, yellow, and red iron oxides manufactured according to "certified standard" to avoid the toxicity of heavy metals; chromium dioxide contributes green shades with different specifications according to the corresponding control organisms [91].

In the search for a healthy and luminous appearance, two types of pigments can be used [92,93]:

- Light-diffusing pigments with soft-focus effect (1–2 μm nylon or silica spheres coated with titanium dioxide and ferric oxide), which reflect light uniformly in all directions, blurring imperfections and highlighting glare.

- Color correcting or interference pigments (mica particles coated with titanium dioxide and/or iron oxide) that act as a prism, that is, they modify the real color of the reflected light toward another color of the spectrum.

To conclude, make-ups should be preparations with a minimum number of ingredients, manufactured in a sterile environment, subjected to tolerance and efficacy tests under dermatological control, and must be functional, that is, covering, easy to apply, unalterable as long as possible, and resistant to water, sweat, and sun.

Types of Products

There are products for the skin, eyes, and lips.

Skin cosmetics: Can have various cosmetic shapes and textures. The concealer sticks are prepared that are applied under makeup in specific areas or on the entire face. They camouflage unsightly changes using the "Newton Chromatic Circle" to disguise the effects of the treatments.

When two colors neutralize each other, they are complementary; that is, they face each other in the color wheel, and a color next to their complement is highlighted. In general, light tones give volume, they stand out and dark tones reduce volume; they give depth. So, the green color is complementary to the red; therefore, it will be used for redness and scars in the reepithelialization phase. The yellow color (beige-yellowish) is complementary to the violet, so it will counteract dark circles and blue or violet tones. Pink will neutralize dark circles and hyperpigmentation; mauve unifies and illuminates the face, mainly on tired or olive skin.

Compact creams are used on scars and hyperpigmentations with the shade that best suits the tone of the skin. Makeup bases

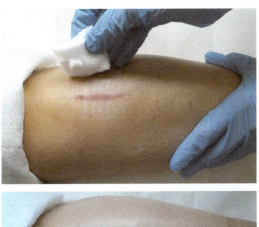
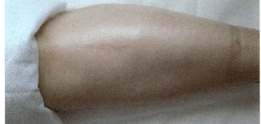
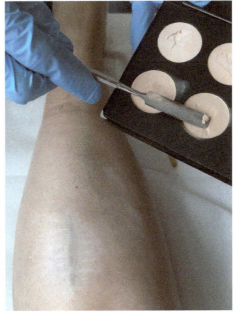

FIGURE 28.1 Camouflage makeup on residual scar after excision of pretibial melanoma.

are emulsions ranging from very fluid with approximately 20% of pigments and corrective purpose, to dense emulsions with a clear camouflage purpose, and a percentage of pigments greater than 30%, which provide luminosity and uniformity to the color of the skin. They can be found in various shades, to enable selection of the one that most closely mimics the skin (Figure 28.1).

Loose or compact powders are used to set makeup and tint skin so it does not shine. It may be convenient to restrict them in cases of skin dehydration to prevent that being increased.

Blush is used to rekindle the skin tone of the face, bringing a blush to the cheeks. It can be presented in powder, liquid, and with a creamy texture that allow its application on cheeks, skin, eyelids, and even lips, allowing natural and easy makeup. It should be chosen in pink tones to minimize a sallow appearance.

Cosmetics for the eye area: Due to the special characteristics of the eye area, this requires totally innocuous cosmetics [94], with a texture that facilitates its application and elimination, remaining unchanged as long as possible.

Eyelid shades are preferably chosen for dry skin with a creamier texture and in brightening tones, taking into account the color of the eyes. Contour eyeliners are used to frame the eye contour, making it larger and concealing missing or deficient eyelashes.

Eyelash masks lengthen, thicken, coat, and color lashes. Easy-to-apply, high-tolerance masks in brown or black tones can be used as long as the treatment does not involve alopecia. If the eyelashes are very weakened, it is better not to apply them, because when removed with a cleaning agent, it can cause the residual eyelashes to break.

Eyebrow pencils and powders are very useful, since eyebrow makeup is essential, especially if total alopecia manifests itself, as they are one of the features that express the face the most by intensifying the look. Either by filling in the existing design or by applying makeup using stencils, hard lead pencils formulated with natural oils and waxes or powders (similar in formulation to eyelid shades) are used in shades of brown or black that mimic natural color or a darker shade, either filling in the existing design or applying makeup using templates.

Cosmetics for the lip area: The use of colored moisturizers or glosses is recommended in order to form an even film, giving color to the lip mucosa and protecting the lips.

Nail cosmetics: Nail modifications from cancer treatments can affect the color, growth, or appearance; they can be concealed from the cosmetic field through the practice of nail polishing. However, there is a direct exposure to ingredients that can cause toxicity and even allergy both in the enamel and in its removal. For example, some nail hardeners and nail polishes may contain formaldehyde, which can cause skin irritation or an allergic reaction. Acrylics, used in some artificial nails and sometimes in nail polishes, can cause allergic reactions [95].

In addition, there may be a possibility of secondary inhalation exposure in the case of cosmetic products containing volatile substances that can be inhaled unintentionally in direct use, for example, toluene in nail polish, various substances included in gels for nail sculpting, such as acrylates, and so on [96]. In short, although the improvement of self-esteem would advise its use,

safety advises against it or, where appropriate, using certified natural products that ensure less toxicity.

Self-Makeup Guide

Cancer patients can improve their appearance by hiding signs of fatigue and camouflaging blemishes with simple, easy-to-apply makeup. However, there are times when hiding injuries requires more complex makeup, requiring the advice and training of professional makeup artists who individually instruct the patient.

The following are recommendations and guidelines for performing a self-makeup respectful of the skin to help camouflage lesions or improve the appearance of the skin.

General Considerations

- Application tools should be clean and sterile and should never be shared.
- Makeup products that have to be removed with fingers or with the use of an applicator should never be shared.
- Carry out a tolerance test of the products, prior to the application of decorative cosmetics.
- Carry out adequate hygiene, toning (thermal water or soothing tonic), and moisturizing, prior to the application of decorative cosmetics.

Study of asymmetries: An imaginary vertical axis is drawn that divides the face; note which eyebrow is highest. This indicates the highest side of the face, and the lines on that side will be the pattern, to achieve greater harmony and balance in the whole. The face is also divided into four horizontal planes (hairline, superciliary arch, base of the nose, and base of the chin) to document the proportions of the face.

Clear corrections give volume and illuminate areas that require it; dark corrections retract and give depth.

There are points to avoid [97]:

- Do not apply false eyelashes, because the glue can irritate the skin. Also, do not use an eyelash curler on existing eyelashes.
- Do not use eyelash mask daily, since it does not facilitate perspiration of the hair, and the additional weight can cause them to fall out.

Table 28.3 indicates some guidelines for easily performing makeup (modified from Gil et al. [97]).

Conclusions

Medical cancer treatments are increasingly effective, but they are not free of side effects. There is currently a general consensus that it is necessary to advise patients on skin care before, during, and after treatment. Dermocosmetic care is therefore essential to minimize cutaneous toxicities and their manifestations, as well as the reactions derived from radiotherapy. There are few studies of the active substances that have demonstrated

TABLE 28.3

Guide to Self-Makeup

1. Sunscreen with a sun protection factor of 50 or more, if doing a day makeup
2. Clear correctors with a latex sponge, brush, or fingers in prominent areas of the face (dark circles, rictus, and nostrils)
3. Color correctors that neutralize and camouflage dyschromias, applied to brush strokes or small touches:
   - Green for redness, such as recent scars, rosacea, etc.
   - Beige-yellowish for bluish or purplish tones, such as bruises and dark circles
   - Pink/coral in dark circles and hyperpigmentation
   - Mauve to unify and illuminate the face, mainly on tired or olive skin
4. Fluid or moisturizing foundation with color; a natural tone is selected; extend it without rubbing, degrading the color on the mandibular edge and at the origin of the scalp
5. If the makeup is worn at night, it supports performing a light-dark technique, optimizing the volumes
6. Translucent powders if sensitivity and dryness allow it
7. Eye makeup:
   - *Matte eyeshadow*: Apply a light color from the eyelid to the arch under the eyebrow and, optionally, a medium color from the eyelid to the crease and blend.
   - *Eyeliner*: Draw a line or tap just above the lower eyelashes line without getting close to the tear duct, with a black pencil/eyeliner for dark skin and gray or dark brown for light and medium skin. It can be blurred.
   - *Mascara*: Apply two to three coats both on top and bottom gently, filling back and front.
   - *Eyebrow makeup*: It is advisable to take a photograph before any alopecia to see the design and then reproduce it.

their ability to calm or regenerate the damaged epidermal barrier, although they have been shown to be effective for emolliency, moisturizing, and protection against external agents that can worsen the alterations. Vegetable oils and butters, vitamins, omega series fatty acids, various algae and botanical extracts, clays, peloids and hot springs, among others, are useful to alleviate the side effects and sequelae of oncological treatments, but it is necessary to carry out clinical studies that show its efficacy and clarify the cases in which it can be used. Likewise, it is essential to prepare guides for health professionals who, frequently, must be guided by the indications of the commercial companies. Collaboration between professionals would allow the elaboration of recommendations and guides where dermatological, nursing, and wellness care are integrated, including qualified aestheticians, who can provide comprehensive skin care, trying to personalize, as far as possible, the skin care. Implementing informative and demonstrative sessions to train patients in self-care and camouflage of injuries can be of great help in improving the self-esteem and quality of life of the cancer patient, resulting in satisfying experiences for all participants.

REFERENCES

1. Titeca G, Poot F, Cassart D et al. Impact of cosmetic care on quality of life in breast cancer patients during chemotherapy and radiotherapy: An initial randomized controlled study. *JEADV.* 2007;21:771–6.
2. Oliveri S, Faccio F, Pizzoli S et al. A pilot study on aesthetic treatments performed by qualified aesthetic practitioners: Efficacy on health-related quality of life in breast cancer patients. *Qual Life Res.* https://doi.org/10.1007/s11136-019-02133-9. Published online. February 20, 2019.
3. Bensadoun R-J, Humbert P, Krutman J et al. Daily baseline skin care in the prevention, treatment, and supportive care of skin toxicity in oncology patients: Recommendations from a multinational expert panel. *Cancer Management and Research.* 2013;5:401–8. http://dx.doi.org/10.2147/CMAR.S52256.
4. Lacouture M, Sibaud V. Toxic side effects of targeted therapies and immunotherapies affecting the skin, oral mucosa, hair, and nails. V. *Am J Clin Dermatol.* 2018;19(1):31. https://doi.org/10.1007/s40257-018-0384-3
5. Sibaud V, Delord J-P, Robert C. *Dermatología de los tratamientos contra el cáncer. Guía Práctica.* Toulouse: ed. Privat; 2015:101–10.
6. Galimont-Collen AF, Vos LE, Lavrijsen AP et al. Classification and management of skin, hair, nail and mucosal side-effects of epidermal growth factor receptor (EGFR) inhibitors. *Eur J Cancer.* 2007;43(5):845–51.
7. Reyes-Habito CM & Roh EK. Cutaneous reactions to chemotherapeutic drugs and targeted therapies for cancer. Part II. Targeted therapies. *J Am Acad Dermatol.* 2014;71:217e1–217e11. DOI: https://doi.org/10.1016/j.jaad.2014.04.013
8. Jatoi A, Green EM, Rowland KM et al. Clinical predictors of severe cetuximab-induced rash: Observations from 933 patients enrolled in north central cancer treatment group study N0147. *Oncology.* 2009;77(2):120–3.
9. Robert C, Soria JC, Spatz A et al. Cutaneous side-effects of kinase inhibitors and blocking antibodies. *Lancet Oncol.* 2005;6(7):491–500.
10. Linsley C & Aziz M. A Case of Azacitidine-Induced Toxic Erythema of Chemotherapy. *The National Society for Cutaneous Medicine.* 2019; 3(1).
11. Bolognia JL, Cooper DL, Glusac EJ. Toxic erythema of chemotherapy: A useful clinical term. *J Am Acad Dermatol.* 2008;59(3):524–9.
12. Martorell-Calatayud A, Sanmartin O, Botella-Estrada R et al. Chemotherapy-related bilateral dermatitis associated with eccrine squamous syringometaplasia: Reappraisal of epidemiological, clinical, and pathological features. *J Am Acad Dermatol.* 2011;64:1092–103.
13. Sibaud V. Toxic erythema of chemotherapy. *Ann Dermatol Venereol.* 2015;142(2):81–4.
14. Larson VA, Tang O, Ständer S et al. Association between itch and cancer in 16,925 patients with pruritus: Experience at a tertiary care center. *J Am Acad Dermatol.* 2019;80(4):931–7.
15. D'Epiro S, Salvi M, Luzi A et al. Drug cutaneous side effect: Focus on skin ulceration. *Clin Ter.* 2014;165 (4):e323–329.
16. Naveed S, Thappa DM, Dubashi B et al. Mucocutaneous adverse reactions of cancer chemotherapy and chemoradiation. *Indian J Dermatol.* 2019;64:122–8.
17. Miller KK, Gorcey L, McLellan BN. Chemotherapy-induced hand-foot syndrome and nail changes: A review of clinical presentation, etiology, pathogenesis, and management. *J Am Acad Dermatol.* 2014;71:787–94.
18. O'Brien P. Lymphedema in Cancer Patients. In: Olver I. (eds) *The MASCC Textbook of Cancer Supportive Care and Survivorship.* Springer, Cham; 2018: 323–35.

19. Anupama C, Anuradha HV, Vinayak VM. Trastuzumab induced radiation recall dermatitis: An interesting case. *Int J Basic Clin Pharmacol.* 2018 Dec;7(12):2465–7.

20. Spasić B, Jovanović M, Golušin Z et al. Radiodermatitis - review of treatment options. *Serbian Journal of Dermatology and Venereology* 2018;10(3):71–81.

21. Antepazo E & Mourelle ML. *Estética Reparadora. Especialización en cuidados postraumáticos y posquirúrgicos,* Estética & Wellness, Madrid; 2017:141–60.

22. Mourelle ML, Gómez CP, Legido JL. The Potential Use of Marine Microalgae and Cyanobacteria in Cosmetics and Thalassotherapy. *Cosmetics.* 2017;4:46.

23. Sabater I & Mourelle, ML. *Cosmética aplicada a Estética Integral y Bienestar,* 2nd edn. Estética & Wellness, Madrid; 2016: 19–32.

24. Chirinos R, Zuloeta G, Pedreschi R et al. Sacha inchi (Plukenetia volubilis): A seed source of polyunsaturated fatty acids, tocopherols, phytosterols, phenolic compounds and antioxidant capacity. *Food Chem.* 2013;14(3):1732–9. https://doi.org/10.1016/j.foodchem.2013.04.078

25. Miko ET, Johnson T, Peterson N et al. Combination glutathione and anthocyanins as an alternative for skin care during external-beam radiation. *Am J Surg.* 2005;189:627–31.

26. Burke KH. Protection From Environmental Skin Damage With Topical Antioxidants. 2018. *Clin Pharmacol Ther.* 2018;105(1) https://doi.org/10.1002/cpt.1235

27. Krautheim A & Gollnick HPM, Vitamins and skin. In: Vahlquist A & Duvic M, eds, *Retinoids and Carotenoids in Dermatology.* New York: Informa healthcare; 2005: 291–308.

28. Tanno O, Ota Y, Kitamura N et al. Nicotinamide increases biosynthesis of ceramides as well as other stratum corneum lipids to improve the epidermal permeability barrier. *Br J Dermatol.* 2000;143:524–31.

29. Wohlrab J, Bangemann N, Kleine-Tebbe A et al. Barrier protective use of skin care to prevent chemotherapy-induced cutaneous symptoms and to maintain quality of life in patients with breast cancer. *Breast Cancer.* 2014;6:115–22.

30. Ebner F, Heller A, Rippke F et al. Topical use of dexpanthenol in skin disorders. *Am J Clin Dermatol.* 2002;3(6):427–33.

31. Censabella S, Claes S, Orlandini M et al. Retrospective study of radiotherapy-induced skin reactions in breast cancer patients: Reduced incidence of moist desquamation with a hydroactive colloid gel versus dexpanthenol. *Eur J Oncol Nurs.* 2014;18(5):499–504. http://dx.doi.org/10.1016/j.ejon.2014.04.009

32. Chen M, Zhang L, Wang Q et al. Pyridoxine for Prevention of Hand-Foot Syndrome Caused by Chemotherapy: A Systematic Review. *PLOS ONE.* 2013;8(8):e72245.

33. Denda M, Inoue K, Fuziwara S et al. P2X Purinergic Receptor Antagonist Accelerates Skin Barrier Repair and Prevents Epidermal Hyperplasia Induced by Skin Barrier Disruption. *J Invest Dermatol.* 2013;119:1034–40.

34. Szuster M, Uram L, Filipowicz-Rachwał A et al. Evaluation of the localization and biological effects of PAMAM G3 dendrimer-biotin/pyridoxal conjugate as HaCaT keratinocyte targeted nanocarrier. *Acta Biochim Pol.* 2019 Apr 9. https://doi.org/10.18388/abp.2018_2767

35. Pinnell SR. Topical L-ascorbic acid: Percutaneous Absorption Studies. *Dermatol Surg.* 2001;27:137–42. https://doi.org/10.1046/j.1524-4725.2001.00264.x

36. Arnold F, Mercier M, Luu MT. Metabolism of Vitamin D in Skin: Benefits for Skin Care Applications. *Cosmetic & Toiletries.* 2009;124:40–6.

37. Bikle, D. Vitamin D, Calcium, and the Epidermis. In Feldman D et al. eds, *Vitamin D (Volume 1): Biochemistry, Physiology and Diagnostics* 4th edn. London: Academic Press; 2018: 527–44.

38. Nasser NJ, Fenig S, Ravid A et al. Vitamin D ointment for prevention of radiation dermatitis in breast cancer patients. *NPJ Breast Cancer.* 2017;3:10.

39. Thiele JJ & Ekanayake-Mudiyanselage S. Vitamin E in human skin: Organ-specific physiology and considerations for its use in dermatology. *Mol Aspects Med.* 2007;28(5–6):646–67.

40. Aykin-Burns N, Pathak R, Boerma M et al. Utilization of Vitamin E Analogs to Protect Normal Tissues While Enhancing Antitumor Effects. *Semin Radiat Oncol.* 2019;29(1):55–61.

41. Weindl G, Schaller M, Schafer-Korting M et al. Hyaluronic acid in the treatment and prevention of skin diseases: Molecular biological, pharmaceutical and clinical aspects. *Skin Pharmacol Physiol.* 2004;17(5):207–13.

42. Primavera G, Carrera M, Berardesca E et al. A Double-Blind, Vehicle-Controlled Clinical Study to Evaluate the Efficacy of MAS065D (XClair™), a Hyaluronic Acid-Based Formulation, in the Management of Radiation-Induced Dermatitis, *Cutan Ocul Toxicol.* 2006; 25 (3):165–171.

43. Elmashad NH, Fatma Zakaria Hussen FZ, Eltatawy RA. Efficacy of Topical Hyaluronic acid during adjuvant Breast Cancer Radiotherapy for radiation dermatitis prophylaxis. *Life Sci.* 2015;12(6). http://www.lifesciencesite.com

44. Guerrero D & Garrigue E. Eau thermale d'Avène et dermatite atopique. *Ann Dermatol Venereol.* 2017;144:S27–34.

45. Mourelle ML & Gómez CP. Cosmética termal. Aplicaciones en el ámbito de la salud y la belleza. *Proceedings 1st International Congress on Water Healing SPA and Quality of Life (Spain),* 23–24 September 2015:389–98.

46. Meijide R & Mourelle ML. Afecciones dermatológicas y cosmética dermotermal. En: Hernández Torres, A. (Coord.). *Técnicas y Tecnologías en Hidrología Médica e Hidroterapia. Agencia de Evaluación de Tecnologías Sanitarias.* Madrid: Instituto Carlos III, Madrid; 2006:175–94.

47. Meijide R, Mourelle ML, Vela A et al. Aplicación a pacientes: Peloterapia en patologías dermatológicas. In: Hernández Torres A (coord.). *Peloterapia: Aplicaciones médicas y cosméticas de fangos termales.* Madrid: Fundación Bílbilis; 2014: 169–83.

48. Sahu PK, Diri DD, Singh R et al. Therapeutic and Medicinal Uses of Aloe vera: A Review. *Pharmacology & Pharmacy.* 2013;4(08):599–610.

49. Bosley C, Smith J, Baratti P. A Phase III Trial Comparing an Anionic Phospholipidbased (APP) Cream and Aloe vera-Based Gel in the Prevention and Treatment of Radiation Dermatitis. *Int J Radiat Oncol Biol Phys.* 2003;57(2):34–8. http://dx.doi.org/10.1016/S0360-3016(03)01404-4

50. Lakhani R & Mahadalkar P. Effectiveness of topical application of aloe vera gel on radiation induced mucositis in patients receiving radiotherapy for head and neck malignancies. *IJNR.* 2017;3(3):92–8.

51. Hoopfer D, Holloway C, Gabos Z et al. Three-Arm Randomized Phase III Trial: Quality Aloe and Placebo Cream Versus Powder as Skin Treatment during Breast Cancer Radiation Therapy. *Clin Breast Cancer.* 2014;15(3):181–90.e1-4.

52. McQuestion M. Evidenced-based skin care management in radiation therapy. *Semin Oncol Nurs.* 2006;22(3):163–73.

53. McQuestion M. Evidence-Based Skin Care Management in Radiation Therapy: Clinical Update. *Seminars in Oncology Nursing.* 2011;27(2):e1–17.

54. Hall S, Rudrawar S, Zunk M et al. Protection against Radiotherapy-Induced Toxicity. *Antioxidants.* 2016;5(5):3.

55. Mourelle ML, Gómez CP, Legido JL. Role of algal derived compounds in pharmaceutical and cosmetics. In: Rajauria G & Yuan YV eds. *Recent Advances in Micro and Macroalgal Processing: Food and Health Perspectives.* In press.

56. Di Franco R, Sammarco E, Calvanese MG et al. Preventing the acute skin side effects in patients treated with radiotherapy for breast cancer: The use of corneometry in order to evaluate the protective effect of moisturizing creams. *Radiat Oncol.* 2013;8:57. http://www.ro-journal.com/content/8/1/57

57. Kim HS, Hong JT, Kim YS et al. Stimulatory Effect of β-glucans on Immune Cells. *Immune Network.* 2011;11(4):191–5. http://dx.doi.org/10.4110/in.2011.11.4.191

58. Jesenak M, Majtan J, Rennerova Z et al. Immunomodulatory effect of pleuran (β-glucan from *Pleurotus ostreatus*) in children with recurrent respiratory tract infections. *Int Immunopharmacol.* 2013;15(2):395–9.

59. Bai J, Ren Y, Li Y et al. Physiological functionalities and mechanisms of β-glucans. *Trends Food Sci Technol.* 88:57–66. DOI: 10.1016/j.tifs.2019.03.023

60. Di Franco R, Ravo V, Falivene S et al. Prevention and treatment of radiation induced skin damage in breast cancer. *JCDSA.* 2014; 4:16–23 Published Online February 2014 (http://www.scirp.org/journal/jcdsa) http://dx.doi.org/10.4236/jcdsa.2014.41003

61. Kang HC, Ahn SD, Choi DH et al. The safety and efficacy of EGF-based cream for the prevention of radiotherapy-induced skin injury: Results from a multicenter observational study. *Radiat Oncol.* 2014;32(3):156–62. http://dx.doi.org/10.3857/roj.2014.32.3.156

62. Pickart L & Margolina A. Skin Regenerative and Anti-Cancer Actions of Copper Peptides. *Cosmetics.* 2018;5:29.

63. Lee SE, Lee SH. Skin Barrier and Calcium. *Ann Dermatol.* 2018;30(3). DOI: https://doi.org/10.5021/ad.2018.30.3.265

64. De Rauglaudre G, Courdi A, Delaby-Chagrin F et al. Tolerance of the association sucralfate/Cu-Zn salts in radiation dermatitis. *Ann Dermatol Venereol.* 2008;125(1):11–5.

65. Meuleneire F & Rügnagal H. Soft silicones made easy. *Wounds International,* 2013. http://tinyurl.com/ou5bses (accessed 30 May 2019)

66. Morgan K. Radiotherapy-induced skin reactions: Prevention and cure. *Br J Nurs.* 2014 Sep 11-24;23(16):S24, S26–32.

67. Herst PM, Bennet CN, Sutherland AE et al. Prophylactic use of Mepitel Film prevents radiation-induced moist desquamation in an intra-patient randomised controlled clinical trial of 78 breast cancer patients. *Radiother Oncol.* 2014; 110(1):137–43.

68. Paterson DB, Poonam P, Bennett NC et al. Randomised intra-patient controlled trial of Mepilex Lite dressings versus aqueous cream in managing radiation induced skin reactions post mastectomy. *J Cancer Sci Ther.* 2012;4(11):347–56. http://tinyurl.com/ p6k2rga

69. Bonomo P, Desideri I, Loi M et al. Management of severe bio-radiation dermatitis induced by radiotherapy and cetuximab in patients with head and neck cancer: Emphasizing the role of calcium alginate dressings. *Support Care Cancer.* 2018;1–11. https://doi.org/10.1007/s00520-018-4606-2

70. Yang B, Wang X, Li Z et al. Beneficial effects of silver foam dressing on healing of wounds with ulcers and infection control of burn patients. *Pak J Med Sci.* 2015;31(6):1334–9. doi: http://dx.doi.org/10.12669/pjms.316.7734

71. Avino A, Marina CN, Balcangiu-Stroescu AE et al. *Our Experience in Skin Grafting and Silver Dressing for Venous Leg Ulcers.* Revista de Chimie, Bucharest, February 2019.

72. Vuong T, Franco E, Lehnert S et al. Silver leaf nylon dressing to prevent radiation dermatitis in patients undergoing chemotherapy and external beam radiotherapy to the perineum. *Int J Radiat Oncol Biol Phys.* 2004;59(3):809–14 https://doi.org/10.1016/j.ijrobp.2003.11.031

73. Aquino-Parsons C, Lomas S, Smith K et al. Phase III Study of Silver Leaf Nylon Dressing vs Standard Care for Reduction of Inframammary Moist Desquamation in Patients Undergoing Adjuvant Whole Breast Radiation Therapy. *JMIRS.* 2000;41(4):215–21. https://doi.org/10.1016/j.jmir.2010.08.005

74. Villanueva RTI, Alcalá PD, Vega GMT et al. Guía de práctica clínica para prevención y tratamiento de la radiodermatitis aguda. *Dermatol Rev Mex.* 2012;56(1).

75. Haley AC, Calahan C, Gandhi M et al. Skin care management in cancer patients: An evaluation of quality of life and tolerability. *Support Care Cancer.* 2011;19:545–54.

76. Bolderston A, Lloyd NS, Wong RKS et al. The prevention and management of acute skin reactions related to radiation therapy: A systematic review and practice guideline. *Support Care Cancer.* 2006;14:802.

77. Bolderston A, Cashell A, McQuestion M et al. A Canadian Survey of the Management of Radiation-Induced Skin Reactions. *JMIRS.* 2018;4(2):164–72. https://doi.org/10.1016/j.jmir.2018.01.003

78. Theberge V, Harel F, Dagnault A. Use of axillary deodorant and effect on acute skin toxicity during radiotherapy for breast cancer: A prospective randomized noninferiority trial. *Int J Radiat Oncol Biol Phys.* 2009;75(4):1048–52.

79. Greenlee H, DuPont-Reyes MJ, Balneaves LG et al. Clinical practice guidelines on the evidence-based use of integrative therapies during and after breast cancer treatment. *CA Cancer J Clin.* 2017;67:194–232.

80. Grant SJ, Hunter J, Seely D et al. Integrative Oncology: International Perspectives. *Integr Cancer Ther.* 2019;18(1):1–11. https://doi.org/10.1177/1534735418823266

81. De la Riva Grandal A, Santiago-et-Sánchez Mateo JL, Rodríguez Martín CF. Maquillaje terapéutico sobre lesiones dermatológicas faciales. *Revisión Bibliográfica. Enfermería Dermatológica.* 2009;8:28–35.

82. Merial-Kieny C, Nocera T, Mery S. Medical corrective make-up in post-chemotherapy. *Ann Dermatol Venereol.* 2008;1:25–8.

83. Patalano A, Fiammenghi E, Fabbrocini G, Calabrò G. The role of camouflage in the management of skin damages in oncologic patients. *J Plastic Dermatol.* 2013;9(1):5–10.

84. Ortiz-Brugués A, Reparaz S, Castillo C, Valls R. Evaluación sobre el impacto del maquillaje dermatológico corrector en los efectos secundarios de los tratamientos oncológicos. *Póster Publicado en Reunión XXVII GEDET.* 13–4 Noviembre 2015.

85. Levy LL & Emer JJ. Emotional benefit of cosmetic camouflage in the treatment of facial skin conditions: Personal experience and review. *Clin Cosmet Investig Dermatol.* 2012;5:173–82.

86. Curso on-line, Módulo II: Onco-educación y atención dermo-farmacéutica del paciente oncológico. *Avène Dermatological Laboratories.*

87. Prieto L. Cosmética decorativa. Atención farmacéutica en Dermofarmacia. *Formación Continuada del Consejo de Colegios de Farmacéuticos.* 2009:143–83.

88. Galvis González VA. Los pigmentos y su efecto estético, 2012. Available from https://www.inpralatina.com/201205312413/articulos/especialidades-quimicas/los-pigmentos-y-su-efecto-estetico.html

89. The chemistry of cosmetics, November 2018. Available from https://www.science.org.au/curious/people-medicine/chemistry-cosmetics

90. Vieira CO, Grice ZE, Roberts MS et al. ZnO:SBA-15 Nanocomposites for potential use in sunscreen: Preparation, properties, human skin penetration and toxicity. *Skin Pharmacol Physiol.* 2019;32:32–42.

91. CosmEthics, Jan 7, 2015. Avaliable from https://medium.com/@cosmethics/the-world-of-colors-in-cosmetics-964dc165d43

92. Alcalde MT & del Pozo A. Fondos de maquillaje (I). Definición y componentes. *OFFARM.* 2003;22(8):161–2.

93. Alcalde MT. Piel luminosa. Características y productos que la favorecen. *OFFARM.* 2005;24(11):90–6.

94. Use Eye Cosmetics Safely. Available from: https://www.fda.gov/consumers/consumer-updates/use-eye-cosmetics-safely

95. How to Safely Use Nail Care Products? Available from: https://www.fda.gov/consumers/consumer-updates/how-safely-use-nail-care-products

96. 2013/674/EU: Commission Implementing Decision of 25 November 2013 on Guidelines on Annex I to Regulation (EC) No 1223/2009 of the European Parliament and of the Council on cosmetic products Text with EEA relevance. Available from: https://publications.europa.eu/en/publication-detail/-/publication/82ff9107-5686-11e3-a8cb-01aa75ed71a1

97. Gil López C, Ariza López LM, Romero Maldonado N et al. Autocuidado en pacientes oncológicos. Pautas Estéticas. Visto Bueno Equipo Creativo. Madrid, 2008.

98. Fabbrocini G, Romano MC, Cameli N et al. "Il Corpo Ritrovato": Dermocosmetological Skin Care Project for the Oncologic Patient. *ISRN Oncol.* 2011;2011:650482.

99. Pardo Masferrer J, Murcia Mejía M, Vidal Fernández M et al. Prophylaxis with a cream containing urea reduces the incidence and severity of radio-induced dermatitis. *Clin Transl Oncol.* 2010;12(1):43–8.

100. Burtness B, Anadkat M, Basti S et al. NCCN Task Force Report: Management of dermatologic and other toxicities associated with EGFR inhibition in patients with cancer. *J Natl Compr Canc Netw.* 2009;7(1):S5–S21.

101. Segaert S, Chiritescu G, Lemmens L et al. Skin toxicities of targeted therapies. *Eur J Cancer.* 2009;45(1):295–308.

102. Kodiyan J, Kyle T, Amber KT. A review of the use of topical calendula in the prevention and treatment of radiotherapy-induced skin reactions. *Antioxidants* 2015; 4:293–303.

103. Pommier P, Gomez F, Sunyach MP et al. Phase III randomized trial of calendula officinalis compared with trolamine for the prevention of acute dermatitis during irradiation for breast cancer. *J Clin Oncol.* 2004;22:1447–53.

104. Navarro A. Curso de Estética Aplicada a la Salud. El Maquillaje corrector. A.E.E.R.I. (Asociación Española de Estética Reparadora Integral), 12–6 Septiembre 2011. Fundación Ángela Navarro.

29

Micropigmentation Applied to Oncology Patients

Mario Gisbert

Definition

Micropigmentation is the microimplantation of coloring substances to the skin. This result will remain in place between 1 and 3 years, then fading to total disappearance, which is its differential feature with the tattoo [1]. A micropigmentation professional applies these coloring substances by means of needles crossing the epidermal level, being an exception to the limits that define the professionals of the sector of personal image.

Objectives of Oncological Micropigmentation

Oncological micropigmentation can be applied in facial (eyebrows, eyelids, lips, etc.) or body areas (areola, scalp, dyschromia, etc.), and regarding the oncology patient, aims fundamentally to correct, reconstruct, repair, and camouflage some of the aesthetic consequences caused by the different types of cancer.

To that end, we can perform different treatments with the aim of achieving very natural and imperceptible results, which are neutral with respect to passing trends and always with the ultimate goal of embellishing, balancing, and harmonizing [2].

We can apply oncological micropigmentation in both males and females; it is suitable for all ages; and we can adapt it to the tastes, desires, expectations, and needs of the patient.

Eyebrows

With the micropigmentation of eyebrows, we manage to recreate the shape of the eyebrows when they no longer exist or are disappearing due to the effects of chemotherapy. In women, we can create them using techniques of shading or blending with "ombré," "stardust," or "powder," or with hair-by-hair techniques with "hairstyle effect." In men, hair-by-hair techniques with "disheveled hyperrealistic effect" are recommended.

Eyelids

Micropigmentation in eyelids allows an effect of more eyelashes to be achieved or they can be recreated optically when they are nonexistent due to the effects of chemotherapy. We can create them using shade techniques called "smoked," "ombré," "stardust," or "powder," adjusting them to the original line of eyelashes, both in men and women, and can also perform in women a sophisticated "eyeliner" effect.

Lips

Through the application of the different micropigmentation techniques to the lips, we manage to restructure and redefine the labial contour and raise the color of the mucosa, since both are lost as a side effect of the different treatments to which the oncology patient may be subjected. In men, we must apply light-dark techniques to redefine the labial contour, which are imperceptible and improve the appearance of the lip.

Scalp Micropigmentation—Tricopigmentation

With scalp micropigmentation, we can camouflage the effects of hair loss caused by chemotherapy, performing the natural-style shaved-effect treatment. It is especially suitable for men, but it could also be made for women who do not want to cover their head with wigs, scarves, or other accessories and like to wear a more extravagant or sophisticated shaved look.

Areola

The high incidence of breast cancer among the female population puts micropigmentation as the star technique of this speciality, since it allows redrawing and totally recreating the areola, nonexistent since the original ones are removed in the mastectomy. This can be done unilaterally or bilaterally. Ideally the plastic surgeon would have reconstructed the nipple and leveled the two breasts, so that we only have to "color" the areas that need it, thus achieving total realism.

Reparative and Reconstructive Camouflage

Reparative and reconstructive micropigmentation allows the application of micropigmentation in lesions that are already stabilized or in areas that have dyschromia. With micropigmentation we can achieve the following:

- Camouflage scars that are already stabilized and that are not at risk of producing keloids or becoming hypertrophic scars.
- Camouflage donor or recipient areas of skin grafts and other dyschromias, artificially coloring the affected areas using mosaic or watercolor techniques.

Interview and Design Test

Interview

During the interview with the patient, we will explain the offer of the appropriate micropigmentation treatment, reporting all its features and emphasizing its advantages and the expected result. The micropigmentation professional must have the ability to observe and listen, and later, inform and convince. The patient may have erroneous preconceptions on the objectives of a micropigmentation treatment, so the professional must neutralize these expectations.

It is a good idea to carry out a design project that closes the interview process, so that the patient can "experience" the effects proposed by the professional and with which the professional can confirm and ratify the proposal or final project offered.

In this stage, we analyze together with the patient the design, density, and color proposed, taking into account the patient's needs and motivations to agree and approve the final project, communicating with sensitivity and empathy.

Design Project Proportions and Measures

In micropigmentation, it must be taken into account that the effects obtained in shape, color, and intensity must harmonize throughout the period of permanence of the result in the skin. The chosen design should be appropriate for any time of day, in any personal and professional situation of the patient, taking into account their expectations, personality, tastes, and needs. In most cases, no exaggerated changes should be made, the primary objective being to achieve the greatest possible naturalness with the design made.

In the project and design proposal, we must take into account the various factors that determine morphological features, such as ethnicity, structure of bones and muscles, inheritance, age, psychological aspects, lifestyle, and weight gain or loss. We also need to consider certain factors that will change after some years, such as aging processes and flaccidity of the skin, as well as the fashions, needs, and circumstances of the patient.

Facial Design

We must assess the shape, lines, and volumes of the facial oval in order to know which aspects we must disguise or hide and which should be highlighted to provide a better balance to the whole face. To do this, we must seek face balance by correcting asymmetries and defects.

There are different faces with different shapes; that is, more or less oval, elongated, wide, and so on. Also, the elements of the face, such as the eyes or mouth, have different morphologies.

The Hairline

We must evaluate the proportions and anatomical characteristics of the patient's skull to draw the defining silhouette of the design, and the areas of application. We use the tools of measurement and calculation, following the classic canons. Next, we compare the skin tone and the surrounding and/or related hair density to choose the color and intensity, thus determining the proposal for a male and female patient.

Study of Areola and Nipple

In the micropigmentation of an areola and nipple, we undertake the study of adequate measures and proportions. To that end, we observe and explore the area to assess the type of mastectomy performed and the plastic-aesthetic surgery used in the reconstruction of the areola and the patient's nipple. We evaluate the proportions and anatomical characteristics of the patient to draw the shape and size of the areola and nipple, using tools of measurement and calculation, following the classic canons, and considering the characteristics of the skin and musculature concerned. Next, we compare the tonality of the surrounding or related skin to choose the color and intensity of the areola and nipple, drawing them by rules of colorimetry and harmony.

Stages of a Micropigmentation Treatment

The realization of *an allergic sensitivity test* is a mandatory legal requirement only in some countries. It can be done moments before the completion of the treatment.

The *initial treatment* may take 2 hours. The application process is to last about an hour, and we need to devote at least another hour for the information and design processes prior to the procedure. After the first application, the patient undergoes an immediate change, obtaining a result similar to that offered by the professional during the counseling, interview, and design test phase, but modified by the slight inflammation and posttreatment color increase.

The period of *healing* comes immediately after the initial treatment and will last approximately 2 days, where a very noticeable increase in perceived color is observed. A few days after healing, when the mini-scab falls, the perceived color may even disappear almost completely.

The period of *regeneration*, which happens after healing, ends approximately 30 days after the initial treatment. During these 30 days, the perceived color will show variations, and we can conclude that the final color will be the one that can be seen between 30 and 60 days after the initial treatment, depending on the treatment performed.

The *revision* and the *retouch* must be done after 30–60 days, assessing the color fixation, tone, balance, and color deviation, and evaluating the structure of the design, in order to rebalance or reinforce it.

The control of the *revision* and the *retouch* must be done after 30–60 days of the intervention.

After 12 months, it is important to make a new *revision* as well as apply a *maintenance session*, since 1 year after the initial treatment, the color begins to lose its vigor and the design its shape. It is important, therefore, that the professional intervene again to avoid the disappearance of the implanted color and the loss of the original design to keep the micropigmentation in perfect condition.

Total *elimination* will occur after approximately 3 years in the event that the patient rejects maintenance sessions. A well-executed micropigmentation should gradually and homogeneously fade away. We should also inform the patient of the possibility of eliminating the treatment by laser, when the patient so desires, without having to wait for the removal of color by natural processes.

Risks, Precautions, and Care Informed Consent

Before performing any type of micropigmentation treatment, we must make a prior aesthetic diagnosis, applying the appropriate preventive measures and evaluating the existence of contraindications that may prevent such treatment, either totally or temporarily [3]. Some health circumstances lead us to request medical supervision or permission, or to perform micropigmentation with extreme care before, during, and after the treatment.

All these circumstances, warnings, precautions, and usual pre- and postcare will be communicated to the patient and collected both in the informed consent form and in the patient file (together with their morphological analysis, the results of the design test, the proposal-project quote, the photographic file, and even the invoice).

Special Health Circumstances

The knowledge and identification of the most common lesions and alterations of the skin and/or the patient's health status related to micropigmentation processes will ensure the safety of the professional and the patient. A visit to a relevant medical specialist must be advised for the treatment of those circumstances that temporarily prevent the application of micropigmentation. Once cured and treated by a doctor, the patient can return and undergo the desired micropigmentation treatment.

The micropigmentation professional should pay attention to skin condition in the micropigmentation area, to verify that there are no alterations preventing the application of micropigmentation in the desired area, and then informing the patient of the process to follow [4]. Likewise, we must check the general state of health of the patient by asking standard questions to rule out the existence of relative and/or absolute contraindications and, if necessary, refer them to their doctor, detailing the aspects observed in said referral report.

We also analyze, where appropriate, the medical information provided by the patient, to determine the suitability of the application of micropigmentation [5]. We can collect reports from different medical specialities treating the patient's pathology and whose analysis and classification is relevant to identify the aftereffects of the patient's pathology and/or evaluate indications and contraindications of the micropigmentation treatment, then inform the patient of the process to follow.

As a general rule, we establish that in all oncological micropigmentation processes, we must maximize the aseptic conditions before, during, and after treatment, as well as posttreatment care and prior consultation, filling out all this information in both the patient file and the consent report together with pre- and postcare advice where these warnings will be emphasized.

Informed Consent

Current regulations require that people who will undergo micropigmentation treatment must be informed of all the circumstances related to it, before it is carried out. This information is collected in a document called "informed consent," whose contents are specified in said regulations and must be signed by both the patient and the specialist technician who performs the treatment, each one of them keeping a copy. The copy of the informed consent delivered to the patient must include the pre- and posttreatment care that the patient must follow, as well as the advice for the correct maintenance of the treatment.

Pretreatment Care

One week before performing a treatment, the patient will be informed that he or she must carry some specific preventive care, such as the following:

- Prevent cold sores (only in the case of micropigmentation on lips). You should consult with your doctor or apply the preventive measures described earlier.
- Do not sunbathe or be exposed to ultraviolet A (UVA) rays.
- Do not perform aesthetic treatments, or medical-aesthetic or surgical interventions in the area of treatment.

Within the 24 hours before treatment, avoid the following:

- Excitatory substances and vasodilators, such as tea, coffee, energy drinks, vitamin complexes, products for physical exercises, alcohol, and so on
- Food whose intake may cause temporary alterations in the patient's skin (spicy, strongly seasoned, allergens, etc.)

Posttreatment Care

Once the treatment is finished, the patient will be advised that, for at least 7 days, he or she should carry some care in order to have a good healing process and avoid unwanted alterations. This care is as follows:

- Keep the treated area dry, limiting direct contact of the treated area with water during daily showers and avoid saunas, swimming pools, and the beach.
- Avoid excessive sweating from exercise.

- Avoid sunbathing and UVA rays. This way there will be no changes in color and alterations.
- Do not hit the area. Do not scratch or rub, avoiding alteration of the cicatrization.
- Avoid applying normal cosmetics on the area.
- Do not perform aesthetic treatments, or medical-aesthetic or surgical interventions, in the area of treatment, avoiding the application in the treated area of creams, makeup, cleansers, petroleum jelly, and so on, other than those prescribed by the specialist and the medical team.
- Clean the area twice a day in a gentle way with the products prescribed by the specialist and the medical team.
- In the case of lips, hair, and areola, apply the specific products prescribed by the specialist and the medical team in the manner described in their instructions.
- In the case of the areolae, it is very convenient to aerate the treated area, as soon as possible after the application of the treatment [5].
- In the case of the areola, for a week, protect the treated area by means of specific dressings, after the specific cleaning and application of specific products described by the specialist and the medical team.

Tips for Maintaining the Treatment

Whenever a treatment is performed, it is essential to inform the patient that, once the week of posttreatment care has ended, to keep the healing process going well, it is advisable to

- Use sunscreen (full screen) on the area.
- Keep the area hydrated and nourished with appropriate cosmetic products.
- In case of undergoing special medical-aesthetic treatments (acids, lasers, etc.), special care should be taken over the pigmented area, protecting it to avoid color changes.
- Perform an annual review to evaluate its evolution and perform a reapplication to keep the color and design in perfect condition.

Technical Parameters

In order to achieve the desired deposit of color on the skin, we must properly select and execute each technical parameter correctly. With the combination of parameters, we produce a maneuver that will give us a concrete effect.

The choice of each variable within each of the parameters involves the mode, depth, density, quantity, intensity, and dispersion with which the color is deposited on the skin and which, in turn, modifies the trace left by the color applied and its duration in time.

These are the principal parameters:

- Hand displacement speed
- Frequency, speed, and power, and characteristics of the dermograph
- Pressure exerted by the hand

- Needle penetration angle
- Projection of implantation
- Position and trajectory of the dermograph
- Needle penetration depth
- Diameter, taper, tip, visibility, exposure, and course of the needles
- Number and configurations of needles
- Geometric trace pattern described by the path of the dermograph

The selection of several maneuvers together with the selection of certain colors results in a specific technique [6]. A complete treatment of micropigmentation is therefore composed of the successive and chronological application of several specific techniques and different colors to obtain the desired final result [7].

Coloring Preparations: Pigments

All the *coloring preparations* are commonly referred to as "pigments" and combine inorganic and/or organic chemical bases with excipients (vehicles) in various ways. They may be present in hydrophobic or hydrophilic form.

All color bases are internationally named and included in the labeling of coloring preparations with the Colour Index (CI).

For the elaboration of browns and pinks necessary in oncological micropigmentation, we use the *inorganic* bases black iron oxide (Fe_3O_4) CI77499, red iron oxide (FeO_2O_3) CI77491, yellow iron oxide ($FeOH_2O$) CI77492, and white titanium dioxide (TiO_2) CI77891. Regarding the *organic* bases, the options are many more, but among the most used worldwide are Carbon Black CI77266, Red 254 CI65110, and Yellow 74 CI56800, which are mixed with white titanium dioxide (TiO_2) CI77891 (this last is obviously inorganic: an exception to the rule).

Obtaining hydrophobic or hydrophilic preparations depends on the combination of *excipients*. Therefore, the excipients greatly influence the ease of penetration into the skin and the durability and evolution over the years of the perceived color.

Hydrophobic coloring preparations are those that *do not* disperse well in water. They have a lower amount of pigment charge; are creamier and easier and safer to handle; have greater difficulty penetrating the skin; have a greater need for deepening and trauma; have lower retention; have greater usability; have lower effectiveness; and have lower efficiency.

Hydrophilic coloring preparations are those that *do* disperse well in water. They have a greater amount of pigment charge; are more fluid, difficult, and risky to handle; have greater ease of penetration in the skin; have a lower need for deepening and trauma; have greater retention; have lower usability; have greater effectiveness; and have greater efficiency.

Normative Context of Micropigmentation

The European and national regulations that affect micropigmentation mainly regulate materials such as coloring preparations (pigments), appliances, instruments, needles, and accessories.

European and national authorities have published the requirements to grant authorization for coloring preparations, without which it is not possible to proceed with its marketing.

The equipment, needles, heads, tips, and other micropigmentation tools and accessories are regulated by European and national laws on medical devices and must meet the requirements that apply to them regarding safety, efficacy, evaluation, and risk.

The regional and local regulations that affect micropigmentation monitor compliance with European and national regulations. In addition, they regulate and monitor the characteristics of the facilities of the establishment where micropigmentation is applied, the responsibility of the owner of the establishment. They also regulate and monitor the knowledge of the personnel and the person in charge of the establishment in terms of safety, hygienic health risks, prevention of infections and transmission of diseases, as well as hygienic measures and professional protection.

Users who are going to undergo micropigmentation treatment must be informed of the steps and processes that will be performed before, during, and after treatment; of the circumstances relative thereto, before it is carried out, identifying the contraindications that may prevent such treatment, either temporarily or totally; and preventive and posttreatment care; as well as the protocol for carrying out the allergy test.

REFERENCES

1. Gisbert M, Ortega A, and Hofman H. Micropigemntacion: tecnología, metodología y practica. Editorial Videocinco. 2011.
2. Gisbert M. Libro de taller. Editorial Videocinco. 2018.
3. Lafaurie P, and Le-Quang C. Forum: Dermopigmentation or medical tattooing. In practice … how to perform medical tattooing? *Ann Chir Plast Esthet.* agosto de 1992;37(4):402–7.
4. Zhang C, Hu G, Biskup E, Qiu X, Zhang H, and Zhang H. Depression induced by total mastectomy, breast conserving surgery and breast reconstruction: A systematic review and meta-analysis. *World J Surg.* 2018;42(7):2076–85.
5. Waljee JF, Hu ES, Ubel PA, Smith DM, Newman LA, and Alderman AK. Effect of esthetic outcome after breast-conserving surgery on psychosocial functioning and quality of life. *J Clin Oncol.* 10 de julio de 2008;26(20):3331–7.
6. Clarkson JHW, Tracey A, Eltigani E, and Park A. The patient's experience of a nurse-led nipple tattoo service: A successful program in Warwickshire. *J Plast Reconstr Aesthet Surg.* 2006;59(10):1058–62.
7. Ortí Rodriguez RJ. estudio comparativo de las distintas técnicas de dermopigmentación en medicina estética en la reconstrucción del complejo areola-pezón. *Trabajo fin de master calidad de vida y cuidados médico estéticos del paciente oncológico.* 2ª edición. Agosto 2018.

30

Photoprotection in Oncology Patients

María Elena Fernández Martín

Introduction

This chapter concerns how to adapt photoprotection recommendations for oncology patients.

Compared with the general population, oncology patients have increased vulnerability to sunlight (light phototypes, presence of nevus, history of skin cancer, exterior workers and athletes, age, etc.), because sun radiation can aggravate the collateral effects derived from antineoplastics, like photosensitization, pigmentation alterations, acneiform rash, other dermatoses, and the risk of developing ultraviolet A (UVA)–induced skin tumors. Long-term dermatological follow-up of these patients, as well as an adapted chronic photoprotection education, is critical [1]. Furthermore, sunlight suppresses the immune system, and treatments may reduce the skin's natural defensive mechanisms (epidermal and dermal thickening, melanin synthesis, activation of antioxidant molecules, DNA repair systems, and cytokine synthesis), altering the skin barrier (xerosis, erythema, and radiodermatitis) and making them even more susceptible to photocarcinogenesis.

Thorough protection using clothes and avoiding sun exposure reduces the levels of vitamin D, which does not happen by only using a hat and lotions [2]. In this situation, the consensus is to recommend supplements to avoid vitamin D deficiency.

In recent decades, the main cause of increased skin cancer rates has been considered to be the patient's behavior regarding the sun. For this reason, and given oncology patients' added vulnerability to the sun, they need information about photoprotection, especially prior to the start of treatment.

Personalized, relevant information has proven to increase adherence [3] and must be clear [4], avoiding any misunderstandings and confusion between sunscreen users [5]. To this end, education is probably the best method to ensure a patient adopts effective photoprotection measures.

> Being well informed creates adherence and is part of the efficacy of photoprotection measures.

Modern photoprotection for the general population, which has been specifically adapted to oncology patients, is based on three basic pillars (by order of importance): first, avoiding sun exposure and preventing sunburn; second, wearing appropriate clothing (clothes, hat, and sunglasses); and third, using topical and oral photoprotection (Figure 30.1).

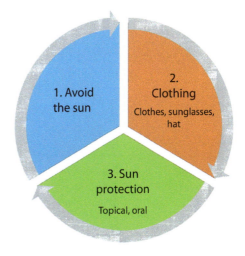

FIGURE 30.1 Basic pillars recommended for photoprotection.

First Line of Photoprotection: Avoid Sun Exposure

It is believed that UV radiation has harmful effects on skin, causing direct cell damage and alterations in the immunological function [6,7].

Tanning must be avoided: according to the International Agency for Research on Cancer (IARC), a tanned skin is a sign of sun damage. The most agreed-upon measure by most health institutions for the general population is to avoid sun exposure during the central hours of the day (10–11 a.m. to 4 p.m.), when sunlight is more intense. The World Health Organization (WHO) recommends physicians use the UV index (which warns about the strength of the sun based on the time of day, season of the year, latitude, altitude, surface reflection, cloud cover, and even environmental pollution) as an educational tool to inform about sun protection and the health risks of UV radiation (sunburn, skin cancer, and aging, or ocular and immune system alterations); the UV index should also encourage the most appropriate protective measures at each time point and change the attitude and behavior of patients who are especially vulnerable to UV radiation exposure. This index is reported by the media through weather agencies.

No doses of maximum sun exposure can be recommended in patients with photosensitivity, nor should exposure times without burning be recommended. Sunscreen should never be used to extend the duration of sun exposure.

Most antineoplastic treatments cause photosensitive reactions, so it is critical to educate these patients on sun photoprotection prior to treatment start, ensuring they know that light exposure also includes indirect exposure (cloudy

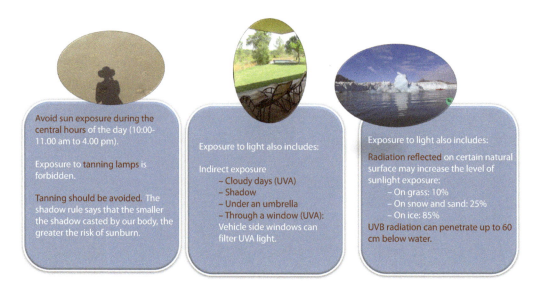

FIGURE 30.2   First line of photoprotection: avoid the sun.

days, shadow, under an umbrella, through a window, below water) and light reflected on certain surfaces (sand, snow, water, grass), because these photosensitivity reactions are mediated both by UVB and UVA radiation, which can go through clouds and windows. Medication can be sensitizing and cause reactions with very little light.

Pigmentation changes caused by antineoplastic treatments can be accentuated by the sun, so prevention must cover visible and infrared spectra of UVA radiation.

The use of sunbeds is forbidden, according to the fourth edition of the European Code Against Cancer.

See further Figure 30.2.

Second Line of Photoprotection: Clothing (Clothes, Hat, and Sunglasses)

After avoiding sun exposure, the second line of photoprotection is to cover the body (clothes) and the head (hat and sunglasses); however, not all fabrics provide the same protection against

the sun. To determine the degrees of efficacy of different sun protection fabrics with accuracy, the ultraviolet protection factor (UPF) is used, which measures blocked UVA and UVB radiation. The higher the UPF, the better the protection against UV radiation. In patients with photosensitivity, it is recommended that they wear clothes with UPF over 40.

The Skin Cancer Foundation suggests wearing clothes and fabrics with tight stitch patterns, no tight clothes, synthetic or semisynthetic fibers (polyester, rayon), as well as bright or dark colors, and with UPF labels. They also warn that wet fabrics open up spaces between fibers, reducing UPF and therefore their protection.

Wide-brimmed hats are recommended (of 7.5 cm or more) to cover the head, the forehead, the cheeks, the nose, and the upper part of the shoulders, as well as sunglasses to protect the skin around the eyes, eyelids, and eyes. Lenses must absorb almost 100% of UV radiation up to 400 nm, and for extra protection of the retina, they must reduce the transmission of blue and violet lights. To protect against UVA, lenses must include plastic films of copper, nickel, and zinc (tinted dark glasses).

See further Figure 30.3.

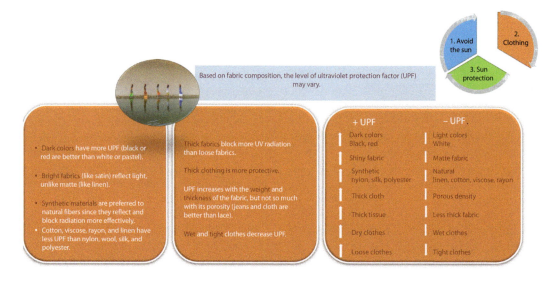

FIGURE 30.3   Second line of photoprotection: clothing (clothes, hat, and sunglasses).

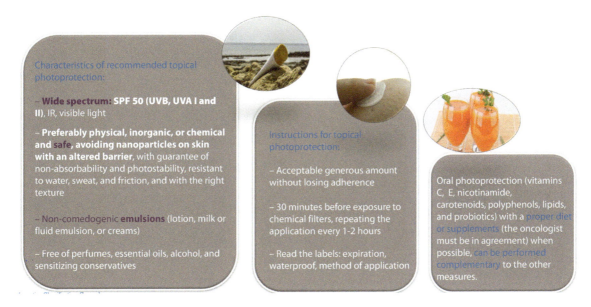

FIGURE 30.4 Third line of photoprotection: topical and oral photoprotection.

Third Line of Photoprotection: Topical and Oral Photoprotection

In general, oncology patients do not tolerate topical photoprotection well, so the first and second lines of photoprotection must be emphasized, especially with the presence of photosensitivity and skin alterations [2].

Oncology patients should use the highest SPF (50+), taking into account that photosensitivity reduces minimal erythematous dose (MED) [1,8]. It must properly cover the UVA spectrum (I and II), which causes most of the photosensitization mechanisms [9,10], protect against infrared (IR) radiation due to its involvement in the formation of free radicals (photocarcinogenesis) and photoaging [2,8,10,11], and protect against visible light involved in certain dermatoses and pigmentation alterations [2]. Its safety must have been proven in *in vivo* studies, particularly for vulnerable patients [12].

Recommended filters must be preferably physical and inorganic (titanium dioxide, zinc oxide) [13], avoiding nanoparticles (NANO forms) on skin with an altered barrier [9,10], with a guarantee of nonabsorbability [8,14] and photostability (nano forms must be film coated) [9,10]; resistance to water, sweat, and friction; and with the right texture (emulsions: lotion, milk or fluid emulsion, or creams) that generates adherence [10,13,15]. Chemical filters may be badly tolerated, but with a bigger problem being photodegradability and the possibility of causing irritation and variable phototoxicity, presenting a higher risk of causing contact reactions compared with mineral screens [8,11]; there is thus a risk of intolerance, especially in sensitized skins after chemotherapy and/or radiotherapy. There are also concerns about the endocrine effect of UV filters that include estrogenic effects. Although high amounts are needed, their long-term effects at low doses have been doubted [9,13,16], thus requiring long-term studies [17]. The products recommended must be followed up.

The alteration of the skin barrier and xerosis will condition the composition of topical photoprotection: patients should avoid alcohol, perfumes, preservatives, and irritant or sensitizing filters [1,18].

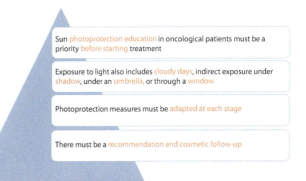

FIGURE 30.5 The importance of informing oncology patients about photoprotection.

Instructions include the application of an acceptable generous amount—without losing adherence—30 minutes before exposure to chemical filters, repeating it every 1–2 hours. Patients must be instructed to read the labels for the expiration date and method of application.

Oral photoprotection (vitamins C, E, nicotinamide, carotenoids, polyphenols, lipids, and probiotics) with a proper diet or supplements may help cover temporary or continuous exposures, but patients need several weeks to reach optimal levels [14], and the oncologist must be in agreement in case of any potential interaction and incompatibility with the oncological treatment. Combining several active compounds has synergic, nonexclusive effects. Based on the circumstances, topical antioxidants may be recommended before sun exposure, which, if they reach sufficient concentrations [8,12], can completely inhibit oxidative stress [19].

See further Figures 30.4 and 30.5.

REFERENCES

1. Sibaud V, Delord J-P, Robert C. *Dermatología de los tratamientos contra el cáncer*. Guía práctica. Editions Privat. 2015.

2. Lim HW et al. Current challenges in photoprotection. *J Am Acad Dermatol.* 2017;76(3S1):S91–9.

3. Robinson JK, Friedewald J, Gordon EJ. Perceptions of risk of developing skin cancer for diverse audiences: Enhancing relevance of sun protection to reduce the risk. *J Cancer Educ.* 2016 March;31(1):153–7.

4. Lin JS, Eder M, Weinmann S. Behavioral counseling to prevent skin cancer: A systematic review for the U.S. preventive services task force. *Ann Intern Med.* 2011;154(3):190–201.

5. Thomas M et al. Physicians involved in the care of patients with high risk of skin cancer should be trained regarding sun protection measures: Evidence from a cross sectional study *JEADV.* 2011;25(1):19–23.

6. González Maglio MG, Pas ML, Leoni J. Sunlight effects on immune system: Is there something else in addition to UV-induced immunosuppression? Hindawi Publishing Corporation. *Bio Med Res Int.* 2016;2016:1934518:10. Disponible en http://dx.doi.org/10.1155/2016/1934518

7. Nishisgori C. Current concept of photocarcinogenesis. *Photochem Photobiol Sci.* 2015 26;14(9):1713–21.

8. Carrascosa JM. El futuro se hace presente en fotoprotección solar. *Piel* Elsevier. 2011;26(7):311–4.

9. Surber C, Ulrich C, Hinrichs B, Stockfleth E. Photoprotection in immunocompetent and immuno compromised people. *Br J Dermatol.* 2012;167(Suppl 2):85–93.

10. Stiefel C, Schwack W. Photoprotection in changing times – UV filter efficacy and safety, sensitization processes and regulatory aspects. *Int J Cosmet Sci.* 2015;37(1):2–30.

11. Skotarczak K, Osmola-Mankowska A, Lodyga M, Polanska A, Mazur M, Admski Z. Photoprotection: Facts and controversies. *Eur Rev Med Pharmacol Sci.* 2015 Jan;19(1):98–112.

12. Valenzuela Landaeta K, Espinoza Piombo M. Estrés oxidativo, carcinogénesis cutánea por radiación solar y quimioprotección con polifenoles. *Piel Elsevier Doyma.* 2012;27(8):446–52.

13. Carvalhi UM. Official publication of the Brazilian Society of Dermatology. *An Bras Dermatol.* 2014;89(6s1):01–74.

14. Simonsen AB et al. Photosensitivity in atopic dermatitis complicated by contact allergy to common sunscreen ingredients. *Contact Dermatitis.* 2016;74(1):56–8.

15. Valentine J, Belum VR, Duran J, Ciccolini K, Schindler K, Wu S, Lacouture ME. Incidence and risk of xerosis with targeted anticancer therapies. *J Am Acad Dermatol.* 2015 Apr;72(4):656–67.

16. Gaspar LR, Tharman J, Maia Campos PM, Liebsch M. Skin phototoxicity of cosmetic formulations containing photounstable and photostable UV-filters and vitamin A palmitate. *Toxicol In Vitro.* 2013 Feb;27(1):418–25.

17. Iannacone MR, Hughes MC, Green AC. Effects of sunscreen on skin cancer and photoaging. *Photodermatol Photoimmunol Photomed.* 2014;30(2–3):55–6.

18. Gilaberte Y, González S. Novedades en fotoprotección. *Actas Dermosifiliogr.* 2010;101(8):659–72.

19. Godic A et al. The role of antioxidants in skin cancer prevention and treatment. *Oxid Med Cell Longev.* 2014; 2014(5):860479.

31

Scar Care after Surgical Treatment in Oncology Patients

Marta Yuste Colom

Introduction

Multidisciplinary treatment is the cornerstone for cancer patient management. Cancer surgery is still the key to control this disease; unfortunately, scarring is part of surgery. A cancer patient's safety always prevails above cosmetic criteria, but this fact does not exclude the surgeon's intention to use the tools that are at his or her disposal to achieve less visible scars, such as incisions along lines of least tension, closure without tension, type of suture, time until sutures are removed, and so on. Nevertheless, cancer scars remain in the patient's day-to-day life, often becoming much more than a skin wound. In this sense, the European Wound Management Association [23] suggests that, with skin scarring, we should not only focus on the physiologic or biological aspects, but also the psychosocial implications. Scarring in more visible areas such as the face, neck, and lower extremities will have a greater impact on the quality of life (QoL) of these patients.

Cancer scarring is a constant reminder of the disease. Sometimes, it becomes a symbol for overcoming the disease, such as the well-known "SCAR Project." In this project, patients with a history of breast cancer are photographed nude in order to raise awareness and share hope, showing their scarred bodies and faces with a new attitude toward life (Figure 31.1). However, for many, visible cancer scarring is stigmatizing. It can be experienced as an aggression toward one's image, revealing an intimate and secret part of oneself. It can affect the patient's self-esteem, affecting their social functioning. In addition, due to the associated surgical aggressiveness, it affects physical comfort (pain, itching, functional deficits, restricted movement), affecting the patient's well-being as a whole.

Therefore, with knowledge of the impact of cancer scarring, it is essential to manage these patients optimally, from the surgical intervention to the immediate and late postoperative care.

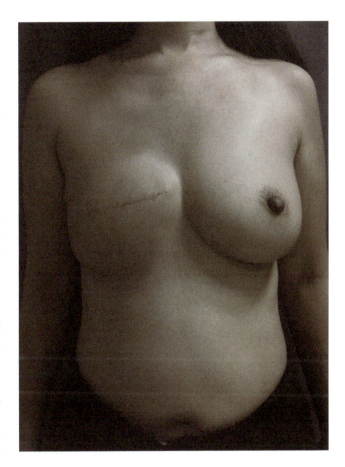

FIGURE 31.1 Female patient, 35 years old, with a history of right breast cancer. Currently in the process of breast reconstruction, although the scar continues to remind us of the disease.

Wound Healing Phases

The scar is the unwanted, although normal, result of surgery. To be able to work on a scar, we must know the different stages of healing. Thus, care and treatments will be adapted in a specific way in each phase.

Wound healing is a complex and dynamic process of replacing devitalized and missing cellular structures and tissue layers. The three stages of wound healing are the inflammatory phase, the proliferative phase, and the maturation and remodeling phase [1].

Inflammatory phase (the first 48–72 hours after the injury) begins with hemostasis and chemotaxis. Both the white cells and thrombocytes speed up the inflammatory process by releasing more mediators and cytokines. Besides platelet-derived growth factor, there are other factors that promote collagen degradation, the transformation of fibroblasts, growth of new vessels, and reepithelialization. All these processes occur at the same time in a synchronized fashion. Mediators like serotonin and histamine are released from platelets and increase cellular permeability. The platelet-derived growth factor attracts fibroblasts and, along with transforming growth factor, enhances the division and multiplication of fibroblasts. The fibroblasts, in turn, synthesize collagen. Inflammatory cells, such as neutrophils, monocytes, and endothelial cells, adhere to a fibrin scaffold that is formed by platelet activation. The neutrophils enable phagocytosis of cellular debris and bacteria, allowing for decontamination of the wound. Proliferative phase or granulation phase does not occur at a discrete time but is occurring all the time in the background. By days 5 through 7, the fibroblasts have started to lay down new collagen and glycosaminoglycans. These proteoglycans form the core of the wound and help stabilize the wound. Reepithelialization starts to occur with the migration of cells from the wound periphery and adjacent edges. Initially, only a thin superficial layer of epithelial cells is laid down, but with time, a thicker and more durable layer of cells will bridge the wound. Neovascularization occurs through both angiogenesis, which is the formation of new blood vessels from existing vessels, and vasculogenesis, which is the formation of new vessels from endothelial progenitor cells (EPCs). Once collagen fibers have been laid down on the fibrin framework, the wound starts to mature. The wound also begins to contract and is facilitated by continued deposition of fibroblasts and myofibroblasts. Maturation phase or remodeling phase starts around week 3 and can last up to 12 months. The excess collagen degrades, and wound contraction also begins to peak around week 3. The maximal tensile strength of the incision wound occurs after about 11–14 weeks. The ultimate resulting scar will never have 100% of the original strength of the wound, and only about 80% of the tensile strength. Despite the long duration of the remodeling phase and the obvious relevance to ultimate appearance, it is by far the least understood phase of wound healing.

Overall, the scars are divided into two types: immature scars (those with less than 12 months) and mature scars (evolution time greater than 12 months). Treatment or prophylaxis on the immature scars is potentially effective; however, the handling of mature scar will involve a more aggressive therapeutic algorithm.

Evaluation of Scars

The healing of postsurgical skin wounds can result in a wide variety of scar types ranging from a fine line to unaesthetic or pathologic scars. Scars can be classified as mature, immature, linear hypertrophic, widespread hypertrophic, and minor and major keloid.

The correct evaluation and classification of scars are essential for choosing the optimal treatment, and in turn, assessing the degree of improvement objectively. The methods for evaluating scars can be divided into two groups: scar scales, which rate the injuries based on descriptions, and tools that analyze one or multiple variables of the injury through technical devices.

An ideal rating scale should be easy to complete and replicate; reliably quantify the magnitude of the measured variables; analyze the impact of the scar on patient activities, social participation, and QoL; include the point of view of both the patient and the observer; and be adequately responsive to individual changes to monitor the effects of interventions over time [2].

In 1978, the first technique to evaluate scars according to three variables was developed—the scar's color (white-pink, purple-red), thickness (flat, slightly raised, protruding), and consistency (soft, moderately hard, hard). More than 20 different scales and modifications have been developed subsequently. The most commonly used scar scales are the Vancouver Scar Scale (VSS), Dermatology Life Quality Index (DLQI), Manchester Scar Scale (MSS), Patient and Observer Scar Assessment Scale (POSAS), Bock Quality of Life (Bock QoL) questionnaire, Stony Brook Scar Evaluation Scale (SBSES), Patient-Reported Impact of Scars Measure (PRISM), and Patient Scar Assessment Questionnaire (PSAQ).

From a strictly clinimetric point of view, the POSAS and PRISM may be preferred over other scales, even if further validation is needed to test their responsiveness, interpret score changes for clinical studies, and adapt them for use in different languages and cultural contexts [2]. It is recommended to use the same scale in all patients; in that way we train ourselves to systematize, and application acquires more weight in the decision and therapeutic assessment.

To determine whether or not a patient benefits from an intervention, instruments that measure how much scars affect function or health-related QoL should also be considered as a clinical outcome. Tools have emerged to allow the highest objectivity, reliability, and reproducibility. Biomechanical techniques allow us to measure the oxygen tension, the degree of elasticity, or the scar thickness. In our practice, we use laser, ultrasound, or three-dimensional imaging techniques, among others.

Factors Affecting Wound Healing

There are certain factors that influence the wound healing process and the cosmetic result of scars. Identifying these factors, we can anticipate the available resources in order to achieve the best result. There is an important systemic involvement in all wound healing phases, and consequently, a correct result will not only depend on local factors.

Smoking is the major modifiable risk factor for wound healing. The nicotine, the carbon monoxide, and the hydrocyanic acid have a direct effect on healing, increasing the risk of wound infection and creating a suboptimal scar. Total cessation of preoperative smoking at least 4 weeks before the intervention should be recommended, and cessation should continue until the surgical wound is completely healed, which means at least 2 weeks [3,4].

The presence of comorbidities such as diabetes mellitus, peripheral vascular disease, pathologies related to collagen synthesis, immunosuppression or malnutrition, among others, will affect the final result of the scar. Severe malnutrition, with weight loss of more than 30% and macro- and micronutrient deficiencies (zinc, magnesium), slows down neovascularization and collagen synthesis and alters the remodeling process. Vitamin A and vitamin C act as cofactors that help to close the wound. It will be important to optimize the cancer patient from a nutritional point of view before beginning the surgical aggression and during the entire scarring process [5,6]. Further research is needed to identify the levels of supplements that will be of benefit to malnourished patients and patients at nutrition risk.

The neoadjuvant treatment that the patients receive may affect the final result of the scar. Ionizing radiations damage stem cell mitotic capacity at the epidermal basal layer, which prevents cell repopulation and weakens the skin's integrity. In the long term, radiated skin becomes fibrotic due to the increase in collagen and loss of vascularization [7]. These effects can become more noticeable with concomitant chemotherapy. Corticoid treatment alters the inflammatory reaction, interferes with epithelialization, and inhibits neovascularization and contraction of the wound. Its effects can be partially reversed with the administration of vitamin A [6].

Local factors that can impair wound healing are pressure, tissue edema, hypoxia, infection, maceration, and dehydration [1]. These can be avoided by accurate surgical technique and systematization of recovery protocol.

The outcome of the application of the same treatment over an identical scar may be different between patients; many individual circumstances can potentially influence the effectiveness of the same treatment. The rate of healing is inversely proportional to the patient's age. In addition, in children, there is a tendency to produce hypertrophic scars. Individuals with darker pigmentation (Fitzpatrick IV, V, VI) are more susceptible to developing pathological scars. There is clearly a genetic component in the tendency to develop suboptimal scars.

Immediate postoperative care with 1% povidone, 0.25% acetic acid, and 3% hydrogen peroxide is extremely lethal for cultivated fibroblasts. This slows down the wound's healing and can affect the final result of the scar. Immobilization favors scarring, which is something to keep in mind with wounds located on extremities and adjacent to joint areas.

When faced with a scar, we must analyze those systemic and local factors intrinsic to the patient that can and cannot be modified, to define a starting point that is as favorable as possible to achieving a normal scar. It will be important to inform the patient of the possible limitations we may find, anticipating treatment when faced with an unpromising starting point.

Nonpathological Scar

The normal scar is mature, flat, nonpigmented, and nonretractable (Figure 31.2). During the first year, the immature scar will be plastic, with an opportunity for improvement before proper treatment. Immature scars are morphologically red and raised and are often associated with slight pain and pruritus (Figure 31.3). The characteristic erythema indicates the creation of a new vascular network, a process that is included in maturation or active remodeling. Having identified the warning signs, an early onset of treatment guarantees better results. According to some studies, between 38% and 70% of scars can alter in their development

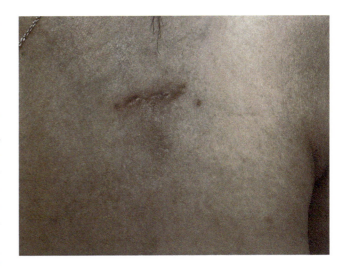

FIGURE 31.3 Immature scars at 3 weeks; central venous access removal.

or evolution [8]. The three major components of scar prevention immediately after wound closure are as follows: tension relief, hydration/taping/occlusion, and pressure garments. Before a scar, there is a wound, so everything will start by taking care of the first lesion (Figures 31.4 and 31.5).

Basic Care

The immature scar with a favorable evolution needs basic care: daily wound washing after 72 hours with soap and water and rigorous drying. During the first 2 weeks, it is recommended to avoid dehydration of the scar, avoid the appearance of scabs, and maintain a semiocclusive dressing. Transepidermal water loss is increased in hypertrophic scars and keloids. The subsequent dehydration of keratinocytes may stimulate the production of cytokines, leading to excessive collagen deposition by fibroblasts, which results in scar formation [9]. An example would be to keep a paper tape enriched in zinc from the immediate postoperative period until the fifth day. Dressings should lightly adhere to irregularly contoured, moist healing tissues and provide a

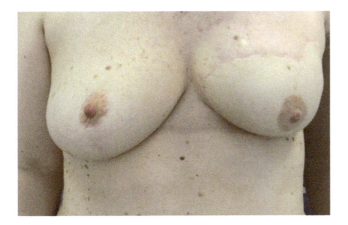

FIGURE 31.2 Lineal normal scar; left breast reconstruction with deep inferior epigastric perforator flap; contralateral symmetrization surgery with periareolar mastopexy.

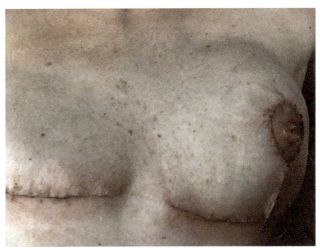

FIGURE 31.4 Before a scar, there is a wound. Immediate right breast reconstruction with tissue expander and nipple; skin-sparing left mastectomy and direct-to-implant breast reconstruction.

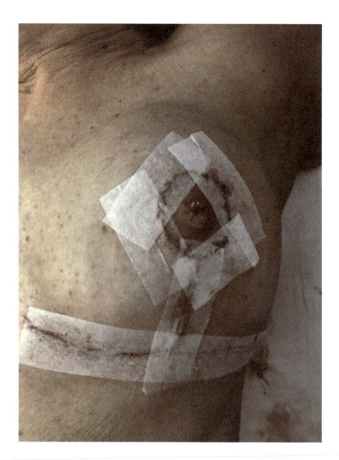

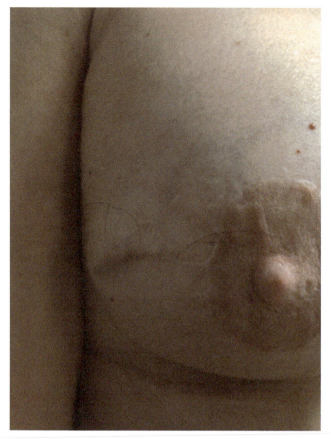

FIGURE 31.5 Postoperative wound management; application of paper tape.

FIGURE 31.6 Hypertrichosis in mature scar.

continuous temporary artificial barrier [10]. There should be early removal of the stitches and placing of adhesive skin closures. The removal of foreign bodies, such as extruded stitches, is performed in a sterile condition, and when a skin continuity solution appears, it is recommended to initiate treatment with topical antibiotic ointment every 24 hours. Daily treatment with povidone-iodine solution should be avoided if the wound shows no signs of infection. It is recommended to avoid physical activity until 10–15 days, as well as bathtubs or spas.

Solar protection will be imperative when managing scars, especially in exposed areas. We recommend daily use of creams that offer maximum sun protection and the use of physical barriers with direct sun exposure.

When epithelialization is complete, continue with daily moisturizing with moisturizer or oils applied to the scar in circular motions, pinching perpendicularly and parallel to the defect. If the patient presents poor prognosis factors such as Hispanic or African ethnicity, Fitzpatrick IV-V-VI phototype, prior pathological scarring, scarring in mobile area or with significant tension, or treatment with neoadjuvant radiotherapy, we recommend commencing with preventive measures of guided treatment, as well as stricter monitoring (e.g., those patients with breast cancer and immediate or delayed breast reconstruction, with adjuvant treatment with radiotherapy, will need stricter monitoring of the scar).

Wound controls should be performed at 6 and 15 days to check the correct epithelialization. After 6 weeks, the detection of warning signs makes it necessary to initiate a physician-directed treatment. The follow-up and assessment of scar changes will be made 3, 6, and 12 months after surgery.

Isolated itching, tightness, and superficial desquamation are normal clinical signs, which can be treated with abundant hydration.

Optimization of the Nonpathological Scar

In the management of dyschromias, micropigmentation can homogenize the final result.

Hypertrichosis within scars has been reported in postoperative patients (Figure 31.6). It is postulated that this phenomenon may be secondary to increased friction, vascularity, and local growth factors [11]. Its management should include minimally aggressive hair removal methods, limiting repeated trauma to the target area.

Certain scars may contribute to local hyper- or hypohidrosis, exacerbating skin irritation and maceration in the setting of scar fragility [11].

It is also possible to observe a nonpathological external scar with deep plane retraction (Figure 31.7); this can occur in the "S" italic mastectomy scar, in its most lateral area. In these cases, the first-choice treatment is fat grafting.

Other tools like tattoos are resources used by patients to completely mask the scar, even if it is linear, not raised (Figure 31.8).

The appearance of the raised, enlarged scar, important erythema or violaceous shade, retraction of adjacent tissue, or pain is a warning sign that should make us consider the start of a physician-directed treatment.

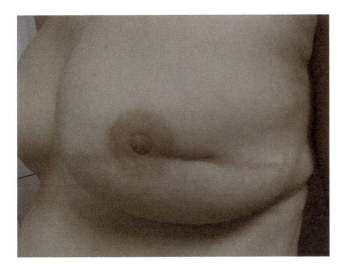

FIGURE 31.7 Mature mastectomy scar with deep plane retraction.

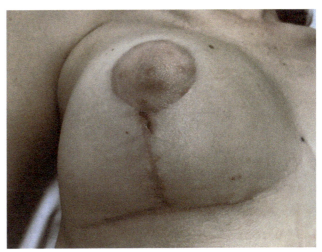

FIGURE 31.9 Adverse effect of silicone therapy: contact dermatitis.

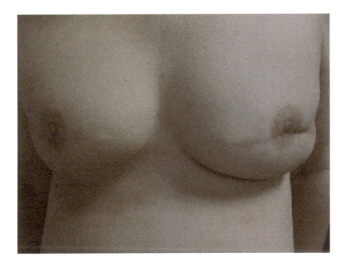

FIGURE 31.8 Tattooing of the nipple-areola complex in breast reconstruction; tattoo on the mature scar.

Prophylaxis

Silicone Therapy

The latest guidelines for scar management advocate silicone therapy as a noninvasive first-line prophylactic and treatment option for both hypertrophic scar and keloids. Of the noninvasive options, silicone sheets and silicone gels are universally considered as the gold standard in scar management and the only noninvasive preventive and therapeutic measure for which there is enough supporting data to make evidence-based recommendations [12]. Silicones may raise the surface temperature of the skin, which can increase collagenase activity leading to collagen breakdown. Furthermore, a negative static electric field between the silicone product and the skin may causa realignment of collagen, resulting in shrinkage of scars. However, occlusion and hydration of the stratum corneum are now universally accepted as the major mechanisms responsible for the action of silicones [9]. Silicone therapy is associated with minimal side effects, such as pruritus, contact dermatitis, and dry skin (Figure 31.9). Its use can be initiated as prophylaxis after complete epithelization, or

after 6 weeks before the appearance of warning signs. Silicone sheets have to be worn over the scar for 12–24 hours each day for 3–6 months. It is important to adapt the silicone to the scar geometry for greater efficiency. For that reason, silicone sheets are not suitable for use on large areas of skin, mobile body parts such as the joints, or in patients living in humid climates, due to sheeting dislodgment. In contrast, the use of silicone gel may be suitable for visible and mobile areas, such as the face or hands. The use of silicone can be combined with other therapies for scar management.

Laser Therapy

In the optimization of the scar result, laser therapy has a key role. Through the "pre-scar," we act on the remodeling phase of the scars, getting the healing of a wound closer to remodeling and away from cicatrization. This treatment increases the number of fibroblasts and elastic fibers and achieves a multidirectional collagen alignment, characteristics of normal skin. The laser of choice to perform the prescar is the nonablative laser, without purpura production, by means of its photobiostimulatory effect [8]. Early onset, after suture removal, has demonstrated excellent results. As is usual with laser therapy, indications, setting, postoperative care, and follow-up must be adapted to the patient's phototype to minimize complications such as scarring or depigmentation. Remember that histological changes are manifested at 3 months of treatment.

Hypertrophic Scar

Hypertrophic scar formation is a complex problem, causing both aesthetic and physical difficulties. Hypertrophic scars are the result of an abnormal wound healing process where an excessive amount of collagen is deposited within the wound area, causing the scar to become raised above the skin surface. Both normal and pathological scars are the result of deposition of collagen types I and III, although collagen synthesis in hypertrophic scar is two to three times as great as in normotrophic scars [13]. These scars often appear red and shiny and cause pain, itching, and

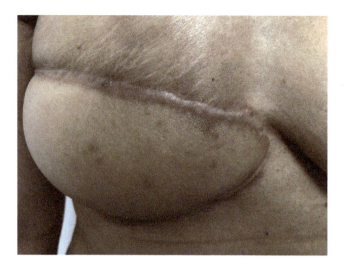

FIGURE 31.10 Hypertrophic scar; latissimus dorsi flap breast reconstruction.

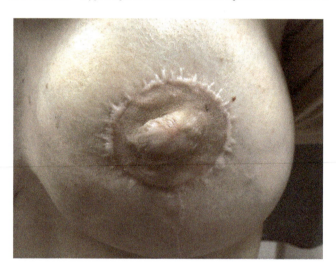

FIGURE 31.11 Hypertrophic scar; hypertrophic periareolar scar in breast reconstruction.

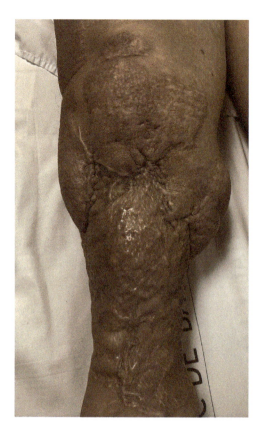

FIGURE 31.12 Widespread hypertrophic scars in a patient with a history of primary lower limb lymphedema; scars secondary to split-thickness skin graft.

The approach to treatment and its goals should be set for the individual patient based on scar evaluation and the patient's characteristics and expectations in order to reduce the scar volume, minimize subjective symptoms, and improve function and aesthetic appearance [13].

Surgical wound complications such as an infection or dehiscence, or wound closure subjected to excessive tension forces, are the situations in which the initiation of prophylactic management of the scar could be indicated. The appearance of warning signs in the checkup at 6 weeks will intensify the treatment; measures implemented should be maintained until the end of 3 months [15].

Treatment

We will perform prophylaxis or the first line of treatment through silicone therapy. In the case of association with alarm signs or in wounds that have taken more than 14 days to heal [8], the combination with compression therapy is recommended. Part of the effect of pressure could involve reduction of oxygen tension in the wound through occlusion of small blood vessels, resulting in a decrease of (myo)fibroblast proliferation and collagen synthesis [15]. A continuous pressure of 20–40 mm Hg must be maintained. Disadvantages of pressure therapy include the cost of treatment, since pressure garments are usually custom made, and poor patient compliance, since the garments are often uncomfortable and have to be worn for most of the day.

In the literature, there is controversy regarding the significant benefit of this therapy. In general, its use in combination with

sometimes even restriction of motion when positioned above a joint, thereby causing significant morbidity (Figures 31.10 and 31.11). Hypertrophic scars are caused by a prolonged inflammatory phase and a delayed onset of epithelialization, which interferes with the resolution of granulation tissue, as reflected by the higher amount of myofibroblasts and collagen present in hypertrophic scars. In addition, remodeling is impaired in excessive scar formation, reflected by a higher amount of immature-type collagen [14]. Hypertrophic scars mostly develop within 1–3 months after deep skin injury [13]. They may stay within the boundaries of the original lesion and may spontaneously regress with time [15]. Studies concerning risk factors for hypertrophic scar formation are young age, bacterial colonization, and skin subjected to stretch. Chemotherapy, statins, and smoking seem to play a protective role in hypertrophic scar formation [14].

Hypertrophic scars are classified into two categories: linear and widespread. Extensive hypertrophic scars present with irregular, highly erythematous surface and have a hardened cord-like appearance. They are typically associated with thermal or chemical burn injuries and are rare in surgical wounds (Figure 31.12).

other therapies is part of first-line management of the hypertrophic scar.

Intralesional Corticosteroids

If the patient presents with pain, significant elevation, and scar tightness, it would be indicated to perform an intralesional infiltration of corticosteroids. Intralesional corticosteroids (e.g., triamcinolone acetonide) remain a mainstay in the treatment of hypertrophic scars and keloids. This is the only invasive management option that currently has enough supporting evidence to be recommended in evidence-based guidelines [15]. The efficacy of corticosteroids for these types of scars is likely secondary to their ability to suppress inflammation, promote collagen degeneration, inhibit collagen production, and limit wound oxygenation and nutrition [11]. Local side effects include skin and subcutaneous tissue atrophy, capillary dilatation, hypopigmentation, and pain on injection. The optimal number of treatments has yet to be determined, and dosing for intralesional scar therapy varies, depending on lesion characteristics and anatomic location. The injection must be administered under sterile conditions. We recommend administering the injection with a 27G needle, with the entry point at the corner of the scar. Place the needle on a superficial plane, in the center of the scar, and administer the injection while removing the needle. We know we are on the right plane when we can whiten the scar skin. Limit the treatment exclusively to the scar, keeping healthy skin intact. The amount of product will be limited by the tissues' low elasticity. We perform successive pricks along the length of the scar (Figure 31.13). Dilution with lidocaine 50 mg/mL (1:1–1:10) may be considered; however, there is pain associated with infiltration, deriving from the tension applied to the tissues. Patients should be warned that they may require painkillers up to 24 hours after the infiltration. We will make an initial assessment 1 month after infiltration and a second checkup to assess clinical improvement in 2–3 months. Between four and five procedures can be performed. We recommend performing the treatment step by step, to avoid the appearance of tissue atrophy. With the corticoid intralesional injection, we will not achieve a lineal scar, but it will be without changes in

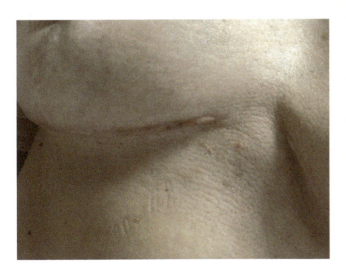

FIGURE 31.13 Intralesional infiltration of corticosteroids in a patient with breast-conserving surgery.

pigmentation and almost indiscernible; the patient will show an improvement in tautness, itchiness, and pain, and we will obtain a flatter scar.

After 6 months, if the hypertrophic scar persists, we can combine infiltration of corticosteroids with other intralesional substances or make use of them in an isolated way. Additional injectable treatment options that may help to treat hypertrophic scars include bleomycin, 5-fluorouracil, and verapamil, although the evidence to support these is currently more limited than for intralesional corticosteroids.

5-Fluorouracil

5-Fluorouracil, a pyrimidine analogue with antimetabolite activity, inhibits fibroblast proliferation in tissue culture and has been shown to be an effective treatment for inflamed hypertrophic scars [15]. The main local side effects associated with 5-fluorouracil injection include pain, purpura formation, and a burning sensation. Systemic 5-FU can cause anemia, leukopenia, and thrombocytopenia. Even though we did not exceed 90 mg 5-FU at each injection session, the use of higher doses has been reported without development of any adverse hematological effects. A combination with triamcinolone acetonide may be more effective at treating scars than are the individual treatments [16].

Bleomycin

Bleomycin is a mixture of cytotoxic glycopeptide antibiotics. The main mode of action is inhibition of DNA synthesis and, to lesser extent, inhibition of RNA and protein synthesis [17]. Bleomycin is thought to work by decreasing collagen synthesis. Occasionally reported complications include atrophy and hyper-hypopigmentation.

Verapamil

Verapamil is a calcium channel antagonist that both decreases collagen synthesis and increases collagen breakdown [15]. A study from 1992 was the first to report the use of the calcium channel blocker verapamil in the treatment of keloids and hypertrophic scars [18]. There is some controversy in the demonstrated efficacy, whether administered by itself or in combination with corticosteroid. A lower rate of local adverse effects associated with its intralesional infiltration has been described, compared to the infiltration of triamcinolone acetonide [19].

Surgical Revision

The detection of a cicatricial contracture that limits the joint range should make us consider the surgical revision of the scar. The prolonged joint limitation could cause changes at the joint level that would make this state chronic. Surgical revision includes the excision of scar tissue to identify a subcutaneous plane free of adhesions. Traditional surgical techniques for contractures include Z- and W-plasties. Our goal will be to achieve wound closure without tension and initiate an early rehabilitation program. Surgical revision is usually associated with aggressive neoplasm and oncological surgery and is frequently associated with lymphadenectomy or sarcomas of the extremities.

Laser Therapy

Laser therapy in this type of scar aims to flatten the scar and remove the significant erythema that usually appears. The possibility of spontaneous regression means that the use of ablative treatments remains in the background. Vascular-type light systems and lasers are a good treatment option for these lesions, since through coagulation of the vessels, the lesion flattens and the erythema diminishes at the same time (e.g., 532Nm KTP, long-pulsed Nd:YAG laser) [8]. In general, systems with purpura induction show better results. The nonablative laser system, pulsed dye laser (PDL) 585 has the most proven scientific evidence for improving hypertrophic scars [20]. The indication for the use of ablative systems is based on the "laser-assisted drug delivery" effect. Its application allows substances to better penetrate the dermis; the combination of fractioned CO_2 ablative laser with intralesional infiltration of triamcinolone acetonide has shown excellent results [21].

Excision Surgery

After 12 months, the mature scar will be difficult to shape with the treatments described. We should consider surgical excision of the scar and the intraoperative or early onset of prophylactic measures (intraoperative intralesional infiltration, use of Z-plasties, silicones) (Figure 31.14).

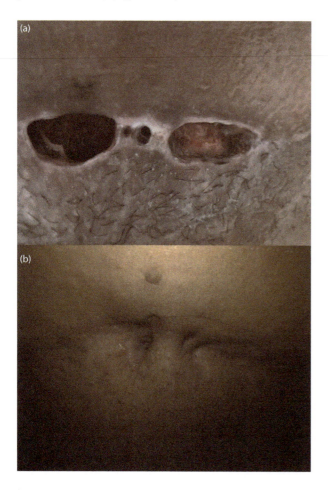

FIGURE 31.14 (a) Wound dehiscence in donor area (deep inferior epigastric perforator flap). (b) Complete healing, in a smoker patient, at 3 months (patient pending surgery for removal of scar tissue).

Botulinum Toxin A

It is recommended that botulinum toxin is given 4–7 days before surgery, perpendicular to the anticipated wound to reduce tensile forces, with doses adjusted according to the muscles involved and to avoid muscular imbalance [9]. Its greatest benefit is found in areas with a high dynamic muscular strength, such as facial injuries. It could be considered in aggressive scars after a mandibular osteosarcoma or a centrofacial squamous carcinoma. Some studies show satisfactory results in the treatment of hypertrophic scar using botulinum toxin [21,22].

Due to the similar underlying pathophysiology, hypertrophic scars and keloids may respond to the same treatment modalities. However, hypertrophic scars are often more responsive and less prone to recurrence, which make them therapeutically less challenging [13].

Keloid

The keloid scar has a low incidence and a lower genetic predisposition than the hypertrophic scar and rarely presents spontaneous regression. Keloids may occur up to 12 months after injury or even develop spontaneously. Some lesions are stable over time, while others have continued growth. The main clinical difference is the excessive scar that grows beyond the boundaries of the original wound (Figures 31.15 through Figure 31.17). Hypertrophic scars contain primarily type III collagen bundles that are oriented parallel to the epidermal surface, arranged in a wavy pattern with abundant nodules containing myofibroblasts expressing alpha-smooth muscle actin (α-SMA) and large extracellular collagen filaments. In contrast, keloid tissue is composed of disorganized type I and III thick, eosinophilic collagen bundles that appear randomly oriented to the epithelial surface with no nodules or excess myofibroblasts. Hypertrophic scars undergo a remodeling phase, while keloids do not enter this final wound healing phase [13].

Keloids can be differentiated into minor (<0.5 cm) and major (>0.5 cm).

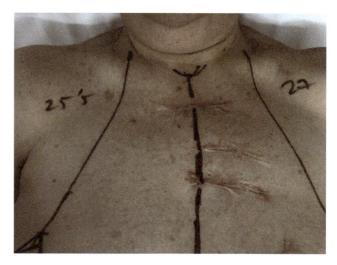

FIGURE 31.15 Presternal keloid secondary to atypical pigmented lesions excision.

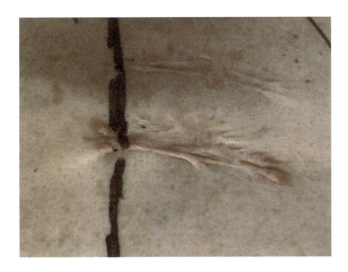

FIGURE 31.16 Presternal keloid: The expansive affectation towards healthy tissue stands out.

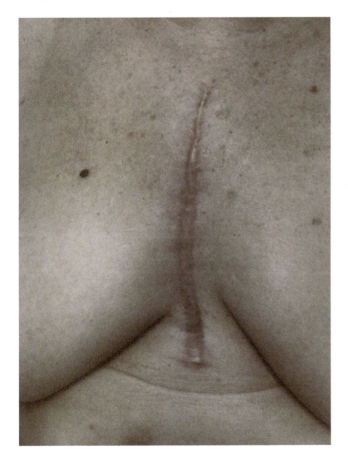

FIGURE 31.17 Presternal keloid secondary to sternotomy scar.

Treatment

The treatment of keloids is a therapeutic challenge.

Combined Treatment

The diagnosis of this pathological scar requires planning a combined treatment: silicone therapy, compression garments, and intralesional infiltrations. No treatment has shown high effectiveness, results maintained over time, and low recurrence rate. In this type of injuries, it is essential to manage patient expectations.

Laser Therapy

Ablative laser therapy decreases scar mass, but it does not stop the process of collagen deposition and extracellular matrix by fibroblasts; it is therefore associated with a high recurrence rate. The combination with intralesional infiltration achieves reduction in this rate. The PDL remains the most used therapy in this type of injury, displaying excellent results maintained over time.

Combined Surgery

The persistence of a keloid scar for 12 months will make us raise the option of surgical exercisis, in combination with adjuvant techniques (intralesional infiltration, brachytherapy, radiotherapy, internal cryotherapy). Some experts recommend that the lateral parts of keloids should not be excised but should be joined together and left *in situ*. However, others have objected to this proposal and consider that the cells from these lateral parts of the keloid are more active in terms of collagen production [15]. The combination of scar resection and immediate postoperative radiotherapy was proposed many years ago, and both electron beam irradiation and brachytherapy with iridium 192 can be used after surgical removal of the keloid to reduce recurrence rates. Disadvantages of this treatment include radiodermatitis, atrophy, and the theorical possibility of carcinogenesis.

Atrophic Scars

Atrophic scars appear as concave recesses in the skin and result from net tissue loss, including collagen [11]. There are frequent lesions in high-mobility areas because of excess tension on the wound at the time of wound closure. They may appear as an adverse effect of intralesional corticosteroids (Figures 31.18 through Figure 31.20).

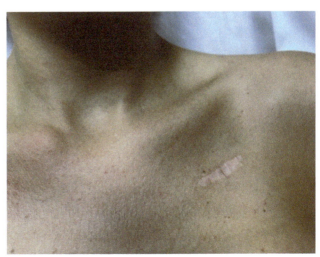

FIGURE 31.18 Atrophic scar; central venous access removal.

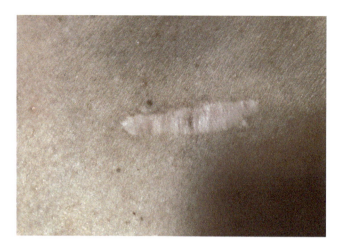

FIGURE 31.19 Atrophic scar: Highlights the thinning of the dermis and the change of skin pigmentation

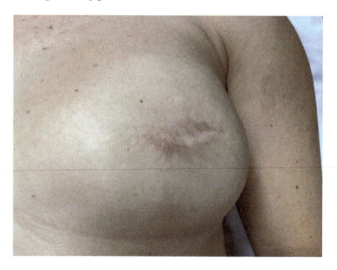

FIGURE 31.20 Atrophic scar; mastectomy scar.

Fat Grafting

To correct the lack of volume, fat grafting techniques can be used. When possible, a donor area close to the wound will be used, in order to obtain fatty tissue of similar characteristics. We recommend avoiding overcorrection, and more than one procedure may be necessary to achieve an optimum result. The presence of stromal vascular fraction and stem cells in the fat graft not only replaces the volume but also stimulates neoangiogenesis, an increase in collagen synthesis, and, in short, the quality of the skin and scar.

Laser Therapy

To correct the associated hypopigmentation and the presence of telangiectasias, laser therapy and micropigmentation can improve the cosmetic result. The main goal of laser therapy will be to reduce the deepness of the edges and stimulate neocollagenesis to fill in the hollows. It is advisable to extend the treatment to the entire cosmetic unit to avoid demarcation lines between the treated and untreated areas. We use lasers within the infrared spectrum, since they act on the mid to deep dermis. The systems of choice are ablative fractioned therapies. Tissue

ablation makes the recovery of the skin layer more uniform, and the heating of the deep dermis promotes the neoformation of collagen [8]. In those cases where a 5- to 7-day recovery time is not possible, and lesions are mild or moderate, we can achieve good results through fractioned-type nonablative systems.

Revision Surgery

In the presence of an atrophic scar, not subject to tension forces at the time of medical control and in areas of low mobility, surgical revision may be considered. We must use an optimal surgical technique, closing depth planes and initiating postoperative care early.

Scar Management in Pediatric Populations

There is a higher incidence in the pediatric population of developing hypertrophic and keloid scars. Pediatric age acts as a risk factor, and therefore, early initiation of prophylaxis is recommended. Therapeutic compliance is usually complicated, so we prefer simple and inconspicuous posologies to noninvasive measures. Pediatric oncological surgery implies a high psychological impact, both for the child and for the parents. The scar, which will change with the child, will be a permanent memory. Diagnoses of joint contractures or major retractions in the eyelid and lip should be addressed early; delayed treatment could involve important functional consequences (limitation of joint range, visual alteration, speech disturbances).

Silicone gel therapy will form the first line of treatment. Intralesional infiltration of corticosteroids is recommended, since the triamcinolone acetonide injectable suspension contains benzyl alcohol, which has been reported to cause toxicity in neonates [11]. It is recommended to prepare the infiltration zone with topical lidocaine cream, which will reduce the pain and fear of later infiltrations. In the pediatric population, autologous fat transfer has been indicated for the improvement of scars and associated malformations. Relatively few safety reports involving fractional laser scar treatment in the pediatric population exist in the literature. Lasers can be associated with significant discomfort during treatment, which is an important consideration for pediatric patients.

Conclusions

Making the scar disappear—a very frequent request among patients—is not possible. We must know the patients' expectations and explain the benefits we can achieve, taking into account individual limitations. There is no set therapeutic plan; we must adapt to each individual and to the characteristics of their scar. We must make the patient participate in decision-making and therapy management. The stigmatization resulting from the "cancer" label makes the scar more relevant, so we must be less tolerant about the result. However, we are talking about aggressive scars, visible in many cases, and located in unfavorable areas, which makes treating them more complicated. Prevention is key to achieve an optimum scar. Detecting risk factors and changes in the scar itself will determine the start of the prophylactic treatment. The use of a combined treatment has proven the most efficient. Patients should be monitored continuously.

REFERENCES

1. Wallace HA, Bhimji SS. *Wound, Healing, Phases. StatPearls [Internet].* Treasure Island, FL: StatPearls Publishing: 2018.

2. Vercelli S, Ferriero G, Sartorio F et al. Clinimetric properties and clinical utility in rehabilitation of postsurgical scar rating scales: A systematic review. *Int J Rehabil Res.* 2015; 38(4):279–86.

3. Pluvy I, Garrido I, Pauchot J et al. Smoking and plastic surgery, part I. Pathophysiological aspects: Update and proposed recommendations. *Ann Chir Plast Esthet.* 2015;60(1):3–13.

4. Sørensen LT. Wound Healing and Infection in Surgery: The Pathophysiological Impact of Smoking, Smoking Cessation, and Nicotine Replacement Therapy. *Ann Surg.* 2012;255(6):1069–79.

5. Roy M, Perry JA, Cross KM. Nutrition and the Plastic Surgeon: Possible Interventions and Practice Considerations. *Plast Reconstr Surg Glob Open.* 2018;6(8):e1704.

6. Stechmiller JK. Understanding the Role of Nutrition and Wound Healing. *Nutr Clin Pract.* 2010;25:61–8.

7. Garrigós Sancristobal X. Manejo de la piel radiada. *Heridas Y Cicatrización.* 2015;19(5): 6–11.

8. Del Pozo Losada J, Vieira Dos Santos V. Láser y cicatrices. *Heridas Y Cicatrización.* 2016;6(3):6–28.

9. Meaume S, Le Pillouer-Prost A, Richert B et al. Management of scars: Updated practical guidelines and use of silicones. *Eur J Dermatol.* 2014;24(4):435–43.

10. Marini L, Odendaal D, Smirnyi S. Importance of scar prevention and treatment. An approach from wound care principles. *Dermatol Surg.* 2017;43:85–90.

11. Krakowski AC, Totri CR, Donelan MB et al. Scar management in the pediatric and adolescent populations. *Pediatrics.* 2016;137(2):2014–65.

12. Tziotzios C, Profyris C, Sterling J. Cutaneous scarring: Pathophysiology, molecular mechanisms, and scar reduction therapeutics. *J Am Acad Dermatol.* 2012;66:13–24.

13. Mokos ZB, Jovic A, Grgurevic L et al. Current Therapeutic Approach to hypertrophic scars. *Front Med.* 2017;4(83):1–11.

14. Butzelaar L, Ulrich MM, Mink van der Molen A et al. Currently known risk factors for hypertrophic skin scarring: A review. *J Plast Reconstr Aesthet Surg.* 2016;69:163–9.

15. Monstrey S, Middelkoop E, Vranckx JJ et al. Update scar management practical guidelines: Non-invasive and invasive measures. *J Plast Reconstr Aesthet Surg.* 2014;6:1017–25.

16. Darougrsheh A, Asilian A, Shariati F. Intralesional triamcinolone alone or in combination with 5-fluorouracil for the treatment of keloid and hypertrophic scars. *Clin Exp Dermatol.* 2009;34:219–23.

17. Aggarwal H, Saxena A, Lubana PS et al. Treatment of keloids and hypertrophic scars using bleom. *J Cosmet Dermatol.* 2008;7:43–9.

18. Lee RC, Doong H, Jellema AF. The response of burn scars to intralesional verapamil. Report of five cases. *Arch Surg.* 1994;129(1):107–11.

19. Li Z, Jin Z. Comparative effect and safety of verapamil in keloid and hypertrophic scar treatment: A meta-analysis. *Ther Clin Risk Manag.* 2016;12:1635–41.

20. Vrijman C, Van Drooge AM, Limpens J et al. Laser and intense pulsed light therapy for the treatment of hypertrophic scars: A systematic review. *Br J Dermatol.* 2011;165(5):934–42.

21. Waibel JS, Wulkan AJ, Shumaker PR. Treatment of hypertrophic scars using laser and laser assisted corticosteroid delivery. *Lasers Surg Med.* 2013;45:135–40.

22. Xiao Z, Zhang F, Cui Z. Treatment of hypertrophic scars with intralesional botulinum toxin type A injections: A preliminary report. *Aesthetic Plast Surg.* 2009;33(3):409–12.

23. European Wound Management Association (EWMA). *Position Documents: Hard-To-Heal Wounds: A Holistic Approach.* London: MEP Ltd, 2008.

32

Cancer and Physical Exercise

Rosa Revert

Introduction

The World Health Organization has published global data on physical activity: the results warn of a fall in physical activity during the twenty-first century and reveal that more than 1.4 billion adults are at risk of cardiovascular disease, type 2 diabetes, dementia, and some cancers because they do not perform enough exercise. The main national and international scientific societies also warn and report about the beneficial effects of physical exercise for health [33].

Cancer is today a chronic disease that can be counteracted to some extent if we maintain healthy habits of life and a good quality of life throughout its duration. Part of that quality of life lies in performing physical exercise before, during, and after the illness. Oncology patients face, in addition to the disease itself, some treatments and terrible consequences (fatigue, asthenia, nausea, changes in body weight, etc.), in which physical exercise is especially recommended. It has been demonstrated that a program of physical exercise of aerobic endurance or strength, combined with another of balance and flexibility, is an effective complementary treatment in multiple chronic diseases, including chronic fatigue syndrome (very common in oncology patients) and cancer itself [7,11,15].

Physical Exercise and Cancer Prevention

Multiple studies have been published that demonstrate an association between the appearance of cancer and a sedentary lifestyle.

With regard to breast cancer, most studies conclude that women who perform more physical exercise throughout their lives have less probability—close to 30%—of developing this type of cancer [20]. The activity has to be at least of moderate intensity (such as walking at a speed of 5 km/h, for 30–60 minutes) or more intense exercise (such as walking at more than 5 km/h, running, cycling, etc., for 7–9 hours per week). This level of activity seems to reduce the risk of breast cancer by up to 37% [14,39,42].

If physical activity is combined with a reduction in other risk factors that can be modified, such as diet, avoiding smoking, or getting rid of hormone therapies, the risk of cancer can decrease by up to 50% [22]. In addition, there are several studies that suggest that regular physical exercise before being diagnosed with breast cancer reduces the risk of mortality from any cause and of recurrence of this cancer.

The realization is that physical exercise causes an increase in energy expenditure and with it a reduction in body fat, which is a risk factor and also a better control of blood glucose levels, causing therefore a lower concentration of plasma insulin. The latter is inversely related to sex hormone–binding globulin. If plasma insulin increases, estrogen and free androgen, that facilitate the development of breast cancer, increase; however, if plasma insulin decreases, the free sex hormones in the blood decrease, thereby decreasing the risk [3].

Physical Exercise during Oncological Disease

Exercise is beneficial if cancer is established but should always be supervised by trained specialists, physiotherapists, or rehabilitative doctors. It can be confirmed that physical exercise could be considered part of the oncological treatment, obviously after the necessary medical or surgical treatment. Sometimes it can be difficult to convince a sick patient to practice exercise, but the benefits are multiple.

If properly done, exercise leads to a significant reduction in cancer mortality, in the recurrence of the disease, and in mortality from any cause [19,29,35]. In the case of breast cancer, this reduction in the risk of mortality can be close to 50% after 2–5 years in patients who exercise by walking at a good rate (close to 5 km/h) for 30 or more minutes per day. (This occurs only by walking.)

The positive effects of a physical training program observed in women diagnosed with breast cancer seem to be due to two reasons [12]:

1. Decrease in base blood levels of breast cancer risk markers (insulin, sex hormones, cytokines, and cholesterol)
2. Increase in blood concentrations of catecholamines, cytokines, and immune cells during exercise and the first hours of recovery

Therefore, performing physical exercise causes both a reduction in harmful factors and an increase in beneficial factors.

All this suggests that aerobic physical training could be an effective adjuvant strategy combined with the antitumor efficacy of chemotherapeutic agents.

Exercise increases the vascularization of the tumor, which usually presents with a disorganized vascular system. This increase in vascularity benefits the arrival of medication and natural killer (NK) cells.

Exercise also causes an increase in immune function. The release to the blood of NK cells, but also of T cells, B cells, and macrophages, allows a greater action of these cells against the tumor due to their greater number and greater destructive capacity [31].

Furthermore, the tumor cells use a lot of glucose and produce a lot of lactate. This high production of lactate can inhibit the immune function on the tumor, but it has been seen that physical training is accompanied by a decrease in the use of glucose and the lactate production of the tumor, so it also can favor the action of cells of the immune system.

Additionally, it seems that muscle contraction produces the release of substances that inhibit the growth of cancer cells [17].

In conclusion, it can be affirmed that frequent physical exercise performed after being diagnosed with cancer is an effective treatment to increase survival and reduce recurrence.

Physical Exercise and Side Effects of Oncological Treatments

The oncological treatments have different mechanisms of action that have in common that their effect is not exclusive on the tumor cell; they are capable of causing the alteration of the cell cycle of cancer cells, but also of healthy cells, so they can damage healthy tissue in addition to destroying cancer cells. This causes a lot of side effects that exert a negative impact on the physical and psychological well-being of patients with the consequent decrease in their quality of life.

In addition to side effects on skin and mucous membranes, oncological treatments can decrease cardiovascular and pulmonary function. General malaise, asthenia, sleep disturbances, nausea and vomiting, and generalized amyotrophy are also among the most striking and frequent side effects in cancer patients.

Although these side effects usually peak during treatment, symptoms related to therapy may persist for months or even years with consequent decline in quality of life.

Both aerobic and strength training programs have been shown to be effective for fatigue, physical condition, energy and vitality, body image, mental health, and quality of life during posttreatment breast cancer care [8,18,32,36].

Fatigue is very common in cancer patients during and after treatment. Traditionally, rest was recommended, but it has been seen that fatigue not only does not improve with rest, but even gets worse. However, supervised exercise, both aerobic and strength, has a positive effect on fatigue [25]. It is observed that these positive effects are greater when the exercise programs last more than 28 weeks, with a frequency of two to three sessions per week of about 40 minutes/session. It may be enough to walk at a good rate.

Oncological treatments can lead to the loss of bone mass, which causes high levels of osteoporosis. In addition, there may be bone involvement due to metastasis, which weakens it. In both cases, the risk of fractures increases, especially in the spine, hip, femur, and/or arms (long bones). In these cases, although the exercise is positive because it increases bone mineral density, or at least partially preserves it, it is essential to prevent falls and

avoid high-intensity exercises, such as running; it is better for these patients to exercise with stationary bicycle or walk. It is believed that the increase of the mechanical load of the bones and the secretion of hormones (parathyroid hormone [PTH] and growth hormone [GH]) during the exercise, together with the increase of the mass and the muscular force that is observed after several weeks of training, supply suitable stimuli for increased bone mineral mass [5,6].

In the specific case of breast cancer, another particularly disabling side effect, lymphedema, is added. It is a sequel that affects about 30% of women treated surgically. Lymphedema is a debilitating condition that causes great anguish in the patient, worsens the performance of ordinary tasks, socially excludes women, and constantly reminds her of the presence of cancer. Controlled and supervised physical activity could have a positive effect on the symptoms of lymphedema, whereas sedentary lifestyle contributes to its deterioration [37]. The performance of aerobic physical exercise can improve the movement of neighboring joints, reverse muscle atrophy, and activate the skeletal muscles that help pump the lymph, resulting in reduction of lymph volume. In addition, the sympathetic tone of the lymphatic vessels is reestablished [23,24]. It is important that the exercises do not cause pain, and they will have to be adjusted to the stage of each patient's disease. In general, the best regimen is to combine stretching and aerobic exercises: swimming (which avoids impact), vigorous walking, cycling, and other disciplines (pilates, yoga, etc.) are *a priori* exercises that can prevent and improve lymphedema.

This disease also produces psychological consequences. It is not easy to face a pathology of this type, and the appearance of depression, anxiety, and stress is frequent. Patients with cancer who perform aerobic exercise have fewer depressive symptoms. The more minutes of aerobic physical exercise performed per week, the greater is the decrease in these symptoms [7].

Even less common exercise programs, such as tai chi or yoga, are accompanied by physical and psychological improvements and improvements in the quality of life of these patients [10,13].

Cancer and Complementary Therapies

People with cancer usually present high levels of anxiety and sleep problems, due both to the emotional and physical impact of the disease, as well as to the cancer treatments themselves [2,25,26]. Anything that can improve the mood of the patient in any way can have a beneficial effect on the development of the disease. The body reacts to physical, mental, or emotional pressure by releasing so-called stress hormones (such as epinephrine and norepinephrine) that increase blood pressure, accelerate heart rate, and elevate serum glucose concentrations. All these reactions weaken the immune system; stressful states are proinflammatory states that could even favor the proliferation of cancer. Extreme anguish is associated with worse predictions and a higher mortality rate, although the mechanism for this to occur is not entirely clear [30,38].

In addition to the direct influence of stress on the cells, there is also the possibility that the person affected by the cancer may give up, feel helpless, and not seek or not follow useful therapy; they can even adopt risky behaviors and not maintain healthy life habits, which could lead to premature death.

Conversely, patients who maintain adequate levels of anxiety have a higher survival rate. The reduction of stress influences markers of immune function, on the regulation of the hypothalamic-pituitary-adrenal axis, and the activity of the autonomic nervous system [38].

Relaxation techniques can help to alleviate some of the most frequent symptoms among people with cancer who are undergoing drug and/or surgical treatments, such as pain, anxiety, and depressive symptoms or sleep disorders. Feeling good helps you on the way to being better.

With regard to this, techniques such as mindfulness and yoga may have their place as a coadjuvant treatment in neoplastic disease [10,16,41]. It seems that yoga can be an alternative to reduce stress levels and is useful for improving sleep problems among survivors, as well as improving mood [9,13,27,40]. Benefits of the regular practice of certain yoga asanas on upper and lower limb lymphedema have also been observed as an adjunct to lymphatic drainage [1,21,28].

Another discipline for combating psychological stress is mindfulness. Mindfulness is a practice related to Buddhist meditation that was created in 1979 by Kabat Zinn, physician and founder of the Clinic of Stress Reduction at the University of Massachusetts. It is a technique that teaches us to live in balance with what we think, feel, and do, focusing on the present. Mindfulness focuses on self-regulation of attention and a state of consciousness that is associated with nonjudgmental, moment-to-moment, awareness, patience, and calmness, nonstriving, letting go, and compassion [4]. The practice of mindfulness contributes mainly to reduce stress, anxiety, and depression. There is evidence that it improves the quality of sleep and fatigue (two serious problems in oncological patients) and also promotes personal growth [34].

With training, relaxation techniques can be a good help to improve the quality of life of the cancer patient, although more work is necessary on this topic.

REFERENCES

1. Aggithaya MG, Narahari SR, Ryan TJ. Yoga for correction of lymphedema's impairment of gait as an adjunct to lymphatic drainage: A pilot observational study. *Int J Yoga.* 2015 Jan;8(1):54–612.
2. Artherholt SB, Fann JR. Psychosocial care in cancer. *Curr Psychiatry Rep.* 2012;14(1):23–9.
3. Bianchini F, Kaaks R, Vainio H. Weight control and physical activity in cancer prevention. *Obes Rev.* 2002;3:5–8.
4. Bishop SR, Lau M et al. Mindfulness: A proposed operational definition. *Clin Psychol Sci Pract.* 2004;11:230–41.
5. Borch KB, Braaten T, Lund E, Weiderpass E. Physical activity before and after breast cancer diagnosis and survival - the Norwegian women and cancer cohort study. *BMC Cancer.* 2015;15:967.
6. Borer KT, Fogleman K, Gross M, La New JM, Dengel D. Walking intensity for postmenopausal bone mineral preservation and accrual. *Bone.* 2007;41(4):713–21.
7. Brown C, Huedo-Medina TB et al. The efficacy of exercise in reducing depressive symptoms among cancer survivors: A Meta-Analysis. *PLOS ONE.* 2012;7:e30955. doi:10.1371/journal. pone.0030955. Epub 2012 Jan 27.

8. Buchan J, Janda M, Box R, Schmitz K, Hayes S. A Randomized Trial on the Effect of Exercise Mode on Breast Cancer-Related Lymphedema. *Med Sci Sports Exerc.* 2016;48(10):1866–74.
9. Buffart LM, van Uffelen JG, Riphagen II, Brug J, van Mechelen W, Brown WJ, Chinapaw MJ. Physical and psychosocial benefits of yoga in cancer patients and survivors, a systematic review and meta-analysis of randomized controlled trials. *BMC Cancer.* 2012 Nov 27;12:559.
10. Chandwani KD, Perkins G et al. Randomized, controlled trial of yoga in women with breast cancer undergoing radiotherapy. *J Clin Oncol.* 2014;32:1058–65.
11. Chomistek AK, Cook NR, Flint AJ, Rimm EB. Vigorous-intensity leisure-time physical activity and risk of major chronic disease in men. *Med Sci Sports Exerc.* 2012;44(10):1898–905.
12. Dethlefsen C, Lillelund C, Midtgaard J, Andersen C, Pedersen BK, Christensen JF, Hojman P. Exercise regulates breast cancer cell viability: Systemic training adaptations versus acute exercise responses. *Breast Cancer Res Treat.* 2016;159(3):469–79.
13. Yagli V, Ulger O. The effects of yoga on the quality of life and depression in elderly breast cancer patients. *Comp Ther Clin Pract.* 2015;21:7–10.
14. Eliassen H, Hankinson SE, Rosner B, Holmes MD, Willett WC. Physical activity and risk of breast cancer among postmenopausal women. *Arch Intern Med.* 2010;170(19):1758–64.
15. Fiuza-Luces C, Garatachea N, Berger NA, Lucia A. Exercise is the Real Polypill. *Physiology (Bethesda).* 2013;28(5), 330.
16. Heidemarie H, Winkler MM et al. Ereview. Mindfulness-based interventions for women with breast cancer: And updated systematic review and meta-analysis. *Acta Oncol.* 2017;56.12:1665–7.
17. Hojman P, Dethlefsen C, Brandt C, Hansen J, Pedersen L, Pedersen BK. Exercise-induced muscle-derived cytokines inhibit mammary cancer cell growth. *Am J Physiol Endocrinol Metab.* 2011;301:E504–10.
18. Zeng Y, Huang M, Cheng ASK, Zhou Y, So WKW. Meta-analysis of the effects of exercise intervention on quality of life in breast cancer survivors. *Breast Cancer.* 2014;21: 262–74.
19. Lahart M, Metsios GS, Nevill AM, Carmichael AR. Physical activity, risk of death and recurrence in breast cancer survivors: A systematic review and meta-analysis of epidemiological studies. *Acta Oncol.* 2015;54(5):635–54.
20. Lee M. Physical activity and cancer prevention. Data from epidemiologic studies. *Med Sci Sports Exerc.* 2003;35:1823–7.
21. Loudon A, Barnett T, Piller N, Immink MA, Williams AD. Yoga management of breast-cancer related lymphoedema: A randomised controlled pilot-trial. *BMC Complement Altern Med.* 2014 Jul 1;14:214.
22. Lyon: International Agency for Research on Cancer. 2008.
23. Lun L, Liqin Y. et al. Current Treatments for breast cancer –related lymphedema: A systematic review. *Asian Pac J Cancer Prev.* 17(11):4875–83.
24. McKenzie DC. Abreast in a boat. A race against breast cancer. *CMAJ.* 1998;159:376–8.
25. Meneses-Echávez F, González-Jiménez E, Ramírez-Vélez R. Effects of supervised exercise on cancer-related fatigue in breast cancer survivors: A systematic review and meta-analysis. *BMC Cancer.* 2015;15:77.
26. Moreno-Smith M, Lutgendorf SK, Sood AK. Impact of stress on cancer metastasis. *Future Oncol.* 2010;6(12):1863–81.

27. Mustian KM. Yoga as treatment for insomnia among cancer patients and survivors: A systematic review. *Eur Med J Oncol.* 2013 Nov 1;1:106–15.

28. Narahari SR, Aggithaya MG, Thernoe L, Bose KS, Ryan TJ. Yoga protocol for treatment of breast cancer-related lymphedema. *Int J Yoga.* 2016 Jul–Dec;9(2):145–55.

29. Zhong S, Jiang T et al. Association between physical activity and mortality in breast cancer: A meta-analysis of cohort studies. *Eur J Epidemiol.* 2014;29(6):391–404.

30. Krizanova O, Babula P, Pacak K. Stress, catecholaminergic system and cancer. *Stress.* 2016;19:4, 419–428.

31. Pedersen L, Christensen JF, Hojman P. Effects of exercise on tumor physiology and metabolism. *Cancer J.* 2015;21(2): 111–6.

32. Pinto B, Frierson G, Rabin C, Trunzo J, Marcus B. Home-based physical activity intervention for breast cancer patients. *J Clin Oncol.* 2005;23:3577–87.

33. Recomendaciones mundiales sobre actividad fisica para la salud. Ginebra, OMS, 2010.

34. Roleau CR, Garland SN, Carlson LE. The impact of mindfulness-based interventions on symptom burden, positive psychological outcomes, and biomarkers in cancer patients. *Cancer Manag Res.* 2015;7:121–31.

35. Schmid D, Leitzmann MF. Association between physical activity and mortality among breast cancer and colorectal cancer survivors: A systematic review and meta-analysis. *Ann Oncol.* 2014;25(7):1293–311.

36. Schmitz H, Holtzman J, Courneya KS, Mâsse LC, Duval S, Kane R. Controlled physical activity trials in cancer survivors: A systematic review and meta-analysis. *Cancer Epidemiol Biomarkers Prev.* 2005;14:1588–95.

37. Schmitz KH, Courneya KS et al. American College of Sports Medicine. American College of Sports Medicine roundtable on exercise guidelines for cancer survivors. *Med Sci Sports Exerc.* 2010;42:1409–26.

38. Segerstrom SC, Miller GE. Psychological stress and the human immune system: A meta-analytic study of 30 years of inquiry. *Psychol Bull.* 2004;130(4):601–30.

39. Sharma M. Yoga as an alternative and complementary approach for stress management: A systematic review. *J Evid Based Complementary Altern Med.* 2014 Jan;19(1):59–67.

40. Si S, Boyle T, Heyworth J, Glass DC, Saunders C, Fritschi L. Lifetime physical activity and risk of breast cancer in pre- and post-menopausal women. *Breast Cancer Res Treat.* 2015;152(2):449–62.

41. Pouy S, Fatemeh A et al. Investigating the effect of Mindfulness-Based Training on Psychological Status an Quality of Life in Patients with Breast Cancer. *Asian Pac J Cancer Prev.* 2018:19.7:1993–8.

42. Thune I, Brenn T, Lund E, Gaard M. Physical activity and the risk of breast cancer. *N Engl J Med.* 1997;336:1269–75.

33

Ozone Therapy in Oncology Patients

Adriana Schwartz

Within the molecular mechanisms of cancer, reactive oxygen species play a fundamental role; they are capable of acting on vital processes such as angiogenesis and apoptosis [1].

Angiogenesis and the inhibition of apoptosis are two processes that favor tumor development. It is known that factors that promote angiogenesis are activated by oxidative stress; for example, when endothelial cells are exposed for 30 minutes to hydrogen peroxide (H_2O_2), a stimulation of angiogenesis is observed. It has now been shown that reactive oxygen species (ROS) such as the superoxide anion radical and H_2O_2 are involved in neovascularization [1].

Apoptosis as known, is programmed cell death, which can occur via receptor activation or the mitochondrial pathway; these mechanisms involve endonucleases as caspases [1]. There have been studies of how H_2O_2 activates caspase 3, reflecting the role of EROS in activating apoptosis. It is further reported that EROS cause overexpression of the tumor necrosis factor receptor CD95 ligand during programmed cell death. All this shows that the control of EROS levels at the tissue and cell level could be important in the treatment of cancer [1–3].

Conversely, tumor cells block the receptor sites of the T lymphocytes causing a failure in the immune system, so adequate modulation of the immune system would be useful in the treatment of cancer [1–6].

Another detail to highlight is that in cancer cells, failure in the metabolism of oxygen leads to a deficient production of antioxidant enzymes, giving rise to an oxidative environment at the level of the tumor tissue [5–7].

A direct effect of O_3 on tumor cells has been described, or as an enhancer of the effect of radiotherapy or chemotherapy. However, these studies were mainly *in vitro*, in the laboratory; some in animals. Therefore, the direct effect has been evidenced in conditions very different from those used clinically during ozone therapy sessions. Clinically, with some exceptions, O_3 does not come into direct contact with tumor cells, and its multiple effects are mediated by second messengers (H_2O_2 and lipoperoxides) [1].

However, just as it is well established in other treatments such as hyperbaric chambers, ozone therapy could not only have a beneficial role as adjuvant during the treatment of some tumors, but could also have a much greater role even in the prevention and treatment of toxicities secondary to oncological treatments.

The basic mechanisms of action rest, in different combinations, on three principles:

- Modulation of the immune system
- Modulation of blood flow, oxygenation, and metabolism
- Modulation of the pro-oxidants/antioxidants balance

Additionally, other effects of O_3 may be beneficial at times, such as its germicidal properties when it is used to treat infected ulcers or wounds (or those at risk of infection).

Mechanism of Action of Ozone

The therapeutic properties of ozone are basically conditioned by two independent mechanisms:

1. *Direct oxidizing capacity*: Its great oxidizing power makes it react directly with microbial walls and exert its germicidal effects or, for example, makes it react directly with mediators of inflammation and pain or cytokine receptors and block biological responses [1,4].

2. *Indirect effects*: These are related to those that take place after the interaction with O_3-biomolecules; in this case, organic peroxides, H_2O_2, ozonides, aldehydes, and other oxidation products generated in adequate and controlled quantities activate endogenous response mechanisms to the stress, managing to rebalance the redox environment that had been altered by the underlying pathology. While the initial mechanism shows the short-term effects of O_3, this second mechanism requires time, which is why the application of a therapeutic cycle is required with several stimuli to achieve most of the effects of O_3 [1,4].

Both mechanisms are responsible for the biological and late therapeutic effects of ozone. The transient presence of elevated H_2O_2 concentrations in the cytoplasm of cells treated with O_3 indicates that H_2O_2 acts as one of the chemical messengers of ozone and that its concentration is critical, which means that it must be above a certain threshold to be effective, but not sufficiently high to cause damage. The small, transient, and calculated oxidative stress that is reached at therapeutic doses (low doses) is necessary to activate a series of inhibited biological functions, without causing adverse effects. It is recognized that H_2O_2 is an intracellular signaling compound, capable of activating thyroxine kinase, which phosphorylates the nuclear transcription factor Nrf2, with the consequent synthesis of different antioxidant proteins. H_2O_2 is capable of acting on mononuclear blood cells, platelets, endothelial cells, and erythrocytes.

It is important to point out that good therapeutic results can be achieved when ozone is applied in adequate doses and via the correct routes. In this way, no adverse reactions or genotoxic injury may occur, and the wide beneficial spectrum of effects it generates makes possible its application in a great diversity of medical specialties and, within these, in a variety of processes.

Ozone in Oxygen Metabolism

The oxygen supply to the tissues improves after ozone therapy. These effects respond to different mechanisms, and there are several experimental pointers to confirm this phenomenon. Ozone therapy reverses the erythrocyte aggregation of occlusive arterial diseases by changes in the electric charges of the erythrocyte membrane. The increase in the rate of glycolysis in the erythrocyte is accompanied by a significant increase in the exchange of sodium and potassium ions, which are responsible for maintaining the membrane electrical potential, normalizing the exchange of such ions. Occlusive arterial diseases are related to the loss of the normal potential of the erythrocyte plasmatic membrane. The normalization of ion exchange by ozone and its products favors the restoration of normal membrane potential. Accordingly, through regeneration of the normal electrical conditions of the membrane, ozone promotes the recovery of the flexibility and plasticity of the erythrocytes, thus improving the rheological properties of the blood and improving oxygen transport. In addition, during the treatment with ozone, a lower settling velocity is observed, with a decrease in viscosity, which explains the improvement in hemorrhagic indicators of these patients [1–5].

Ozone can increase 2,3-DPG (2,3 diphosphoglycerate) in erythrocytes, which produces changes in the dissociation curve of hemoglobin (Hb), shifting the balance HbO_2/Hb to the right ($HbO_2 + 2,3\text{-DPG} \rightarrow \text{Hb-}2,3\text{-DPG} + O_2$). It has been described that this increase could only occur in those patients with decreased baseline levels (pre-O_3) [3]. The production of the Bohr effect could also contribute to this effect on Hb. The final result is that Hb increases the transfer of O_2 to tissues [14].

In addition, ozone improves the flexibility of the erythrocyte and the rheological properties of the blood, decreasing the blood viscosity [4], and it induces the production of NO by vascular endothelial cells, producing vasodilatation at the microcirculation level. These two effects decrease peripheral vascular resistance, which, in the end, leads to an increase in blood flow [4].

Additionally, ozone has effects on cerebral blood flow: there were increases in diastolic velocity in the middle cerebral artery compatible with a decrease in vascular resistance, an improvement in rheological properties, and therefore, an increase in blood flow (corroborated by observed increases in blood flow in the common carotid artery). Some experiments have also observed satisfactory results in the oxygenation of resting muscles after treatment with ozone, especially in those with greater hypoxia [14].

When choosing doses, one must take into account the stage of the disease, the tumor markers, the clinical status of the patient, and the response of the same to conventional therapy.

Although the number of patients with neoplasia treated with ozone is small compared to those for other disease states, it has been observed first that the ozone dose scheme used in these patients has not caused adverse effects and second that it has proved the quality of life of these patients, albeit in a temporary way.

Ozone Therapy as an Immunomodulator Agent

It has also been shown that EROS promotes damage to proteins [8–11]; this damage, if not regulated in time, could decrease the efficiency of DNA repair enzymes, causing conformational changes in affecting replication, resulting in an increase in mutations, breaking the balance between the oncogenes and the tumor suppressor genes, as happens in cancer. As a stimulatory therapy for endogenous antioxidant enzyme systems, by decreasing EROS concentrations, ozone therapy could protect proteins from oxidative damage and thus inhibit this cascade.

Another effect of ozone therapy that could explain improvement in these patients is that under controlled dose schemes, ozone is an immunomodulator via activation-repression of the proinflammatory–anti-inflammatory activity of interleukins in a manner that is concentration-dependent [10–12]; the cancer cell modifies the receptor of the T lymphocyte, leading the patient to immunosuppression. Ozone is able to activate the immunocompetent cells and in this way help to improve the quality of life of the patient with cancer [1,2,10–12].

Finally, there is another effect of ozone therapy that could be taken into account for the treatment of cancer patients—its role as a therapy to increase levels of prostacyclins [13]. Since 1881, prostacyclin has been recognized as an antimetastatic agent [13], and the effect of ozone therapy on the elevation of prostacyclin in blood and urine of different species has been demonstrated in different research works [1,2,13]. This effect of ozone could be beneficial in the treatment of cancer and its complications.

In conclusion, ozone therapy as an adjuvant treatment in oncology patients could improve the results of chemotherapy and radiotherapy in some tumors, as well as serve to prevent or treat some side effects of these treatments. There are a growing number of scientific articles that justify this rationale; however, the final demonstration will depend on properly conducted clinical trials.

REFERENCES

1. Adriana S et al. Manual de Ozonoterapia Clínica, Medizeus S.L., ISBN: 2017: 978–84-617-9394-5.
2. International Scientific Committee of Ozone Therapy. *Madrid Declaration on Ozone Therapy.* 2nd ed. Madrid: ISCO3; ISBN 978-84-606-8312-4; 2015. 50 p.
3. Mattassi R, D'Angelo F, Bisetti P, Colombo R, Vaghi M. Terapia con ozono per via parenterale nelle arteriopatie obliteranti periferiche: Mecanismo biochimico e risultati clinici. *G Chir.* 1987;VIII:109–11.
4. Giunta R, Coppola A, Luongo C et al. Ozonized autohemotransfusion improves hemorheological parameters and oxygen delivery to tissues in patients with peripheral occlusive arterial disease. *Ann Hematol.* 2001;80(12):745–8.
5. Bocci V. *Oxygen–Ozone Therapy. A Critical Evaluation.* AH Dordrecht. The Netherlands: Kluwer Academic Publishers, 2002.
6. Bocci V. Scientific and medical aspects of ozone therapy. State of the art. *Arch Med Res.* 2006;37:425–35.
7. Rodríguez Y, Menendez S, Turrents J, Matos E. Actividad Antitumoral del Ozono. *Rev. CENIC. Ciencias Biológicas* 1998;39(3).

8. Jamieh HH, Berlanga J, Merino N, Sánchez G, Carmona A, Menéndez-Cepero S, Giuliani A, Re L, León OS. Role of protein synthesis in the protection conferred by ozone-oxidative-preconditioning in hepatic ischaemia/reperfusion. *Transpl Int.* 2005;18(5):604–12.

9. Menendez S, Cepero J, Borrego L. Ozone therapy in cancer treatment: State of the art. *Ozone: Science and Engineering* 2008;30:398–404. Copyright 2008 International Ozone Association.

10. Zamora Z, Borrego A, Orlay Y, Delgado R, González R. Effects of ozone oxidative preconditioning on TNFalfa release and antioxidant prooxidant intracellular balance in mice during endotoxic shock. *Mediat Inflamm.* 2005;1:16–22.

11. Hui Chen, Bianzhi X, Xiuheng L, Jiangqiao Z. Ozone oxidative preconditioning inhibits inflammation and apoptosis in a rat model of renal ischemia/reperfusion injury. *Eur J Pharmacol.* 2008;581:306–14.

12. Schulz S, Haussler U, Mandic R, Heverhagen JT, Neubauer A, Dunne AA. Treatment with ozone/oxygen pneumoperitoneum results in complete remission of rabbit squamous cell carcinomas. *Int. J. Cancer.* 2008;122:2360–7.

13. Honn KV, Skoff A. Prostacyclin: A potent antimetastatic agent. *Science.* 12 June 1981:212(4500):1270–2.

14. Clavo B, Catalá L, Pérez JL, Rodríguez V, Robaina F. Ozone therapy on cerebral blood flow: A preliminary report. *eCAM.* 2004;1(3):315–9. doi:10.1093/ecam/neh039

34

Thermal Treatments in Postcancer Care

Ángela García Matas

Thermal Treatments in Postcancer

There are several factors that support thermal waters being used again as a therapeutic resource. There are many relevant publications in scientific journals. More financial support is available to get the treatment (e.g., government programs such as IMSERSO in Spain). Most important, there is a shift in thinking; patients now choose balneotherapy to treat chronic illnesses, especially in cancer patients, in order to treat the aftermath.

It is very important that doctors know the scope of these treatments and their indications and contraindications.

Thermal Treatment Components

First, we have to be aware that thermal cure has three components: thermal water and derived products, the route of administration, and the environment (the thermal place). We should also be aware that the thermal station is a medical facility; therefore, a doctor is needed to decide on the indications for treatments. Doctors, mineral-medicinal water (the drug), and medical facilities are all necessary for an environment conducive to healing.

Cancer patients are perfect candidates, as they have suffered an acute illness that has been turned into a chronic disease. They feel the adverse effects as well as the aftermath of the chemical and physical treatments used against cancer [1–7,17]. We can use thermal water to improve not only the physical treatment but also the psychic problems. The thermal environment is very appropriate for a patient wishing to gain or regain healthy ways of life.

Thermal Water: Concept and Classification

The term *thermal water* means natural mineral water with features that make it suitable for therapeutic use. We can find a lot of different classifications, but most include three parameters: *temperature*, *fixed residue*, and *chemical composition*. Of these, the classification based on chemical composition is the most helpful to understand how a mineral compound can be the principal identifying feature of "mineromedicinal" water, because most of the therapeutic activity is based on that.

The most common classifications are as follows.

Classification According to Temperature

- *Cold*: Below 20°C
- *Hypothermal*: Between 20°C and 30°C
- *Homothermal or thermal*: Between 30°C and 40°C
- *Hyperthermal*: Greater than 40°C

Classification According to Fixed Residue

Fixed residue consists of the total amount of dissolved substances contained in the water. The determination of fixed residue is a very important investigation, because fixed residue is part of the official classification of thermal and bottled waters with healing properties. It is normally expressed as fixed residue in mg/L:

- *Minimally mineralized waters*: Less than 50 mg/L
- *Slightly mineralized waters*: Less than 500 mg/L
- *Mineral waters*: Between 500 and 1000 mg/L
- *Waters rich in mineral salts*: Greater than 1500 mg/L

Classification According to Chemical Composition

Building on the chemical composition of the fixed residue, thermal water takes its name from the element or group of elements from which it is composed. While determining what kind of ionic composition there is in the water, we have to take into account first the prevalent anion (or anions) and then the cation. When an ion is greater than 20 mEq/L, this gives the water its name. According to prevalent ionic composition, mineral waters are classified as

- Bicarbonate waters
- Salt waters or with sodium chloride
- Sulfurous waters
- Arsenical-ferruginous waters
- Sulfated waters
- Radioactive waters

Often, when there are different prevalent ions present at the same time, the water will be called *multi-ionic mineral water*; each mineral has different properties to affect something in the human body (Table 34.1).

TABLE 34.1

Characteristics and Applications of Different Mineral Waters

Type of Mineral Water	Characteristics	Application
Salt waters or with sodium chloride	The chloride anion predominates, and most frequent cations are sodium, calcium, or magnesium. The total mineralization must exceed 1 (g/L). They are stimulating waters with different organic functions.	The principal indications are in rheumatology, dermatology, and upper and lower tract chronic respiratory diseases. They are used in states of exhaustion.
Sulfated waters	The anion sulfate is the most frequent. The total mineralization must exceed 1 (g/L).	Its main uses are in dyspepsia, digestive and biliary dyskinesias.
Sulfur waters	They contain more than 1 mg/L of sulfur bivalent, usually under the forms of hydrogen sulfide and phenyl sulfuric acids. Bivalent sulfur has a high oxidoreduction capacity.	Sulfur waters have their main indication in rheumatic, dermatologic, upper and lower tract chronic respiratory diseases. The skin, the digestive and respiratory mucosa, absorb the bivalent sulfur.
Bicarbonate waters	They are waters where the anion bicarbonate is in a concentration greater than 1 g/L.	This kind of water is usually for drinking. You can recommend if you want to improve pancreatic secretion, bilis secretion, or increase urine pH.
Acid carbonic waters	They are waters that contain a concentration greater than 250 mg/L of carbonic acid free.	Carbonic acid has a preserving side effect and kills bacteria. You can improve the acid secretion and bowel movements. You can use it, if you want to improve vascular and respiratory diseases. It produces arterial vasodilatation.
Radioactive waters	They are waters that contain a concentration greater than 67.3 Bq/L of radon gas.	The main indication for this kind of water is for psychiatric diseases. They are also indicated in rheumatology and respiratory diseases.

Source: Data from Sociedad Española de Hidrología Médica, https://www.hidromed.org, accessed April 2020.

The mineral-medicinal waters most indicated in postcancer care are those with ionic actives in the skin (sulfur, salt waters, selenium waters, and radioactive waters).

Route of Administration

Mineral-medicinal waters are drugs. We have different ways to use them in order to obtain different effects. In general terms, we can use mineral-medicinal waters (crenotherapy) via the oral route (drinking water or the hydroponic cure) or the topical route, depending on the result you wish to obtain.

Drinking water measure has to be defined by doctors (500 mL to 1 L or more). Topical waters could be applied with or without pressure and full body or not.

The following are the most appropriate ways to apply mineral-medicinal water in oncological processes.

Showers

Pressurized mineral-medicinal waters can be applied in a wide variety of types and are distinguished by the means of administration, the degree of pressure, and the temperature.

Circular shower: Low-pressure application of mineral-medicinal waters through multiple orifices arranged in a series of rings at different heights, with the same effect as a whole-body massage (Figure 34.1).

Contrast shower: Application of mineral-medicinal waters at two temperatures in which the water is applied alternately at hot and cold temperatures in order to generate a stimulant effect.

Filiform shower: Application of mineral-medicinal water through numerous holes no larger than a millimeter and at very high pressures (plus 12 atmospheres). It is used mainly in cases of skin diseases.

Vichy shower: Mixed technique combining the relaxing action of a vertical shower, while the patient simultaneously receives a massage according to individual particular needs; the name is Vichy massage.

Jet shower: The balneotherapist directs a high-pressure jet of up to 2.5 kg on the surface of the body according to a technique specifically adapted to each individual patient. This treatment has an effect that is both invigorating and energizing. Muscle tone is increased, the nervous system is balanced, blood circulation is activated, and the skin condition improved.

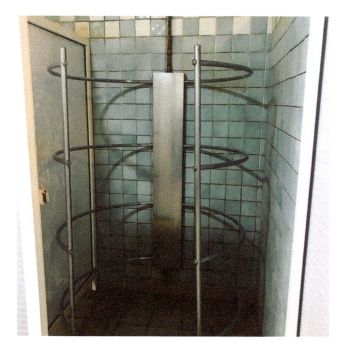

FIGURE 34.1 Circular shower.

Baths

The term *bath* is given to all those techniques based on the immersion of the body or any of its parts in mineral-medicinal waters. The temperature and duration of a bath depends on the treatment prescribed.

A temperature range of 37°C–39°C (10–30 minutes) has a relaxing effect. For a stimulating bath, a temperature of 34°C or less is required. These immersions can be total or partial, individual or collective, and can take place in baths, tanks, or pools.

Whirlpools: Baths pumped with air or thermal gas by means of an underwater programmable jet, applied either locally to the specific area to be treated or generally in order to achieve a relaxing effect.

Hydromassage baths: Baths with the addition of current waters by means of an underwater programmable jet, designed to produce an overall massaging effect and have a relaxing action.

Respiratory Therapy (Mucositis)

Thermal water can be directly applied to the respiratory mucous membranes using specific medical devices, which break the water into tiny droplets and allow them to be inhaled through the mouth and nose, reaching the higher and lower respiratory tracts (Figure 34.2).

Products Derived from Thermal Water: Peloids

Peloid therapy consists of mud used therapeutically, as part of balneotherapy, or therapeutic bathing (Figure 34.3). Peloids consist of humus and minerals formed over many years by geological and biological, chemical, and physical processes. The water-soluble peat substances pass transdermally in sufficient quantities to induce a biological effect; the "human skin possesses a selective permeability for the water-soluble fulvic and ulmic acids and derivative fraction isolated as peat extract" [18]. The bacteriostatic and bactericidal activities of humic acid have a positive effect on mucous membranes [19]. The anti-inflammatory and antioxidant effects are key in postcancer patient treatment.

Oncology Massage (Figure 34.4)

Oncology massage is an approach to massage therapy based in both compassion and specialized massage treatments to help people manage their experience with cancer. Thermal stations are the most indicated places to begin this therapy.

Thermal Environment

There is much scientific evidence to demonstrate that thermal treatment has a very important psychological component; rest in a place that invites you to relax has the effect of reducing stress hormones and improving patients' well-being.

Additionally, thermal stations can offer diet programs and exercise programs adapted to postcure cancer patients.

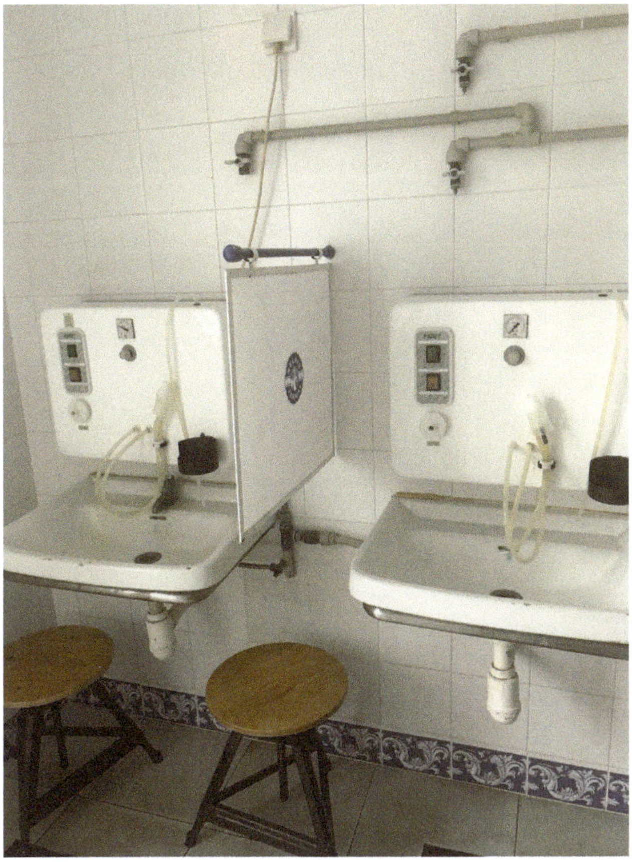

FIGURE 34.2 Installations for respiratory treatment and inhalations.

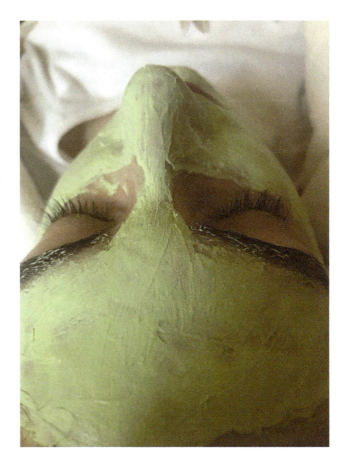

FIGURE 34.3 Pelotherapy face mask.

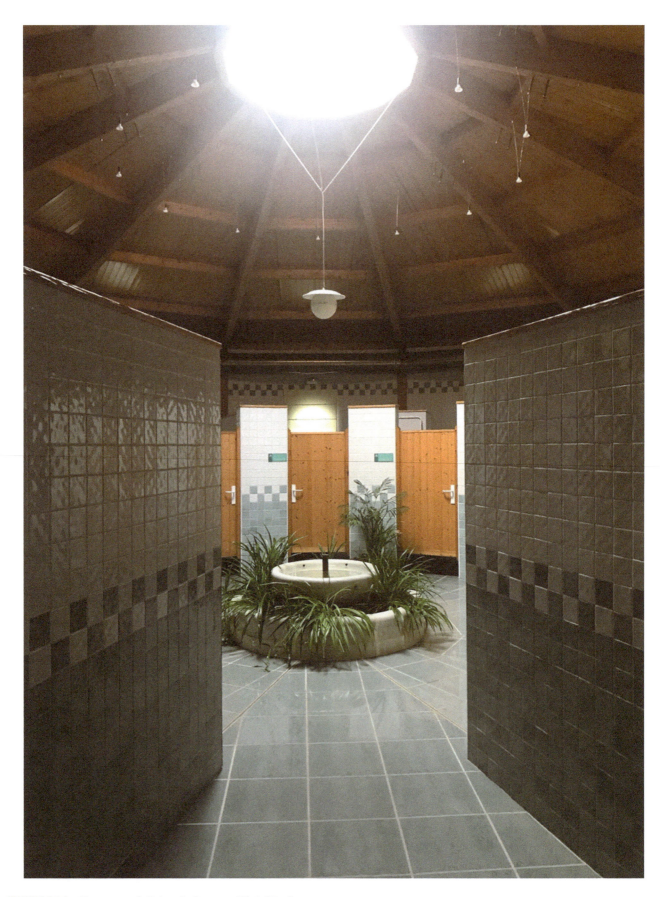

FIGURE 34.4   Massage area in Balneario Cervantes (Ciudad Real).

Scientific Evidence

Although all kinds of cancer are susceptible to treatment with thermal treatment, it has been most used for the sequels derived from *breast tumor* due to its high incidence, prevalence, and, above all, advances in curative treatments, which have often turned it into a chronic disease after the acute treatment period. After the end of the acute treatment, patients want to return to their lives in the best possible conditions. In a thermal environment, using thermal water, we can improve skin diseases and any loss of quality of life (QoL), and in general, restore everything they need to recover their old life (in terms of working and physical and social activity).

That is why, although clinical studies are under way on other types of cancer, breast cancer is currently the goal of thermal treatments. Research to date includes the following:

- A multicenter, randomized controlled trial has demonstrated how the spa treatment is a cost-effective strategy to improve resumption of occupational and nonoccupational activities and the abilities of women in breast cancer remission [8].
- A randomized controlled study has concluded that specific hydrotherapy is an effective supportive care for highly prevalent and long-lasting dermatologic adverse events occurring after early breast cancer treatment, including chemotherapy, and leads to improvement in QoL and dermatologic toxicities [9].
- Hydrotherapy as part of an integrated physical rehabilitation program has been found to sustainably improve symptoms and QoL in breast cancer survivors [10].
- A specific hydrotherapy program has been demonstrated to benefit patients with severe skin conditions such as atopic dermatitis, psoriasis, and inherited ichthyosis and might therefore be of interest as a supportive treatment in breast cancer patients [11].

France is the leader in thermal research, and La Roche Posay has been a pioneer in this respect. They have developed a very wide research program where they have demonstrated that 3 weeks of thermal treatment could increase the QoL in patients with breast cancer, in a program including water techniques, massage, psychological treatment, and different workshops (makeup, cream application, etc.) [12].

Avene Thermal Station has also published a report showing how chemotherapy and radiotherapy side effects diminish with 3 weeks of thermal cure with rates of 100% for dry skin, 61% for pruritus, and 43% for lymphoedema [13].

Postcancer Thermal Programs

Each thermal station has a different kind of water and its own special treatment; see further Table 34.1. Most aim to improve skin injuries because of radiotherapy or chemotherapy. Scars after surgery are another target for treatment. In some European countries (France and Germany), treatments are supported by the public health system.

Each thermal station may offer different programs, but they all use the same tools: thermal water and derived products, daily diet, an exercise program, and workshops on different aspects [14–16].

REFERENCES

1. Hernández Torres A, Ramón JR, Casado Á, Cuenca Giralde E, Polo De Santos MM, García Matas Á. Aguas minero medicinales y efectos antioxidantes en el envejecimiento.; 2009. Disponible en: http://fundacionbilbilis.es/pdf/aguas_minero_medicinales_y-efectos_antioxidantes_en_el_envejecimiento_capit_23.pdf, último (acceso 08. 01.2015).
2. Martín Cordero JE et al. *Agentes físicos-terapéuticos*. Ed. Ciencias Médicas–La Habana; 2008.
3. Hernández A et al. *Técnicas y tecnologías en hidrología médica e hidroterapia. Informe de Evaluación de Tecnologías Sanitarias*. Madrid: Instituto de Salud Carlos III, 2006.
4. Maraver F, Aguilera López L, Armijo Castro F, Martín Megías AI, Meijide Failde R, Soto Torres J. *Vademécum de aguas mineromedicinales españolas*. Instituto de Salud Carlos III, 2004.
5. Pérez Fernández M. *Principios de hidroterapia y balneoterapia*. Madrid: McGraw-Hill Interamericana, 2005, MA. Glosario de hidrología médica. Madrid, Universidad Europea CEES Ediciones; 2001.
6. Arbués E. Crenoterapia. Características de las aguas mineromedicinales y sus usos terapéuticos. Revista Electrónica de Portales Médicos, 18/04/2012, URL disponible en. http://www.portalesmedicos.com/revista/-index.htm, último (acceso 16.12.2014).
7. Hanh T, Seroy P. One year effectiveness of a 3-week balneotherapy program for the treatment of overweigh and obesity. *Evid Based Complementary Altern Med.* 2012;Artc IA 150838:7. Doi. 10.1155/2012/150839.
8. Mourgues C, Gerbaud L, Leger S. *Eur J Oncol Nurs.* Oct 2014;18(5):505–11.
9. Danlec F et al. Efficacy of a global supportive skin care programme with hydrotherapy after non-metastatic breast cáncer treatment: A randomised, controlled study. *Eur J Cancer Care.* January 2018;27(1).
10. Kwiatkowski F et al. Long term improved quality of life by a 2-week group physical and educational intervention shortly after breast cancer chemotherapy completion. *Eur J Cancer.* 2013 May;49(7):1530–8.
11. Bodemer C et al. Short- and medium-term efficacy of specific hydrotherapy in inherited ichthyosis. *Br J Dermatol.* 2011 Nov;165(5):1087–94.
12. Gire J, Automassage cicatriciel et gestion des œdèmes; at: https://www.thermes-larocheposay.fr/wp-content/uploads/2019/11/AUTO-MASSAGE-CICATRICIEL-GESTION-OEDEMES 2020.pdf (accessed April 2020).
13. Dalenc F et al. Efficacy of a global supportive skin care programme with hydrotherapy after non-metastatic breast cancer treatment: A randomised, controlled study. *Eur J Cancer Care.* 2017;e12735. https://doi.org/10.1111/ecc.12735
14. Dax Thermal Station: Rosavite Cure. https://www.thermes-berot.com/cures-dax/cure-post-cancer/traitements-soins-post-cancer/ (accessed April 2020).

15. La Bourboule Thermal Station. https://www.grandsthermes-bourboule.com/cure-post-cancer-dermatologie.html (accessed April 2020).
16. Thalasso Atlantique centre: https://www.talasoatlantico.com/blog/cuidados-integrales-a-personas-afectadas-por-cancer/, accessed April 2020.
17. Sociedad Española de Hidrología Médica. www.hidromed.org (accessed April 2020).
18. Beer A, Juginger HE, Lukanov J. Evaluation of the permeation of peat substances through human skin in vitro. *Int J Pharma.* 2003 May;253(1–2):169–175.
19. Shehab AL, Mohammed RA. Antibacterial effect of some mineral clays in vitro. *Egypt. Acad. J. Biol. Sci., G Microbiol.* 2011;3(1):75–81, Article 10.

Index